The Health Professional's Guide to Diabetes and Exercise

Editors   Neil Ruderman, MD, DPhil
John T. Devlin, MD

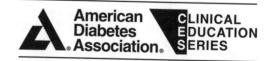
American Diabetes Association. CLINICAL EDUCATION SERIES

Chief Scientific and Medical Officer
Richard Kahn, PhD

Publisher
Susan H. Lau

Editorial Director
Peter Banks

Acquisitions Editor
Susan Reynolds

Book Editor
Karen Lombardi Ingle

Production Director
Carolyn R. Segree

The health professional's guide to diabetes and exercise/editors,
    Neil Ruderman, John T. Devlin
        p.   cm.
    ISBN 0-945448-52-X
    1. Diabetes—Exercise therapy—Handbooks, manuals, etc.
I. Ruderman, Neil.   II. Devlin, John T.   III. American Diabetes Association.
    [DNLM: 1. Diabetes Mellitus—therapy—handbooks. 2. Exercise Therapy—handbooks.
WK 39 H434 1995]
RC661.E94H36   1995
616.4'620624—dc20
DNLM/DLC
for Library of Congress   95-31497
                                                                          CIP

American Diabetes Association, Inc., 1660 Duke Street, Alexandria, VA 22314

Contents

Contributors

Editors

NEIL RUDERMAN, MD, DPhil
Boston University School of Medicine
Boston, MA

JOHN T. DEVLIN, MD
Maine Medical Center
Portland, ME

Associate
Editors

BARBARA N. CAMPAIGNE, PhD, FACSM
American College of Sports Medicine
Indianapolis, IN

W. GUYTON HORNSBY, Jr, PhD, CDE
West Virginia University School of Medicine
Morgantown, WV

JOHN L. IVY, PhD
University of Texas
Austin, TX

STEPHEN H. SCHNEIDER, MD
Robert Wood Johnson Medical School
New Brunswick, NJ

International
Advisory
Committee

MICHAEL BERGER, MD
Heinrich-Heine University of Düsseldorf
Düsseldorf, Germany

EDWARD S. HORTON, MD
Joslin Diabetes Center
Boston, MA

ERIK RICHTER
August Krogh Institute
Copenhagen, Denmark

MLADEN VRANIC, MD, PhD
University of Toronto
Toronto, Ontario, Canada

JOHN WAHREN, PhD
Karolinska Hospital
Stockholm, Sweden

BERNARD ZINMAN, MD
University of Toronto
Toronto, Ontario, Canada

Authors

LLOYD M. AIELLO, MD
Beetham Eye Institute
Joslin Diabetes Center
Boston, MA

LLOYD P. AIELLO, MD, PhD
Beetham Eye Institute
Joslin Diabetes Center
Boston, MA

ERIK BAEKKLUND, PhD
Nakskov, Denmark

EVAN M. BENJAMIN, MD
Baystate Medical Center
Tufts University School of Medicine
Springfield, MA

MICHAEL BERGER, MD
Heinrich-Heine University Düsseldorf
Düsseldorf, Germany

GREGORY L. BRADEN, MD
Baystate Medical Center
Tufts University School of Medicine
Springfield, MA

MELANIE J. BRUNT, MD, MPH
Boston City Hospital
Boston University School of Medicine
Boston, MA

SVEN-ERIK BURSELL, PhD
Beetham Eye Institute
Joslin Diabetes Center
Boston, MA

BILL CARLSON
Diamond Bar, CA

JERRY CAVALLERANO, OD, PhD
Beetham Eye Institute
Joslin Diabetes Center
Boston, MA

STUART R. CHIPKIN, MD
Boston City Hospital
Boston University School of Medicine
Boston, MA

S. TZIPORAH COHEN, BA
Mental Health Unit
Joslin Diabetes Center
Boston, MA

JOHN T. DEVLIN, MD
Maine Medical Center
Portland, ME

ERIC P. DURAK, MSc
Medical Health & Fitness
Santa Barbara, CA

WILLIAM J. EVANS, PhD
Pennsylvania State University
University Park, PA

CYNTHIA FERRARA, PhD
Ohio State University
Columbus, OH

BETTY FINNEGAN
Bryn Mawr, PA

CARL FOSTER, PhD
Sinai Samaritan Medical Center
Milwaukee, WI

MARION J. FRANZ, MS, RD, CDE
International Diabetes Center
Minneapolis, MN

OM P. GANDA, MD
Joslin Diabetes Center
Boston, MA

NEIL J. GOLDBERG, MD
Culver City, CA

NEIL F. GORDON, MD, PhD, MPH
Presbyterian Hospital of Dallas
Dallas, TX

CLAUDIA GRAHAM, CDE, PhD, MPH
Long Beach, CA

JEAN-JACQUES GRIMM, MD
Moutier, Switzerland

ROBERT J. HANISCH, MA, CDE
Sinai Samaritan Medical Center
Milwaukee, WI

PAULA HARPER, RN, CDE
International Diabetic Athletes Association
Phoenix, AZ

W. GUYTON HORNSBY, Jr, PhD, CDE
West Virginia University School of Medicine
Morgantown, WV

JOHN L. IVY, PhD
University of Texas
Austin, TX

ALAN M. JACOBSON, MD
Mental Health Unit
Joslin Diabetes Center
Boston, MA

LOIS JOVANOVIC-PETERSON, MD
Sansum Medical Research Foundation
Santa Barbara, CA

JOY KISTLER, MS, CDE
Joslin Diabetes Center
Boston, MA

RICHARD M. LAMPMAN, PhD
St. Joseph Mercy Hospital
Ann Arbor, MI

MARVIN E. LEVIN, MD
Washington University School of Medicine
St. Louis, MO

JOANN E. MANSON, MD, DrPH
Harvard Medical School
Brigham and Women's Hospital
Boston, MA

CARL ERIK MOGENSEN, MD
Aarhus Kommunehospital
Aarhus, Denmark

RICHARD W. NESTO, MD
Deaconess Hospital
Harvard Medical School
Boston, MA

STEVE PROSTERMAN
University of the Virgin Islands
St. Thomas, U.S. Virgin Islands

NEIL RUDERMAN, MD, DPhil
Boston University School of Medicine
Boston, MA

BARBARA SCHNEIDER, MS
Ohio State University
Columbus, OH

STEPHEN H. SCHNEIDER, MD
Robert Wood Johnson Medical School
University of Medicine and
    Dentistry of New Jersey
New Brunswick, NJ

W. MICHAEL SHERMAN, PhD
Ohio State University
Columbus, OH

ANGELA SPELSBERG, MD, SM
Harvard School of Public Health
Boston, MA

ULRIKE THURM, MD
Heinrich-Heine University Düsseldorf
Düsseldorf, Germany

AARON I. VINIK, MD, PhD, FCP, FACP
The Diabetes Institutes
Eastern Virginia Medical School
Norfolk, VA

GARY I. WADLER, MD, FACP, FACSM,
    FACPM
Cornell University Medical College
North Shore University Hospital
Manhasset, NY

DAVID H. WASSERMAN, PhD
Vanderbilt University School of Medicine
Nashville, TN

SERGIO WAXMAN, MD
Deaconess Hospital
Harvard Medical School
Boston, MA

RENA R. WING, PhD
University of Pittsburgh School of Medicine
Pittsburgh, PA

BERNARD ZINMAN, MD
University of Toronto
Toronto, Ontario, Canada

Reviewers

Albert, S.G.
Andres, R.
Balady, G.J.
Barrett, E.J.
Bernard, D.B.
Blair, S.N.
Braden, G.
Breckenridge, B.
Brink, S.
Brown, D.
Brownell, K.
Campaigne, B.N.
Carpenter, M.
Clapp, J.F.
Davidson, J.
Davidson, M.B.
DeFronzo, R.
Devlin, J.T.
Drash, A.
Freeman, R.
Gabbe, S.
Garg, S.
Goldberg, A.P.
Greene, D.
Habershaw, G.M.
Hagberg, J.
Halter, J.
Harkless, L.B.
Holloszy, J.O.
Hornsby, W.G.

Horton, E.S.
Ivy, J.L.
Kaufmann, F.R.
Kelley, D.B.
Kistler, J.
Kriska, A.
Manson, J.E.
Micheli, L.
Nesto, R.W.
Raglen, J.
Rand, L.
Reaven, G.
Richter, E.
Ruderman, N.B.
Salant, D.
Sanders, L.J.
Scheiner, G.
Scheuer, J.
Schneider, S.H.
Schwartz, R.S.
Sims, E.A.
Skyler, J.S.
Stephens, M.
Vranic, M.
Wahren, J.
Weiner, D.
Wilmore, J.H.
Wing, R.R.
Young, J.C.
Zinman, B.

Foreword

Exercise is an important component of diabetes management and may be useful in enhancing the health and quality of life for patients with diabetes. *The Health Professional's Guide to Diabetes and Exercise* reflects a strong commitment by the American Diabetes Association to increase professional knowledge about the use of exercise in the management and care of individuals with diabetes. On behalf of the members, fellows, officers, and trustees of the American College of Sports Medicine, I extend a hearty thank-you to the American Diabetes Association for supporting the important role of physical activity in maintaining health. I congratulate the editors, authors, reviewers, and organizers of *The Health Professional's Guide to Diabetes and Exercise*. It will undoubtedly be an invaluable resource for a host of professionals, including clinicians, nurse practitioners, nutritionists, and exercise physiologists, who treat and counsel patients with diabetes.

Steven P. Van Camp, MD
President
American College of Sports Medicine

Preface

The concept for this book was developed by the American Diabetes Association's Council on Exercise to fill an important niche in the diabetes and exercise literature; namely, the need for a comprehensive, yet practical, resource for health-care professionals involved in the management of physical activity in patients with diabetes. We recognized early the dual loyalties of many of our members and readers in the diabetes/metabolism and sports medicine communities. Thus, this book was conceived as a joint effort with the American College of Sports Medicine, and the guidelines in it represent a consensus opinion written by the two organizations. It is our hope that this effort will lay the foundation for future cooperation between these organizations in the preparation of Position Statements, Technical Reviews, and other important publications.

Throughout the book, our aim has been to provide "hands-on" advice to health-care providers in their daily clinical practices. The intended audience includes clinical and research scientists, physicians, nurses, dietitians, physical therapists, and exercise physiologists, among others. With these considerations in mind, we have included voices usually silent in diabetes and exercise manuals, namely, those of the diabetic athletes themselves. The section "Sports: Practical Advice and Experience" includes individual descriptions of therapeutic regimens used by successful, competitive athletes. Although this information may not be applicable to the general population of patients with diabetes, the insights gained from a difficult trial-and-error process, the "tricks of the trade," are a unique part of this volume.

In assembling the contents of this book, it became clear to us how far our knowledge of diabetes and exercise has advanced in the past several years and how much additional work is still needed. This seems to be especially true for such areas as the effects of exercise on the microvascular complications of diabetes, the incorporation of an exercise routine into intensive insulin treatment regimens (in increasing demand following publication of the Diabetes Control and Complications Trial results), and the effects of exercise in special patient populations, such as diabetic women. Although specific recommendations can now be made in these areas, it is equally clear that current, seemingly prudent, recommendations will need to be modified as ongoing scientific research sheds new light on these subjects.

Also included in this book are topics that are presently the focus of very active investigation. One of these is the role of exercise in the possible prevention of diabetes mellitus in high-risk groups. Ongoing large collaborative trials, such as the National Institutes of Health–sponsored multicenter Diabetes Prevention Trial-Type II, should provide valuable insights into the ability of physical exercise programs to reduce the incidence rate of diabetes. The results could have potentially far-reaching implications from a public health standpoint. Other chapters deal with topics that have received far too little attention, such as the psychological effects of exercise in patients with diabetes. Much of the previous research effort in the field of diabetes and exercise has been devoted to characterizing the metabolic benefits of increased levels of physical activity, especially in patients with NIDDM. Now that the benefits have been identified, more research is needed to define techniques for motivating the desired lifestyle changes (i.e., exercise and diet) and increasing the likelihood of maintaining these healthier behaviors over the lifetime of the patient.

The editors intend this book to reflect the broad range of interests and opinions and the numerous disciplines represented by the ADA Council on Exercise and the American College of Sports Medicine. If this book serves as a catalyst for ongoing discussion and debate and stimulates new scientific endeavors by these groups, our efforts will have been well worth it.

The individual chapters were written over the past 2 years, reviewed by outside experts, and then revised by the authors and edited. The editors gratefully acknowledge these efforts and those of a number of other people who made this possible: at Boston University, Joan Judge and Maryse Roudier, who provided secretarial and administrative assistance, and Aimee Montoya and Linda Abraham, who assisted them in these tasks; at Maine Medical Center, Diane Devlin, who typed manuscripts, and Judy Barrington, who assisted with figures; at the American Diabetes Association, Christine Welch and Sherrye Landrum, who guided the book through its formative stages, Laurie Guffey, who helped with copyediting and rewriting, and Karen Ingle, who expertly edited the manuscript and shepherded it through publication. Our thanks also to Barbara Campaigne of the American College of Sports Medicine and Lois Lipsett of the American Diabetes Association, who made the interactions between the two organizations, with respect to this book and other exercise-related matters, both pleasant and productive; and to Dr. Bernie Zinman of the book's International Advisory Committee, whose services above and beyond the call of duty freed up the editors to complete the book.

NEIL RUDERMAN, MD, DPhil and
JOHN T. DEVLIN, MD

I. Basic Considerations

1. Diabetes and Exercise: The Risk-Benefit Profile

JOHN T. DEVLIN, MD, AND NEIL RUDERMAN, MD, DPhil

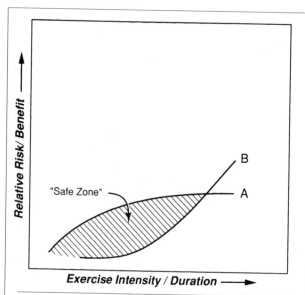

Figure 1.1. A hypothetical risk/benefit profile of a typical 40-year-old woman with recent-onset type II diabetes controlled with diet alone and no chronic complications. Curve A = benefit; curve B = risk.

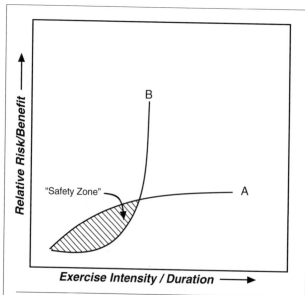

Figure 1.2. A hypothetical risk/benefit profile of a person with proliferative retinopathy. Curve A = benefit; curve B = risk. The risk curve is shifted to the left in this individual.

Exercise can play an important role in the therapy of patients with diabetes. On the other hand, the motivations to exercise, the specific concerns about its use, and the types of exercise that are acceptable may differ considerably between groups and among individuals.

An exercise prescription needs to be tailored to each person's unique set of circumstances. Exercise recommendations may differ widely based on the type of diabetes (type I, type II, or pre-diabetes), age-group or special characteristics of the patient (e.g., adolescent, female), and the presence or absence of chronic diabetic complications.

In each individual, the prescription should reflect an effort to optimize the anticipated benefits and minimize the risks from exercise. Benefits may include cardiovascular risk reduction, improved strength and physical energy, a better quality of life, and a psychological sense of well-being. Risks will vary with the presence and degree of microvascular and macrovascular complications, metabolic control, and adjustments to the treatment regimen (medications, caloric intake) required because of increases in physical activity.

The likelihood of maximizing the benefits and minimizing the risks of exercise will be greatest when the exercise prescription is developed jointly by the patient and health-care team. Education of patients and their families, as well as their health-care professionals, appropriate medical evaluations, and development and use of well-informed and judicious guidelines are all important for achieving exercise goals.

As an example of the potential application of exercise guidelines to an individual patient, consider a typical 40-year-old woman with recent-onset type II diabetes controlled with diet alone and no chronic complications. On the assumption that she will have the same benefits and risks from an exercise training program as a nondiabetic, otherwise healthy, individual, we have drawn a hypothetical risk/benefit profile as shown schematically in Fig. 1.1. The construct uses existing data (1,2) to estimate cardiovascular risk reduction with habitual increases in physical activity levels and increases in cardiovascular risk during a single bout of strenuous exercise. The maximal benefit versus risk occurs at exercise workloads below a certain point (x) in the shaded area (labeled "Safe Zone"), above which the risk of exercise exceeds the expected benefit.

In contrast to the example in Fig. 1.1, a person with proliferative retinopathy is clearly at greater risk of an adverse event (retinal hemorrhage) at low workloads than someone without this complication. As shown in Fig. 1.2, the risk curve (curve B) is shifted to the left in this individual. Optimization of the risk/benefit ratio (below point x) occurs at lower workloads in this patient than in the patient without complications.

Similar analyses can be made for other groups of patients, e.g., women, adolescents, and the elderly. Benefits and risks and optimal types and intensities of exercise may vary widely among these different groups. Unfortunately, we often are still not in a position to make totally informed recommendations about physical activities for specific individuals. On the other hand, we are far more able to do so than was possible only a few years ago.

REFERENCES

1. Mittleman MA, Maclure MPH, Tofler GH, Sherwood JB, Goldberg RJ, Muller JE: Triggering of acute myocardial infarction by heavy physical exertion. *N Engl J Med* 329:1677–83, 1993
2. Willich SN, Lewis M, Löwel H, Arntz H-R, Schubert F, Schröder R: Physical exertion as a trigger of acute myocardial infarction. *N Engl J Med* 329:1684–90, 1993

2. Exercise Physiology and Adaptations to Training

Highlights

Introduction

Physical Fitness

Cardiorespiratory Endurance
Muscle Fitness
Flexibility

Energy Systems

Anaerobic Energy Systems
Aerobic Energy System

Skeletal Muscle and Motor Units

Muscle Contraction
Motor Unit Recruitment

Cardiopulmonary Adjustments to Exercise

Pulmonary Ventilation
Cardiac Function
Peripheral Changes

Fatigue

Fatigue and Anaerobic Exercise
Fatigue and Aerobic Exercise

Exercise Training Adaptations

Aerobic Training
Anaerobic Adaptations

The Role of Exercise in the Possible Prevention and Treatment of Non-Insulin-Dependent Diabetes Mellitus (NIDDM)

Exercise and the Possible Prevention of NIDDM
Exercise and the Treatment of NIDDM
Possible Mechanisms of Action

Highlights
Exercise Physiology
and Adaptations to Training

- Regularly performed exercise can be used for disease prevention and rehabilitation.
- A major component of one's health is physical fitness, and regularly performed exercise is required to remain physically fit.
- Both aerobic (with oxygen) and anaerobic (without oxygen) processes provide energy for muscle contraction during exercise.
- Skeletal muscles are composed of three basic muscle fiber types that have distinct contractile, biochemical, and morphological properties.
- A motor unit (a motor neuron and the muscle fibers it innervates) is composed of the same muscle fiber types, and its activation is exercise intensity specific.
- The responses of the cardiovascular and pulmonary systems during exercise increase oxygen delivery to the exercising musculature.
- The cause of fatigue during exercise is determined by the type and intensity of the exercise performed.
- Adaptations to exercise training follow the principles of specificity and overload.
- Adaptations to training optimize the physiological and metabolic systems being stressed and are specific to the systems being stressed.
- Exercise training has been found to be effective in the treatment of impaired glucose tolerance and non-insulin-dependent diabetes mellitus (NIDDM) and may prove useful in their prevention.
- Improvements in glucose tolerance and NIDDM appear to be manifested through physiological, biochemical, and morphological changes in insulin-regulatable tissue.

Exercise Physiology and Adaptations to Training

JOHN L. IVY, PhD

INTRODUCTION

Physical activity can be defined as any form of body movement that results in an increase in metabolic demand (1). Therefore, physical activity encompasses work-related tasks, normal daily activities, leisure-time pursuits, and recreational and competitive sports. Exercise may be considered the voluntary component of the overall physical activity performed. When a program of exercise is performed on a regular basis in order to achieve a goal, such as to improve cardiorespiratory fitness, it is referred to as physical training or exercise training. Generally, exercise training is considered in the context of athletic training, in which chronic exercise is performed to enhance athletic ability and improve physical performance. However, in actuality, most exercise training is performed for therapeutic purposes. It is used to promote physical fitness, reduce the risk of disease, to rehabilitate orthopedic injuries, and to strengthen muscles to prevent the reoccurrence of such injuries. It is also performed to rehabilitate from disease. Exercise training has been shown to reduce the risk of heart disease, lower blood pressure, slow bone mineral loss that occurs with advancing age, relieve lower back pain and stress, and to be a major asset in the control of body weight. Recent evidence also suggests that regular exercise helps regulate carbohydrate metabolism and is beneficial in the treatment and management of both type I and type II diabetes (2,3).

PHYSICAL FITNESS

A major component of one's health is physical fitness. Physical fitness is the ability to perform the routine tasks of daily life with vigor and alertness, without undue fatigue, and to maintain sufficient energy to enjoy leisure-time pursuits and to be able to respond to unforeseen emergencies (4). Physical fitness is comprised of three basic components; cardiorespiratory endurance, muscular fitness, and flexibility.

Cardiorespiratory Endurance

Cardiorespiratory endurance is the ability of the heart, lungs, and circulatory system to efficiently supply oxygen and nutrients to working muscles. One of the most valid measures of functional capacity of the cardiorespiratory system is maximum oxygen consumption (VO_{2max}). VO_{2max} represents the maximum rate at which oxygen can be used by the body for energy production. As exercise intensity increases, oxygen uptake increases in direct proportion. Eventually, maximal oxygen delivery to the active muscle tissue is achieved, and oxygen uptake will plateau even with a continued increase in exercise intensity. Improvements in cardiorespiratory endurance are achieved by performing exercises that require rhythmic use of a large muscle mass. The exercises should be performed 3–4 times a week for a minimum of 15–20 min continuously at an intensity that elevates the heart rate and respiration but does not cause undue discomfort (5). These types of exercises are normally referred to as aerobic exercises. Aerobic means requiring oxygen for energy production. Examples of aerobic exercises are brisk walking, jogging, cycling, swimming, rowing, aerobic dance, and cross-country skiing. Exercises of short duration that can be supported by the energy sources stored in the muscles and that do not require oxygen are referred to as anaerobic exercises. Examples of anaerobic exercises are running, cycling, and swimming at very fast speeds (sprinting) and weight lifting. Aerobic exercises are generally better in terms of overall health benefits and result in fewer contraindications.

Muscle Fitness

Muscle fitness includes both muscle strength and muscle endurance. Muscle strength is the maximum force or tension that can be performed by a particular muscle group. Muscle contractions may be static or dynamic in nature, depending on the resistance encoun-

7

tered by the muscle. If the resistance is immovable, the muscle contraction is static or isometric; there is no change in the muscle length as tension develops. Dynamic contractions, in which the muscle changes length and in which there is visible joint movement, are either concentric, eccentric, or isokinetic (6). During concentric contraction, the force generated by the muscle is greater than the resistance allowing the muscle to shorten, resulting in movement of the bony lever system. The muscle is also capable of exerting tension while lengthening. This is known as eccentric contraction, which typically occurs when the muscles produce a braking force to decelerate rapidly moving body segments or to resist gravity, such as when lowering the body during a pull-up. It is the eccentric phase of a muscle contraction that causes muscle soreness. Sometimes the term isotonic contraction is used in the same context as dynamic contraction. This is a misnomer. The word isotonic means same (iso) tension (tonic). However, tension produced by a muscle group fluctuates greatly when the resistance is constant throughout the range of motion of a joint (i.e., curling a barbell). This is due to the change in mechanical and physiological advantage brought about by a change in the muscle length and joint angle as the limb is moving. An isokinetic contraction is defined as a contraction in which the tension developed by the muscle while shortening or lengthening at a constant speed is maximal over the full range of motion. The speed of contraction is controlled mechanically so that the limb rotates at a set velocity. Electromechanical or hydraulic devices vary the resistance to match the muscular force produced at each point in the range of motion of a joint. Thus, the isokinetic devices allow the muscle groups to encounter variable maximum resistances throughout the movement. The isokinetic contraction is most commonly used for diagnostic tests of muscle strength and endurance and for rehabilitation of muscle groups following injury or surgery to a limb.

Muscle endurance is defined as the ability of a muscle group to exert submaximal force for extended periods. Muscle endurance can be assessed for both sustained (static) and repeated (dynamic) contractions. An exercise program of weight lifting and calisthenics is the most efficient way to improve muscle fitness.

Flexibility

Flexibility is the capacity of a joint to move smoothly through its full range of motion. Lack of flexibility is associated with musculoskeletal injury and lower back problems. Flexibility progressively decreases with aging because of changes in the elasticity of the soft tissues of the body and a decrease in the physical activity level. Thus, flexibility exercises should be incorporated in all exercise training programs, particularly those of older people. A good time to perform these exercises is during the warm-up and warm-down phases of an exercise program. This will help prevent serious injury to the muscles and soft tissues around the muscles. When performing flexibility exercises, avoid bouncy, jerky movements. Slowly stretch the muscle until the muscle feels tight and then hold that position for 15–30 s. Repeat several times while gradually increasing the length the muscle is stretched.

ENERGY SYSTEMS

The energy for muscle contraction is derived directly from the breakdown of adenosine triphosphate (ATP) by the enzyme myosin ATPase. When acted on by myosin ATPase, a high-energy phosphate group (inorganic phosphate [Pi]) is split away from the ATP molecule, thereby releasing the energy necessary to drive muscle contractions (7.6 kcal/molecule of ATP). As the force and frequency of contraction increases, the rate of ATP breakdown increases. During muscle contraction, it is important that the ATP concentration of the muscle not decrease to any substantial degree, because this would decrease the rate of free energy change and ultimately inhibit further contraction by the muscle. The free ATP concentration of the muscle is, however, quite limited and sufficient for a maximal contraction of only 2–3 s in length. To maintain the ATP concentration during contraction, the muscle relies on both anaerobic and aerobic metabolic processes. The proportion of energy provided by these processes is intensity related. The higher the intensity of the contraction, the greater the reliance on anaerobic energy production. Conversely, the lower the intensity of contraction, the greater the reliance on aerobic energy production.

Anaerobic Energy Systems

The immediate and rapid replenishment of ATP during muscle contraction is supported by the breakdown of the high-energy phosphate compound phosphocreatine (PCr). Because both ATP and PCr are high-energy phosphate compounds, they are referred to as phosphagens, and the metabolic system in which these compounds are used for the liberation of energy for muscle contraction is referred to as the "phosphagen system." The end products of PCr hydrolysis are creatine and Pi. The energy released is immediately available and is biochemically coupled to the resynthesis of ATP, but the capacity to maintain levels of ATP from the energy derived from PCr is limited. The stores of ATP and PCr can only sustain the energy needs of the muscle during an all-out effort, such as sprinting for 8–12 s. Without this system, however, fast, powerful movements could not be performed.

A second anaerobic system in which ATP is produced within the muscle, anaerobic glycolysis, involves the breakdown of carbohydrate stored within the muscle cell (glycogen) to lactic acid. Glycolysis generates ATP when there is inadequate oxygen supplied to the muscle to meet metabolic demands. Unfortunately, this system of energy production is relatively inefficient, providing only three molecules of ATP from the anaerobic breakdown of one molecule of glycogen. A second limitation of this system is the produc-

tion of lactic acid, which, if accumulated in high concentrations, will interfere with muscle metabolism and contraction and adversely affect performance. However, anaerobic glycolysis, like the phosphagen system, is extremely important at the onset of exercise, when oxygen availability is limited, and during exercise of high intensity, when the energy demand exceeds the energy-producing capability of the aerobic energy system.

Aerobic Energy System

In order for the muscles to continuously produce the force needed during long-term physical activity, they must have a steady supply of energy. In the presence of oxygen, the muscle fiber is able to break down carbohydrates and fats, and protein if necessary, for generation of ATP. This process is referred to as aerobic metabolism or cellular respiration. As discussed, the anaerobic production of ATP is quite inefficient and inadequate for exercise lasting more than a few minutes. Consequently, aerobic metabolism is the primary method of energy production during endurance exercise.

Within each muscle fiber, there are special structures called mitochondria, which are capable of using fats and carbohydrates to produce large amounts of ATP. The reactions of the aerobic system can be divided into three main series: 1) substrate preparation, 2) Krebs cycle, and 3) the electron transport chain. Substrate preparation can occur in the cytoplasm or mitochondria of the cell, depending on the substrate being used. Carbohydrates are broken down in the cytoplasm by glycolytic enzymes to form pyruvate before entry into a second series of reactions in the Krebs cycle of the mitochondria. Fatty acids are transported directly into the mitochondria by a membrane carrier and prepared to enter the Krebs cycle by a series of reactions called beta oxidation. Both reactions result in the formation of acetyl coenzyme A, which condenses with oxaloacetate to form citrate in the first reaction of the Krebs cycle. Citrate then enters a series of

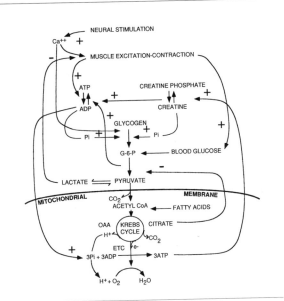

Figure 2.1. Energy systems responsible for replenishment of adenosine triphosphate (ATP) to support muscle contraction. Neural stimulation results in the initiation of excitation and contraction of muscle, which, in turn, causes the hydrolysis of ATP to adenosine diphosphate (ADP) and inorganic phosphate (Pi). The immediate and rapid replenishment of ATP during muscle contraction is supported by the hydrolysis of phosphocreatine (PCr). A second system for rapid replenishment of ATP is glycolysis, which is activated by elevated levels of intracellular ADP and Pi. Glycolysis involves the incomplete breakdown of carbohydrates to lactate. High levels of intracellular lactate can cause muscle fatigue. Predominant sources of carbohydrate for glycolysis are muscle glycogen and blood glucose. Blood glucose uptake by muscle is stimulated by muscle contraction. The hydrolysis of PCr and glycolysis are anaerobic processes. A third source of ATP production is aerobic respiration. Aerobic respiration occurs in the mitochondria and requires the presence of oxygen (O_2). In the mitochondria, acetyl coenzyme A (acetyl CoA), produced from pyruvate or the beta oxidation of fatty acids, condenses with oxaloacetate (OAA) to form citrate. Citrate then enters a series of reactions that result in the reformation of OAA, the liberation of carbon dioxide (CO_2) and hydrogen. The hydrogen atom is split into a proton (H^+) and electron (e^-), with the e^- entering the electron transport chain (ETC). Once in the ETC, the e^- is transported to O_2 in a series of enzymatic reactions. At the final reaction of the ETC, the e^- is reunited with the H^+ and combined with O_2 to form water. For each pair of e^- carried down the ETC, enough energy is released to produce three molecules of ATP. +, activation of reaction; –, inhibition of reaction.

reactions controlled by oxidative enzymes that result in the reformation of oxaloacetate, the liberation of CO_2 and hydrogen. The CO_2 produced diffuses into the blood and is carried to the lungs, where it is eliminated from the body. The hydrogen atom splits into a hydrogen ion (H^+) and an electron (e^-), which subsequently enters the electron transport chain of the mitochondria. Once in the electron transport chain, the e^- is transported to oxygen in a series of enzymatic reactions. At the final reaction of the electron transport chain, the e^- is reunited with the H^+ and combined with oxygen to form water. As the e^- is carried down the electron transport chain, energy is released, and ATP is resynthesized. For each pair of e^- carried down the electron transport chain, enough energy is released to produce three molecules of ATP.

The efficiency of aerobic energy production can be illustrated by comparing the ATP production from the breakdown of muscle glycogen to lactate during anaerobic glycolysis and the breakdown of muscle glycogen to CO_2 and H_2O during aerobic respiration. From one molecule of muscle glycogen, three molecules of ATP will be formed during anaerobic glycolysis. On the other hand, if the glycogen is completely broken down to CO_2 and H_2O, 37 molecules of ATP will be formed. The obvious advantage of aerobic respiration over anaerobic processes is the efficiency with which ATP can be resynthesized. However, the rate of ATP production is limited by the availability of O_2, which must be transported from the lungs to the active muscle (Fig. 2.1).

SKELETAL MUSCLE AND MOTOR UNITS

Skeletal muscle is composed of two basic types of muscle fibers, slow twitch or Type I fibers and fast twitch or Type II fibers (7). The fast twitch fibers can be subdivided into Type IIa and Type IIb. In general, the Type I fibers have a high oxidative capacity and capillary density, have a relatively

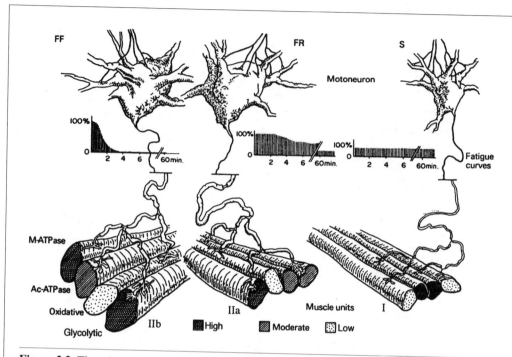

Figure 2.2. Three basic motor units found in human skeletal muscle. Axon diameter is directly related to conduction velocity. The muscle fibers (I, IIa, and IIb) have been stained for different biochemicals: myosin ATPase, acid ATPase, oxidative enzyme, glycolytic enzyme. Note the differences in fatigue curves: FF, fast, fatigable; FR, fast, fatigue-resistant; S, slow, fatigue-resistant.

Modified from Edington and Edgerton (42).

slow contraction and relaxation time, and are fatigue resistant. The Type IIb fibers have a low oxidative capacity and capillary density, a high glycolytic capacity, a relatively fast contraction and relaxation time, and fatigue rapidly. The morphological and physiological characteristics of the Type IIa fibers are intermediate to those of the Type I and IIb fibers. Type IIa fibers have a high oxidative and a high glycolytic capacity, a fast contraction and relaxation time, and are somewhat fatigue resistant (Fig. 2.2).

Muscle fibers of similar morphological and physiological characteristics are grouped into motor units. A motor unit is composed of a motor neuron and the muscle fibers it innervates. When a motor neuron is activated, all the muscle fibers within the motor unit will contract. However, like the three basic muscle fiber types, motor units differ with regard to speed and force of contraction, metabolic characteristics, and fatigability. Differences in contractile properties among motor units are due to differences in the motor neurons that innervate the muscle fibers as well as the contractile differences among the muscle fibers themselves.

Muscle Contraction

Muscle contraction is initiated by a neural impulse from a motor nerve. The impulse from the motor nerve causes the release of acetylcholine at the neuromuscular junction, resulting in the depolarization of the sarcolemma (plasma membrane) of the innervated muscle fibers. Depolarization spreads from the sarcolemma deep into the muscle fiber via the transverse tubules (T-tubules). The T-tubules connect with the sarcoplasmic reticulum, a system of chan-

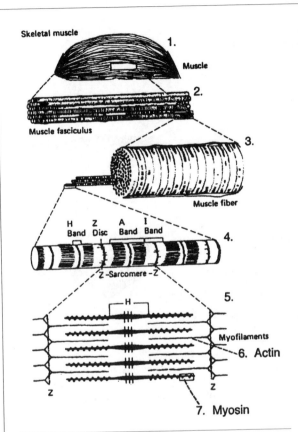

Skeletal muscle

1.

Muscle

2.

Muscle fasciculus

3.

Muscle fiber

H   Z   A   I
Band Disc Band Band   4.

Z –Sarcomere– Z

5.

H

Myofilaments

6. Actin

Z

Z

7. Myosin

Figure 2.3. Organization of skeletal muscle. 1, muscle; 2, fasciculus (muscle fiber bundles); 3, muscle fiber (muscle cell); 4, myofibril; 5, sarcomere (runs from Z-line to Z-line); 6, actin filament (attaches to Z-line); 7, myosin filament.

Modified from Bloom and Fawcett (41).

nels that run in parallel with the major contractile proteins, myosin and actin. At the junction where the T-tubule and sarcoplasmic reticulum meet, called the triad, calcium is stored in a large quantity. Upon depolarization of this region, calcium is released into the cytoplasm where it binds with the regulatory protein troponin. This results in a conformational change in troponin and causes tropomyosin, a second regulatory protein, to shift its orientation along the actin filament exposing myosin binding sites. With adenosine diphosphate (ADP) + Pi bound to myosin, myosin will form cross-bridges with actin. This causes the release of the ADP and Pi and a conformational change in the myosin cross-bridge (Fig 2.3). As the myosin cross-bridge changes position (the power stroke), it pulls the actin filament over the myosin filament resulting in a shortening of the muscle fiber. ATP then binds to the myosin head causing detachment of the myosin cross-bridge. ATP is then hydrolyzed by the enzyme myosin ATPase to form ADP + Pi, and the cross-bridge cycle is repeated in the presence of Ca^{2+} (Fig. 2.4).

Motor Unit Recruitment

The force and speed of muscle contraction is governed by the type, number, and frequency of motor unit recruitment (7). Fiber recruitment is based on the size of the motor neuron, its threshold for activation, and its conduction velocity. Type I fiber motor units are innervated by small, low threshold, slowly conducting motor nerves, while Type II motor units are innervated by large, higher threshold, fast-conducting motor nerves. In actuality, rather than discrete differences in motor neurons, there is a continuum of thresholds for activation. This allows for the systematic mobilization of motor units to accommodate the specific tension, speed, and metabolic requirements of the muscle contraction (8). In general, Type I motor units are recruited during low-intensity exercise. This is followed by activation of the more powerful, higher threshold Type II motor units as the muscle force requirements increase. When low-intensity activity is prolonged, Type I motor units are initially recruited. As the exercise duration increases and the Type I motor units start to fatigue, there is a progressive involvement of Type II motor units with the Type IIa units being recruited before the Type IIb units. If the exercise is performed to exhaustion, practically all motor units may be recruited.

The differential control of the motor unit recruitment pattern is a major factor in determining success in various athletic activities. For example, weight lifters are capable of recruiting a high number of both Type I and Type II motor units in a synchronous pattern. This synchronous pattern of motor unit recruitment aids the weight lifter in generating high amounts of force quickly. Conversely, the endurance athlete recruits motor units asynchronously, depending heavily on the high oxidative Type I and Type IIa motor units. The asynchronous recruitment pattern is advantageous because it provides a recovery period for the motor units during the activity.

CARDIOPULMONARY ADJUSTMENTS TO EXERCISE

Along with an increase in physical activity comes an increased demand for oxygen to support aerobic energy production. This requires an increase in oxygen delivery to the active muscle tissue by the cardiopulmonary system. At the onset of exercise, pulmonary ventilation and heart rate increase rapidly. The increase in pulmonary ventilation is due to an increase in both the frequency and depth of breathing. During exercise, ventilation may be 20–25 times greater than at rest. The increase in ventilation is proportional to oxygen consumption up to 60–70% VO_{2max}. Thereafter, it becomes disproportionately greater than the rise in oxygen consumption. The point of delineation between oxygen consumption and pulmonary ventilation is referred to as the ventilatory threshold and is associated with the onset of blood lactate accumulation or lactate threshold. The lactate threshold is important because it represents the maximal exercise intensity that can be sustained for a prolonged period of time. Typically, the majority of training performed by endurance athletes is at or around the lactate threshold (9) (Fig. 2.5).

Pulmonary Ventilation

The increase in pulmonary ventilation during exercise provides an increased supply of oxygen to the alveoli of the lungs, where it diffuses into the circulatory system and binds to the hemoglobin of the red blood cells. One gram of hemoglobin can transport 1.34 ml of

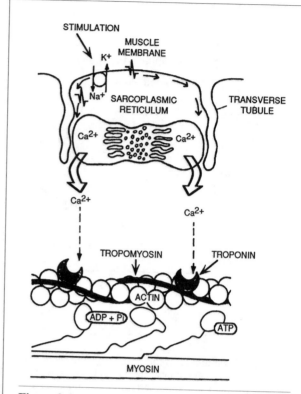

Figure 2.4. Excitation-contraction coupling of skeletal muscle. See text under MUSCLE CONTRACTION.

Modified from Fitts (14).

oxygen. In men, there are 15 g of hemoglobin in each 100 ml of blood. The value is less for women, averaging about 14 g/100 ml. The increase in pulmonary ventilation also, results in an increased removal of CO_2 from the circulatory system. Generally, hemoglobin is 95–98% O_2 saturated as it leaves the lungs, even during maximal exercise. Therefore, oxygen consumption is not limited by pulmonary ventilation except in the case of lung disease or under conditions of low atmospheric pressure, such as at altitude.

Cardiac Function

Under normal conditions, cardiac output increases primarily to match the increased need for O_2 by the working muscles, and it is maximum cardiac

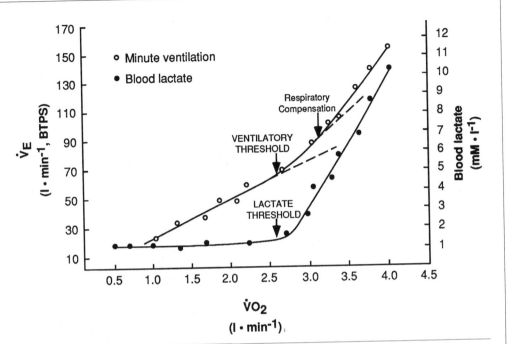

Figure 2.5. Pulmonary ventilation ($\dot{V}_E$) and blood lactate response to increasing workload expressed as oxygen consumption ($\dot{V}O_2$). Dashed line, the extrapolation of the linear relationship between $\dot{V}_E$ and $\dot{V}O_2$ observed during submaximal exercise. Lactate threshold is the point at which blood lactate begins to increase above the resting value and generally corresponds with the ventilatory threshold, or the point at which the relationship between ventilation and $\dot{V}O_2$ deviate from linearity. Respiratory compensation is a further increase in ventilation to counter the falling blood pH due to the rise in blood lactate.

Modified from McArdle et al. (43).

output that determines VO_{2max}. Cardiac output is the product of heart rate and stroke volume. Stroke volume is the amount of blood ejected from the heart per beat. At rest, cardiac output is 5 l/min. Cardiac output increases directly with increasing exercise intensity to 20–40 l/min. The absolute value will vary with body size and aerobic conditioning (10).

The increase in exercise heart rate is proportional to exercise intensity until near the point of exhaustion, when it begins to level off and maximum heart rate is obtained. When the rate of work is held constant at submaximal levels of exercise, heart rate increases fairly rapidly until it reaches a plateau. This is referred to as the steady-state heart rate, and it is the optimal heart rate for

meeting the circulatory demands at that specific rate of work or exercise intensity. The concept of steady-state heart rate forms the basis for several physical fitness tests. Individuals in better physical condition, based on their cardiorespiratory endurance capacity, will have lower steady-state heart rates at a submaximal exercise intensity than individuals who are less fit.

Stroke volume also increases with an increase in physical activity. However, maximal stroke volume is thought to be reached at exercise intensities between 40 and 60% of VO_{2max}. At this point, stroke volume plateaus, remaining essentially unchanged up to and including the point of exhaustion. Stroke volume is controlled by the volume of venous blood returned to the heart, ventricular capacity, ventricular contractility, and aortic artery pressure. The first two factors regulate the end diastolic volume, or the amount of blood accumulated in the ventricle during diastole. The last two factors influence the ability of the ventricle to empty, determining the force with which blood is ejected and the pressure against which it must flow in the arteries. The blood remaining in the ventricle after cardiac contraction is termed the end systolic volume. Therefore, stroke volume is equal to the end diastolic volume minus the end systolic volume.

Several mechanisms account for the increase in stroke volume during exercise, but the most important is an increase in venous return. This results in a greater left ventricular filling placing more stretch on the ventricular wall and increasing force of contraction. This is referred to as the Frank-Starling law. The increase in venous return is due to rapid redistribution of blood by sympathetic activation of arteries and arterioles in inactive areas of the body and a general sympathetic activation of the venous system. A second factor is the increased pumping action of the active muscles that assists in venous return. Also, there are greater differences in intra-abdominal and intrathoracic pressures because of increased breathing, which creates a more optimal flow gradient from the abdominal cavity to the thoracic cavity. An increase in stroke volume is also manifested by an increase in ventricular contractility, resulting from increased sympathetic nervous system activity. Aside from accelerating heart rate during exercise, an increase in sympathetic activity can increase the strength of myocardial contraction two to threefold.

Peripheral Changes

An essential response to increased physical activity is the redistribution of blood flow. This is necessary to provide sufficient oxygen to the working muscles. Blood is redirected through the action of the sympathetic nervous system and locally produced metabo-

lites, away from areas where it is not essential, to those areas that are active during exercise. Only 15–20% of the resting cardiac output goes to muscle, but during exhaustive exercise, the muscles receive 80–85% of the cardiac output. This shift in blood flow to the muscles is accomplished primarily by reducing blood flow to the splanchnic area.

With aerobic-type exercise, systolic blood pressure increases in direct proportion to increased exercise intensity. Systolic blood pressure can exceed 200 mmHg at exhaustion. Increased systolic blood pressure results from the increased cardiac output that accompanies increasing rates of work. Its rise is necessary to drive the blood through the vasculature. Conversely, diastolic blood pressure decreases slightly or does not change during aerobic exercise. Increases in diastolic pressure of 15 mmHg or more are considered abnormal responses to aerobic exercise and are one of several indicators for immediately stopping a diagnostic exercise test.

Blood pressure responses to resistance exercise, such as weight lifting, can be quite high. Blood pressures in excess of 450/300 mmHg have been measured during intense resistance training (11). This is partly due to an increase in intrathoracic pressure resulting from the use of the Valsalva maneuver. A Valsalva is performed when exhalation is attempted against a closed glottis.

The blood pressure response to the same absolute rate of energy expenditure is determined by the amount of muscle mass being used (12). The greater the muscle mass involved, the lower the blood pressure, or the less the muscle mass used, the greater the blood pressure. The use of a smaller muscle mass requires a greater percentage of available muscle fibers to be recruited at one time with a greater frequency of recruitment that results in a high intramuscular pressure. Coupled with a smaller vasculature, blood pressure must rise to overcome the high intramuscular pressure to deliver an adequate supply of blood to the active muscles.

During rest, the amount of oxygen extracted from the blood by the muscles is relatively small. At rest, arterial blood contains about 20 ml of O_2 per 100 ml, while venous blood contains about 14 ml of O_2 per 100 ml. The difference between these two values is referred to as the arterial-venous oxygen difference (a-vO_2diff). The value represents the extent to which oxygen is extracted from the blood by the tissues as it passes through the body. With increasing exercise intensity, the a-vO_2diff increases progressively. The a-vO_2diff can increase approximately threefold from rest to maximal levels of exercise. This reflects a decreasing venous oxygen content. The venous oxygen content can drop to values approaching zero in the active musculature, but the mixed venous blood in the right atrium of the heart rarely drops below 2–4 ml of oxygen per 100 ml of blood. This is due to the mixing of blood from the active tissues with blood from the inactive tissues as it returns to the heart.

FATIGUE

Fatigue may be defined as the inability to maintain a given level of muscle force during sustained or repeated contractions. The causes of fatigue are generally exercise intensity specific and appear to be due to either substrate depletion or metabolic by-product inhibition of muscle contractile activity. At the onset of exercise, there is a rise in the free intracellular ADP concentration of the muscle due to the hydrolysis of ATP. The rise in ADP stimulates the hydrolysis of PCr, resulting in an increase in Pi. The increase in Pi, as well as an increase in the cytosolic Ca^{2+} concentration of the muscle, signals an increase in glycogen breakdown through activation of the enzyme glycogen phosphorylase. The anaerobic metabolism of PCr and muscle glycogen as substrate for ATP resynthesis is used at the start of exercise and will continue to be used if the energy demand is higher than can be met by aerobic respiration. For the average man, the maximum rate of energy

release from the phosphagens (ATP and PCr) is between 35 and 50 kcal/min. The maximum rate of energy release by anaerobic glycolysis is 30 kcal/min. At exercise intensities lower than maximum aerobic power, i.e. VO_{2max}, the relative importance of blood glucose and free fatty acids as substrates increases relative to the muscle PCr and glycogen stores. The lower the exercise intensity, the greater the percent contribution from aerobic respiration. The maximum rate of carbohydrate oxidation for an individual with a VO_{2max} of 3.5 l/min is 17 kcal/min, and for fat oxidation it is 10 kcal/min. From the above discussion, it can be seen that exercise of different intensities requires different energy systems and substrate.

Fatigue and Anaerobic Exercise

During exercise of maximum effort, such as sprinting, PCr use proceeds rapidly. The duration of this exercise intensity, however, is limited to seconds, as a result of the low muscle PCr stores that cannot be replaced as rapidly as they are used. Studies of human thigh muscle and isolated muscle preparations have shown that exhaustion during repeated maximal contractions coincides with the depletion of PCr (13).

During high-intensity exercise that lasts more than a few seconds, muscle glycogen becomes a primary source of energy for the synthesis of ATP. As with PCr use, the rate of hydrolysis of muscle glycogen is directly related to the intensity of the exercise. An increase in the rate of work results in an increase in muscle glycogen utilization. When the rate of muscle glycogen utilization is very rapid, as during the mile run, lactic acid accumulates in the muscle. The accumulation of lactic acid can result in severe acidosis within the muscles and throughout the body. Such changes in pH have a negative effect on energy production and the contraction process within the muscle (14). Substantial reductions in intracellular pH have been found to inhibit the activities of key glycolytic enzymes, thereby slowing the rate of ATP production via the glycolytic pathway. In addition, hydrogen ions will compete with calcium ions for binding to troponin, interfering with the interaction of myosin and actin and causing a decline in the contractile force of the muscle.

Fatigue and Aerobic Exercise

Under many circumstances, the cause of fatigue during aerobic exercise cannot be readily identified. However, for aerobic activities that require a substantial amount of carbohydrate for ATP production, the muscle glycogen concentration appears critical. Research has found that during aerobic activities that can be sustained from 60 to 90 min, fatigue is related to total muscle glycogen depletion or depletion within specific muscle fibers, such as the Type II fibers (15). At lower exercise intensities, in which time to fatigue is 90 min or longer, blood glucose can be taken up by the muscles at a rate fast enough to compensate for low muscle glycogen and meet the carbohydrate requirements for energy production. During exercises of this type, such as marathon running, fatigue appears due to a general depletion of the carbohydrate stores in the body. That is, fatigue is associated with a depletion of muscle glycogen and a low blood glucose level due to liver glycogen depletion. If carbohydrate is consumed during the exercise, the decline in blood glucose can be delayed and exercise can be sustained for a considerably longer period of time (16).

EXERCISE TRAINING ADAPTATIONS

The adaptations to exercise training follow two principles: the principle of training specificity and the overload principle (17). The principle of specificity implies that the biological adaptations to training are specific to the training program, and therefore, improvements are restricted to the energy systems, muscle groups, and other biological systems stressed during training. Skill activities are best improved when the training includes the muscle groups and simulates the movement patterns most often used during the actual execution of a particular skill. Simply stated, the overload principle postulates that for a biological system to adapt it must be stressed beyond its normal use. Continuous improvement, therefore, requires that the level of training increase as the system being trained improves. For example, if a continuous increase in muscle strength and hypertrophy are desired, the resistance against which the muscle works will have to be increased throughout the course of the training program. Overload can be increased by changing the intensity, duration, and/or frequency of the exercise.

Aerobic Training

After several weeks of endurance training, individuals are generally capable of exercising at higher workloads while maintaining sufficient energy production aerobically. They are capable of exercising for prolonged periods of time at exercise intensities that had previously resulted in early fatigue. They also demonstrate an increased ability to oxidize free fatty acids and to use carbohydrate stores more effectively during exercise. The adaptations that result in an improved aerobic power and endurance reside both in the cardiorespiratory system and within the skeletal muscle. Aerobic power or VO_{2max} is limited by oxygen delivery to the active muscle tissue. Although aerobic exercise training stimulates adaptations in the respiratory system, it is the adaptations within the cardiovascular system that generally result in an improved aerobic power. Aerobic endurance, however, is increased primarily through biochemical and morphological adaptations in skeletal muscle.

Pulmonary Ventilation
With exercise training there is a tendency for vital capacity to increase and residual volume to decrease, but these changes are minor and there is no significant change in total lung capacity. Pulmonary ventilation and ventilation rate, however, are lower after training

when exercise is performed at the same submaximal standardized exercise task. Exercise training generally results in a substantial increase in maximal pulmonary ventilation. For men, the increase can range from 120 l/min in the untrained state to 150 l/min in the trained state. Highly trained aerobic athletes may actually exceed pulmonary ventilations of 200 l/min. In addition, maximal pulmonary blood flow is increased, resulting in increased perfusion of the lungs. Along with the increase in maximal ventilation, the increased perfusion of the lungs provides a larger and more efficient surface area for gas exchange. Maximal ventilation, or the rate of gas exchange across the lungs, is not considered to be limiting for VO_{2max}. Typically, hemoglobin oxygen binding is close to 100% at VO_{2max} before and after training. However, exceptions have been noted. Extremely highly trained individuals have been observed to have hemoglobin oxygen binding below 92% during maximal exercise, suggesting that VO_{2max} is limited by O_2 diffusion in the lungs (18). These observations are rare, however, and VO_{2max} is generally considered to be limited by the cardiovascular system.

Cardiovascular Adaptations

As a result of endurance training, heart weight and volume increase. There may also be an increase in left ventricular septal and posterior wall thickness. Like skeletal muscle, cardiac muscle will undergo hypertrophy, and this hypertrophy is a normal adaptation to endurance training. The increase in chamber size allows for a greater end diastolic volume. An increase in chamber filling places a greater stretch on the cardiac muscle fibers, and this, in conjunction with an increase in ventricular wall thickness, will result in an increase in contractile force that can be generated by the heart during systole.

Resting heart rate decreases markedly as a result of endurance training. Heart rates of sedentary individuals average between 70 and 80 beats/min. Highly conditioned endurance athletes often have resting heart rates of 40 beats/min or lower. Following aerobic training, heart rate is reduced at the same absolute submaximal work rate. The reduction is proportional to the improvement in aerobic conditioning. Therefore, monitoring changes in submaximal exercise heart rate is a simple and easy means of monitoring improvement in aerobic conditioning (19). The decrease in resting and submaximal exercise heart rate also indicates that the heart has become more efficient through training. That is, it requires less energy in the trained condition for the heart to do the same amount of work. Maximal heart rate shows little change with aerobic training. If it does change, it will generally decline slightly.

A major adaptation to endurance training is an increase in stroke volume. Stroke volume is increased at rest and during both submaximal and maximal exercise. In the untrained condition, resting stroke volume ranges from 55 to 75 ml and maximal stroke volume from 80 to 110 ml. After training, resting and maximal stroke volume may increase 40–60%. Exceptionally well-trained individuals have been reported to have resting stroke volumes of 100–120 ml and maximal stroke volumes of 160–220 ml (20).

The increase in stroke volume is due, in part, to an increase in ventricular filling. This is a consequence of an increase in blood volume and ventricular chamber size. A longer diastole, due to a slower heart rate at rest and submaximal exercise, also contributes, because this provides more time for adequate ventricular filling to occur. The net result is an increase in end diastolic volume. This increases the stretching of the ventricular walls and by the Frank-Starling law, results in an increased force of contraction during systole. An increase in rate of Ca^{2+} influx during depolarization of the myocardium as well as an increase in ventricular mass may also contribute to a more forceful contraction. Therefore, the increases in ventricular filling and force of contraction combine to increase stroke volume in the trained heart.

Resting cardiac output and cardiac output during a standardized submaximal exercise task are unchanged or slightly lower following aerobic training. With the reduction in heart rate under these conditions, cardiac output is maintained by an increase in stroke volume. While the changes in submaximal cardiac output are minor following training, maximal cardiac output is increased significantly. This results from the increase in maximal stroke volume, because maximal heart rate does not increase. Maximal cardiac output ranges from 15 to 20 l/min in untrained people, 20–30 l/min in trained people, and as much as 40 l/min or more in large highly trained endurance athletes. The increase in VO_{2max} is directly related to the increase in cardiac output.

After aerobic training, muscle blood flow per gram muscle is lower than in the untrained state during a standardized submaximal exercise task. However, recent animal research suggests that there is better redistribution of the muscle blood flow so that there is actually an increase around the most active muscle fibers (21). That is, muscle blood flow is distributed differently among and within muscles after training so that the active high oxidative fibers receive elevated blood flows and the inactive low oxidative fibers receive reduced flows. Blood flow to visceral tissues, such as the kidney, spleen, and intestines is also increased. This is possible because of an increase in total blood volume. The increase in blood volume is due to both a greater plasma volume and a greater red blood cell volume. The change in plasma volume, however, is greater than the change in red blood cell volume, so that the ratio of cell volume to total blood volume (hematocrit) decreases slightly.

The total muscle O_2 delivery at a given submaximal exercise intensity should decrease after training because of the decrease in total muscle blood flow. Since VO_2 at a given submaximal exercise intensity is similar before and after training, the a-vO_2diff across the total musculature must be greater. The increased O_2 extraction may be related to the increase in muscle capillary density that occurs with training. This would maintain adequate capillary mean transit times in the active muscles and provide a greater capillary sur-

face area for O_2 exchange. The increased O_2 extraction could also be facilitated by a redistribution of blood, as previously mentioned, and an increase in mitochondrial volume in the active muscles.

During exercise at VO_{2max}, total muscle blood flow is increased after training, with little change in the amount of blood flow redirected from non-muscular organs. Thus, the increase in total cardiac output is quantitatively equal to the elevation in muscle blood flow that is due, in part, to an increase in total blood volume. As with submaximal exercise, it appears that the majority of increase in muscle blood flow during maximal exercise occurs in the active musculature.

With regard to the cardiovascular system, the overall effect of aerobic exercise training is to increase O_2 delivery to the active muscles. This occurs by increasing cardiac output, increasing blood flow in the active musculature, and providing better O_2 diffusion from the capillary to the muscle fiber by increasing the volume and surface area of the capillaries. Increases in maximal pulmonary ventilation and lung blood flow prevent the respiratory system from becoming rate limiting for VO_{2max} (Fig. 2.6).

Cellular Adaptations of Skeletal Muscle

One of the major changes in skeletal muscle with exercise training is an increase in the number of capillaries around each muscle fiber. In the untrained state, the number of capillaries around Type I fibers averages four per fiber and the number around Type II fibers about three per fiber. With aerobic training, the number of capillaries around each fiber has been seen to increase by 20–30% and parallels the increase in the oxidative capacity of the muscle (20). The increase in capillarity allows for greater exchange of gases, nutrients, waste products, and heat between the blood and active muscle tissue.

Another major morphological change with aerobic training is a shift in fiber type composition. In untrained individu-

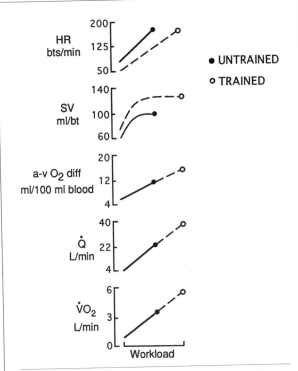

HR
bts/min
200
125
50

SV
ml/bt
140
100
60

a-v O$_2$ diff
ml/100 ml blood
20
12
4

● UNTRAINED
○ TRAINED

Q̇
L/min
40
22
4

V̇O$_2$
L/min
6
3
0

Workload

Figure 2.6. The effects of aerobic exercise training on the cardiovascular responses to increasing workloads to a maximum. Solid lines, submaximal responses in untrained subjects. Dashed line, submaximal responses in trained subjects. HR, heart rate; SV, stroke volume; a-vO$_2$diff, tissue oxygen extraction; Q̇, cardiac output; V̇O$_2$, total body oxygen consumption.

Modified from Rowell (44).

a higher percentage of Type I fibers, and that the percentage of Type I fibers in these athletes is directly related to the number of years of training (23). It therefore appears that if aerobic exercise training can cause the conversion of Type II fibers to Type I fibers it occurs over many years of training.

Aerobic training has a substantial impact on the metabolic pathways of skeletal muscle (24). The major adaptation is an increase in the size and number of mitochondria. Isolated mitochondrial preparations and muscle homogenates from trained muscle show an increased ability to oxidize pyruvate, fatty acids, and ketones. The ability for enhanced oxidation of substrate is associated with an increase in enzymes responsible for the activation, transport, and ß-oxidation of long-chain fatty acids, the enzymes involved in ketone oxidation, the enzymes of the Krebs cycle, and the components of the electron transport chain. The mitochondria from trained muscle exhibit a high level of respiratory control and tightly coupled oxidative phosphorylation, indicating that these adaptations in the mitochondrial metabolic pathways are functional and are associated with an increased capacity for ATP production via oxidative phosphorylation. Other metabolic adaptations include an increase in the insulin regulatable glucose transporter, GLUT4, and an increase in hexokinase and glycogen synthase. These proteins control the rate of glucose uptake, phosphorylation, and storage, respectively. There is also an increase in the malate-aspartate shuttle, which is responsible for transferring the reducing equivalents (H$_2$) from cytoplasmic NADH formed during glycolysis into the mitochondria where they enter the electron transport chain. If cytosolic NAD$^+$ is not replenished in this manner, then the NADH is oxidized in the cytoplasm by reducing pyruvate to form lactate. Thus, the increase in the rate of NAD$^+$ regeneration via the malate-aspartate shuttle is of significant importance in the control of lactate formation during exercise.

These biochemical adaptations of the skeletal muscle result in marked

als, the Type IIb fibers may compose 25–35% of the total Type II fibers. After several weeks of training, there is an obvious decline in the number of low oxidative Type IIb fibers and an increase in moderate oxidative Type IIa fibers, suggesting that Type IIb fibers are being converted to Type IIa fibers (22). Muscles of highly trained individuals may not show any Type IIb fibers, but upon detraining for several weeks IIb fibers become apparent. The conversion of Type II fibers to Type I fibers by aerobic training has not been established. Short-term training studies have failed to identify this conversion. Cross-sectional studies, however, have found that the more successful endurance athletes have alterations in the metabolic response to exercise that require a submaximal aerobic effort and are primarily responsible for the substantial improvements in aerobic endurance that follow aerobic training. The major metabolic adaptations are an increase in the workload that results in an accumulation of blood lactate, a sparing of stored carbohydrates, and an increase in fatty acid oxidation.

In the trained as opposed to the untrained state, blood lactate is lower at both the same absolute and relative (intensity based on a percentage of $\dot{V}O_{2max}$) workloads. Thus, the workload at which blood lactate starts to accumulate, the lactate threshold, is increased. A rise in blood lactate is secondary to an increase in lactate in the exercising muscles. Therefore, the increase in the lactate threshold is significant in that individuals are able to exercise at a higher relative exercise intensity for a given time period in the trained compared with the untrained state.

Depletion of carbohydrate stores is directly associated with fatigue. Studies comparing individuals before and after training have demonstrated a reduced respiratory exchange ratio at the same relative workload. This indicates a reduced reliance on carbohydrate for fuel and an increase in fatty acid oxidation. Studies in which muscle biopsies were taken to evaluate the rate of muscle glycogen utilization during a standardized exercise bout clearly indicate that the rate of muscle glycogen utilization is slowed after training (25). Although it has not been demonstrated directly in humans, rat studies indicate that training has a sparing effect on liver glycogen as well (26). Thus, for the same absolute workload, the trained individual will have a slower rate of decline in both muscle and liver glycogen, which will also result in a reduced rate of decline in blood glucose. It is well documented that depletion of carbohydrate stores and the onset of hypoglycemia can be related to the development of fatigue. The increased reliance on fatty acid oxidation and the sparing of carbohydrate stores during prolonged exercise

most likely play a major role in the increase in aerobic endurance after training.

Anaerobic Adaptations

Anaerobic training can be divided into two major categories: *1*) sprint training, in which the training is of high intensity and of short duration with adequate time to recover between intervals, and *2*) strength training, which requires work against a high resistance for short durations. Although they are both considered forms of anaerobic training, they result in substantially different neurological, physiological, and biochemical adaptations (27).

Cardiovascular Adaptations
With anaerobic training, such as high-resistance strength training and sprint workouts, there are few adaptations by the cardiovascular system. This is because there is little increase in venous return and therefore no volume overload on the heart. There are a few cardiovascular adaptations to strength training, however, because of the pressure overload that occurs due to the increase in mean arterial blood pressure. Strength training can result in cardiac hypertrophy. The cardiac hypertrophy, however, is limited to an increase in ventricular wall thickness and not an increase in ventricular chamber size (28). There is no change in maximal heart rate, stroke volume, cardiac output, or $\dot{V}O_{2max}$.

Neuronal Adaptations
During the first 2–3 months of strength training, the major gains in strength occur because of changes in the central and peripheral nervous systems (29). Whether a motor unit will be activated depends on the algebraic sum of the excitatory and inhibitory impulses. Inhibitor mechanisms are in place to prevent the muscles from exerting more force than can be tolerated by the bones and connective tissues. When the tension of the tendon and internal connective tissue of a muscle becomes overly stressed, a reflex inhibition of motor neuron discharge occurs to prevent excessive motor unit recruitment. This

process is referred to as autogenic inhibition, and it is activated when the tension on the tendon and connective tissue supporting the muscle exceeds a threshold level. With strength training, there is an increase in tendon, ligament, and internal connective tissue strength and a facilitation of motor unit recruitment by reducing autogenic inhibition. There also appears to be an increased coordination of motor unit recruitment and general neural trafficking, which results in better synchronization of motor unit firing, which results in an increase in force development. Synchronization of motor unit firing will also occur with high-intensity training, such as sprint training.

Myogenic Adaptations

After the first few months of strength training, there is generally a noticeable increase in muscle mass. This is due to hypertrophy of individual muscle fibers through increases in cytoplasmic volume, myofibrils, and filaments (30). Muscle fiber hypertrophy is typically greatest in Type II fibers. The increase in muscle mass may also be caused by hyperplasia, which is an increase in the number of muscle fibers. Although hyperplasia has not been directly demonstrated in humans, it has been demonstrated to occur in muscle of experimental animals taught to lift weights for rewards (31). It has also been observed that the muscle fiber sizes of some body builders are the same as those of individuals of average size and muscle mass. While strength training causes muscle hypertrophy and possibly hyperplasia, it does not appear to cause fiber type conversion.

The enzymatic changes that occur with strength training are small. There is a small increase in the activities of some glycolytic enzymes, such as phosphofructokinase, glycogen phosphorylase, and lactate dehydrogenase (32). There may also be a decrease in aerobic enzyme activities due to a decreased mitochondrial density subsequent to an increase in myofibrils and cytoplasmic volume.

Myogenic training adaptations to high-intensity exercise are very specific to the intensity and duration of the training and the energy requirements of the training (17). Sprint training will result in elevations in ATP and PCr stores and increased anaerobic power. The activities of enzymes that catalyze the rapid replenishment of ATP and PCr, myokinase, and creatine kinase also increase. If the duration of exercise training results in high muscle and blood lactate accumulation, an increased tolerance to lactate will develop because of an increase in muscle proteins that buffer lactate. If Type IIb fibers are recruited substantially, they may be converted to Type IIa fibers. However, high-intensity exercise generally has little effect on muscle fiber type composition.

THE ROLE OF EXERCISE IN THE POSSIBLE PREVENTION AND TREATMENT OF NON-INSULIN-DEPENDENT DIABETES MELLITUS (NIDDM)

Despite years of advocating that physical activity is beneficial in the prevention of insulin resistance and NIDDM, until recently, there was little scientific evidence to support this contention. In fact, a National Institutes of Health Consensus Development Conference on Diet and Exercise in NIDDM in 1987 concluded that the impact of exercise on control of NIDDM is small and ineffective. However, during the last several years considerable evidence has accumulated from epidemiological studies, exercise training studies, and community health programs that increased physical activity can be an effective intervention in the treatment of insulin resistance and NIDDM and possibly in their prevention.

Exercise and the Possible Prevention of NIDDM

For individuals with normal insulin function, prolonged aerobic exercise training results in lower plasma insulin concentrations both during fasting and following glucose ingestion. Despite a markedly blunted insulin response to a glucose challenge, glucose tolerance is normal or improved, providing evidence that the effectiveness of insulin to control blood glucose is improved. Such results strongly suggest that regularly performed aerobic exercise can reduce the risk of insulin resistance and may prevent the development of impaired glucose tolerance and NIDDM. This contention is strongly supported by recent epidemiological studies indicating that individuals who maintain a physically active lifestyle are much less likely to develop NIDDM than individuals who have a very sedentary lifestyle (33,34). Furthermore, it was found that the protective effect of physical activity was strongest for individuals at highest risk for NIDDM (34). This included individuals who were overweight, had high blood pressure, and had a family history of NIDDM. Reducing the risk of insulin resistance and NIDDM by regularly performed exercise is also supported by several aging studies. Glucose tolerance generally deteriorates as one ages because of the development of insulin resistance. However, older individuals who vigorously train on a regular basis exhibit a greater glucose tolerance and a lower insulin response to a glucose challenge than sedentary individuals of similar age and weight (35). Older physically active individuals also demonstrate a glucose tolerance similar to that of young untrained individuals while maintaining a lower insulin response to an oral glucose load.

Exercise and the Treatment of NIDDM

While the evidence is substantial that endurance exercise training can reduce the risk of glucose intolerance and NIDDM, the evidence that exercise training is beneficial in the treatment of NIDDM is not particularly strong. Many of the early studies investigating the effects of exercise training on NIDDM could not demonstrate improvements in glucose tolerance or plasma insulin levels. The adequacy of the training programs in many of these studies, however, is questionable. More

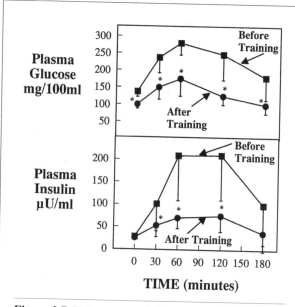

Figure 2.7. Values are means ± SE for five patients. Plasma glucose and insulin responses to a 100-g oral glucose load in patients with mild NIDDM before and after 12 months of vigorous aerobic exercise training. The after-training glucose tolerance test was performed ~18 h after the patients' most recent bout of exercise.

Modified from Holloszy and colleagues (37).

recent studies using prolonged, vigorous exercise training protocols have produced more favorable results. For example, Reitman et al. (36) reported a significant improvement in glucose tolerance and insulin action in Pima Indians with recent-onset NIDDM who exercised vigorously 5–6 days/week for an average of 8 weeks. Also, Holloszy and colleagues (37) found that 12 months of vigorous exercise training 3–4 times/week normalized the glucose tolerance while markedly lowering the plasma insulin response of patients classified as glucose intolerant or NIDDM (Fig. 2.7). However, because exercise decreases insulin secretion to counter an improvement in insulin sensitivity, it is generally not effective as the sole treatment of NIDDM in patients who have moderate to marked insulin deficiency.

Possible Mechanisms of Action

Adaptations that could contribute to an improvement in glucose intolerance and NIDDM are an increase in the action of insulin on the peripheral tissues, an increased rate of liver glucose clearance, and a reduced rate of liver glucose production. Of the three, the most important is an increase in insulin action on peripheral tissue. Exercise training increases peripheral glucose clearance in the presence of insulin. This is primarily due to an increase in skeletal muscle insulin action. The increased insulin action is associated with an increase in insulin-responsive glucose transporters (GLUT4) and enzymes that regulate the storage and oxidation of glucose in skeletal muscle. Changes in muscle morphology may also be important after training. As previously discussed, with aerobic exercise training, there is an increase in the conversion of Type IIb fibers to Type IIa, as well as an increase in the muscle capillary density. Type IIa fibers have a greater capillary density, have a higher concentration of glucose transporters, and are more insulin responsive than Type IIb fibers. Evidence has been provided that morphological changes in muscle, particularly the capillary density of the muscle, are associated with changes in fasting insulin concentrations and glucose tolerance. Furthermore, significant correlations between glucose clearance and muscle capillary density and fiber type have been found in humans during a euglycemic clamp (38).

An increase in muscle mass may also improve the insulin-resistant state by increasing glucose storage space. In support of this hypothesis is the finding that weight lifters have lower blood glucose and insulin responses to an oral glucose load than sedentary age-matched control subjects or endurance-trained athletes (39). Also, Miller et al. (40) reported that the decline in the plasma insulin response to an oral glucose load following several months of weight training was significantly related to the increase in muscle mass achieved by the subjects. Such findings may be particularly pertinent to the elderly, who generally experience a large reduction in muscle mass as well as a deterioration in insulin sensitivity and glucose tolerance.

An increase in insulin-stimulated liver glucose clearance following exercise training has not been documented. However, the liver does appear to become more sensitive to insulin, resulting in better control of liver glucose production. Exercise training may also improve control over liver glucose production by increasing insulin's control over blood free fatty acid concentration. An elevated blood free fatty acid level, which is associated with obesity and NIDDM, stimulates gluconeogenesis, which, in turn, stimulates liver glucose production. An elevated blood free fatty acid level may also attenuate skeletal muscle glucose uptake and storage. Therefore, an increased control over the blood free fatty acid concentration may serve to increase peripheral glucose clearance as well as reduce liver glucose production.

REFERENCES

1. Caspersen CJ, Powell KE, Christenson GM: Physical activity, exercise, and physical fitness: definitions and distinctions for health-related research. *Public Health Rep* 100:126–31, 1985
2. Kriska AM, Blair SN, Pereira MA: The potential role of physical activity in the prevention of non-insulin-dependent diabetes mellitus: The epidemiological evidence. In *Exercise and Sport Sciences Reviews*. Vol. 22. Holloszy JO, Ed. Baltimore, Williams & Wilkins, 1994, p. 121–43
3. Wallberg-Henriksson H: Exercise and diabetes mellitus. In *Exercise and Sport Sciences Reviews*. Vol. 20. Holloszy JO, Ed. Baltimore, MD, Williams & Wilkins, 1992, p. 339–68
4. Clarke HH: *Application of Measurement to Health and Physical Education*. Englewood Cliffs, NJ, Prentice-Hall, 1967, p. 14
5. American College of Sports Medicine: The recommended quantity and quality of exercise for develop-

ing and maintaining cardiorespiratory and muscular fitness in healthy adults (Position Statement). *Med Sci Sports Exercise* 22:265–74, 1994

6. Berger RA: *Applied Science Physiology.* Philadelphia, Lea & Febiger, 1982

7. Burke RE, Edgerton VR: Motor unit properties and selective involvement in movement. In *Exercise and Sport Sciences Reviews.* Wilmore J, Krogh J, Eds. New York, Academic, 1975, p. 31–83

8. Henneman E, Mendell LM: Functional organization of motoneurone poll and its inputs. In *Handbook of Physiology.* Sec. I, vol II. Brooks VB, Ed. Bethesda, MD, American Physiology Society, 1981, p. 423–507

9. Farrell PA, Wilmore JH, Coyle EF, Billing JE, Costill DL: Plasma lactate accumulation and distance running performance. *Med Sci Sports Exercise* 11:338–44, 1979

10. Åstrand PO, Cuddy TE, Saltin B, Stenberg J: Cardiac output during submaximal and maximal work. *J Appl Physiol* 19:268–74, 1964

11. MacDougall JD, Tuxen D, Sale DG, Moroz JR, Sutton JR: Arterial blood pressure response to heavy resistance exercise. *J Appl Physiol* 58:785–90, 1985

12. Lewis SF, Snell PG, Taylor WF, Hamra M, Granham RM, Pettinger WA, Blomqvist CG: Role of muscle mass and mode of contraction in circulatory responses to exercise. *J Appl Physiol* 58:146–51, 1985

13. Karlsson J: Lactate and phosphagen concentrations in working muscle of man. *Acta Physiol Scand Suppl* 358:1–72, 1971

14. Fitts RH: Mechanisms of muscular fatigue. In *Resource Manual for Guidelines for Exercise Testing and Prescription.* Blair SN, Painter P, Pate RR, Smith LK, Taylor CB, Eds. Philadelphia, PA, Lea & Febiger, 1988, p. 76–82

15. Ahlborg B, Bergström J, Ekelund EG, Hultman E: Muscle glycogen and muscle electrolytes during prolonged physical exercise. *Acta Physiol Scand* 70:129–42, 1967

16. Coyle EF, Coggan AR, Hemmert MK, Ivy JL: Muscle glycogen utilization during prolonged strenuous exercise when fed carbohydrates. *J Appl Physiol* 61:165–72, 1986

17. Fox EL, Matthews DK: *The Physiological Basis of Physical Education and Athletics.* 3rd ed. New York, CBS College Publishing, 1981

18. Dempsey JA, Vidruk EH, Mitchell GS: Is the lung built for exercise? *Med Sci Sports Exercise* 18:143–55, 1986

19. Wilmore JH, Costill DH: *Training for Sport and Activity: The Physiological Basis of the Conditioning Process.* 3rd ed. Dubuque, IA, Brown, 1988

20. Saltin B, Rowell LB: Functional adaptations to physical activity and inactivity. *Fed Proc* 39:1506–13, 1980

21. Armstrong RB: Influence of exercise training on O_2 delivery to skeletal muscle. In *The Lung: Scientific Foundations.* Crystal RG, West JB, Eds. New York, Raven, 1991, p. 1517–24

22. Saltin B, Henriksson J, Nyaard E, Andersen P, Jansson E: Fiber types and metabolic potentials of skeletal muscles in sedentary man and endurance runners. In *The Marathon: Physiological, Medical, Epidemiological, and Psychological Studies. Ann NY Acad Sci.* Vol. 301. Milvy P, Ed. New York, 1977, p. 3–29

23. Coyle EF, Feltner ME, Kautz SA, Hamilton MT, Montain SJ, Baylor A, Abraham LD, Petrek GW: Physiological and biomechanical factors associated with elite endurance cycling performance. *Med Sci Sports Exercise* 23:93–107, 1991

24. Holloszy JO: Biochemical adaptations to exercise: aerobic metabolism. In *Exercise and Sport Sciences Reviews.* Vol. 1. Wilmore JH, Ed. New York, Academic, 1973, p. 44–71

25. Hermansen L, Hultman E, Saltin B: Muscle glycogen during prolonged severe exercise. *Acta Physiol Scand* 71:129–39, 1967

26. Fitts RH, Booth FW, Winder WW, Holloszy JO: Skeletal muscle respiratory capacity, endurance, and glycogen utilization. *Am J Physiol* 228:1029–33, 1975
27. Gollnick PD, Hermansen L: Biochemical adaptations to exercise: anaerobic metabolism. In *Exercise and Sport Sciences Reviews.* Vol. 1. Wilmore JH, Ed. New York, Academic, 1973, p. 1–43
28. Schaible TF, Scheur J: Cardiac adaptation to exercise. *Prog Cardiovasc Dis* 27:297–324, 1985
29. Sale DL: Influence of exercise and training on motor unit activation. In *Exercise and Sport Sciences Reviews.* Vol. 15. Pandolf KB, Ed. New York, Macmillan, 1987, p. 95–152
30. MacDougall JD: Morphological changes in human skeletal muscle following strength training and immobilization. In *Human Muscle Power.* Jones NL, McCartney N, McComas AJ, Eds. Champaign, IL, Human Kinetics Books, 1986, p. 269–88
31. Gonyea WJ, Sales DG, Gonyea FB, Mikesky A: Exercise-induced increases in muscle fiber number. *Eur J Appl Physiol* 55:137–41, 1986
32. Costill DL, Coyle EF, Fink WF, Lesmes GR, Witzmann FA: Adaptations in skeletal muscle following strength training. *J Appl Physiol* 46:96–99, 1979
33. Manson JE, Rim EB, Stampfer MJ, Colditz GA, Willett WC, Krolewski AS, Rosner B, Hennekens CH, Speizer FE: Physical activity and incidence of non-insulin-dependent diabetes mellitus in women. *Lancet* 338:774–78, 1991
34. Helmrich SP, Ragland DR, Leung RW, Paffenbarger RS Jr: Physical activity and reduced occurrence on non-insulin-dependent diabetes mellitus. *N Engl J Med* 325:147–52, 1991
35. Seals DR, Hagberg JM, Allen WK, Hurley BF, Dalsky GP, Ehsani AA, Holloszy JO: Glucose tolerance in young and older athletes and sedentary men. *J Appl Physiol* 56:1521–25, 1984
36. Reitman JS, Vasquez B, Klimes I, Nauglesparan M: Improvement of glucose homeostasis after exercise training in non-insulin-dependent diabetes. *Diabetes Care* 7:434–41, 1984
37. Holloszy JO, Schultz J, Kusnierkiewic J, Hagberg JM, Ehsani AA: Effects of exercise on glucose tolerance and insulin resistance. *Acta Med Scand Suppl* 711:55–65, 1986
38. Lillioja S, Young AA, Cutler CL, Ivy JL, Abbott WGH, Zawadzki JK, Yki-Järvinen H, Christin L, Secomb TW, Bogardus C: Skeletal muscle capillary density and fiber type are possible determinants of in vivo insulin resistance in man. *J Clin Invest* 80:415–24, 1987
39. Cüppers HJ, Erdmann D, Schubert H, Berchtold P, Berger M: Glucose tolerance, serum insulin, serum lipids and athletes. In *Diabetes and Exercise.* Berger M, Christacopoulus P, Wahren J, Eds. Bern, Han Huber, 1982, p. 115–65
40. Miller WJ, Sherman WM, Ivy JL: Effects of strength training on glucose tolerance and post-glucose insulin response. *Med Sci Sports Exercise* 16:539–43, 1984
41. Bloom W, Fawcett DW: *A Textbook of Histology.* Philadelphia, Saunders, 1975
42. Edington DW, Edgerton VR: *The Biology of Physical Activity.* Boston, Houghton Mifflin, 1976
43. McArdle WD, Katch FI, Katch VL: *Exercise Physiology, Energy, Nutrition, and Human Performance.* 3rd ed. Philadelphia, Lea & Febiger, 1991
44. Rowell LB: *Human Circulation, Regulation During Physical Stress.* New York, Oxford Press, 1986

3. Fuel Homeostasis

Highlights
Fuel Homeostasis

- Energy requirements of muscular work require increased fuel mobilization and utilization.
- Changes in glucagon and insulin levels stimulate the release of glucose from the liver during moderate-intensity exercise.
- Catecholamines and insulin are important in the mobilization of extrahepatic fuels (muscle glycogen and fats).
- High-intensity exercise results in a disproportionate increase in carbohydrate metabolism and hyperglycemia.
- Glucose uptake and oxidation by the working muscle is increased because of an increase in insulin action as well as an acceleration in insulin-independent mechanisms.
- The exercise response in insulin-dependent diabetes mellitus (IDDM) patients is highly variable and depends on many factors, including the absorptive state, insulinization, and the type of exercise.

- IDDM patients who are overinsulinized risk hypoglycemia during exercise, while those who are underinsulinized risk a worsening of the diabetic state.
- Overinsulinization of IDDM patients during exercise can result from a mismatching of insulin dose to needs, accelerated insulin absorption from its subcutaneous depot, and increased insulin action.
- The deleterious effects of too little insulin in IDDM patients can be amplified by an accelerated counterregulatory hormone response.
- Weight loss and increased glucose tolerance that results from regular exercise is beneficial in the treatment of non-insulin-dependent diabetes mellitus (NIDDM).
- Diet, insulin therapy, fitness, and any specific pathology must be considered when prescribing exercise to any individual with diabetes.

Fuel Homeostasis

DAVID H. WASSERMAN, PhD, AND BERNARD ZINMAN, MD

INTRODUCTION

The increased metabolic demands that accompany exercise require an increase in fuel mobilization from sites of storage and an increase in fuel oxidation within the working muscle. The needed increment in fuel metabolism is controlled by a precise endocrine response. The importance of the endocrine system is readily apparent in individuals with insulin-dependent diabetes mellitus (IDDM) in whom the normal endocrine response to exercise is often lost. When a person with IDDM undertakes exercise with too little circulating insulin, an excessive counterregulatory hormone response may occur, and the already elevated blood glucose and ketone body levels can become even greater. In contrast, too much insulin can attenuate the exercise-induced increase in hepatic glucose production and lipolysis, causing hypoglycemia. Modification of insulin therapy in anticipation of exercise can be used to avoid states of under- or overinsulinization. In addition, increased carbohydrate ingestion may be used to compensate for the hypoglycemic effects of inappropriately high circulating insulin. In contrast to individuals with IDDM, individuals with non-insulin-dependent diabetes mellitus (NIDDM) treated with diet do not have the same risk of metabolic deterioration with exercise. Note that the presence of advanced diabetic complications can dramatically limit exercise in people with IDDM and NIDDM. In this chapter, we describe the regulation of fuel metabolism during exercise and how this regulation is affected by diabetes. Segments of this chapter were reproduced from our recent technical review (1). Please refer to it for more detailed referencing.

PHYSIOLOGY OF FUEL METABOLISM DURING EXERCISE

Individuals with IDDM must overcome obstacles in metabolic regulation during each acute bout of exercise to enjoy exercise benefits. The metabolic adaptations to moderate exercise in the nondiabetic individual are designed to meet the energy needs of the working muscle, while at the same time maintaining glucose homeostasis. To understand the difficulties individuals with IDDM face and address possible approaches by which defects in fuel metabolism can be corrected, it is necessary to understand the normal means by which the regulation of fuel utilization is intended to occur. This section describes the utilization of fuels during exercise and provides an overview of the central role hormones play in regulating these processes.

The metabolic response to exercise will vary in accordance with factors such as nutritional state, age, general health, and work capacity. Variables that influence the metabolic response to exercise are summarized in Table 3.1. Nevertheless, the precise mix of fuels that are used will always be a function of the exercise duration and intensity. During the transition from rest to exercise, the working muscle shifts from using mainly nonesterified fatty acids (NEFAs) to using a blend of NEFAs, blood glucose, and muscle glycogen. During the initial stages of exercise, muscle glycogen is the chief source of energy. With increasing exercise duration, the contributions of circulating glucose and, particularly, NEFAs become of increasing importance as muscle glycogen depletes gradually. In addition, the origin of the blood glucose shifts from hepatic glycogenolysis to the gluconeogenic pathway. The greater reliance on gluconeogenesis is facilitated by adaptations that increase gluconeogenic precursor supply to the liver and the use of these precursors within the liver.

Fuel mobilization and utilization during exercise is governed by changes in hormone levels and sympathetic nerve activity (2). Generally, arterial insulin levels decrease and arterial glucagon, cortisol, epinephrine, and norepinephrine levels increase. Usually

Table 3.1. Factors That Influence the Exercise Response

General population (including those with diabetes)
- Exercise intensity, duration, and type
- Fitness level
- Nutritional state
- Temporal relationship to meal
- Calories and content of meal

Factors specific to individuals with diabetes
- Temporal relationship to insulin injection
- Type of insulin administered and site of administration
- Metabolic control
- Presence of complications

the magnitude of these changes is greater with increasing exercise duration and intensity. Ascribing metabolic effects to hormone action based on concentration changes in peripheral blood can be misleading to some extent, particularly for the pancreatic hormones and norepinephrine, because their levels at the liver and synaptic cleft, respectively, will not necessarily be reflected. The events that lead to the exercise-induced hormone responses remain to be fully elucidated. The endocrine response may be triggered by the stimulation of afferents from the working muscle, subtle deviations in blood glucose, and/or feedforward mechanisms originating in the hypothalamus (3).

Regulation of Hepatic Glucose Production

Despite the increase in muscle glucose uptake, arterial glucose levels change very little during moderate-intensity exercise, because the sum of increments in hepatic glycogenolysis and gluconeogenesis is similar to this increase. The importance of the close tracking of glucose utilization by hepatic glucose production is illustrated by the precipitous fall in circulating glucose that would otherwise result. Glucose utilization may rise by 3 mg·kg^{-1}·min in response to just moderate-intensity exercise. If the liver did not respond to

exercise, blood glucose would decrease at a rate of ~1.5 mg·dl^{-1}·min^{-1}, and overt hypoglycemia would be present in 30 min.

Studies in healthy humans (4) and dogs (5,6) have shown that the fall in insulin (4,5) and rise in glucagon (4,6) are the major determinants of glucose production during moderate exercise. The fall in insulin is necessary for the full increase in hepatic glycogenolysis, while the rise in glucagon is required for the full increment in both hepatic glycogenolysis and gluconeogenesis (5). When the rise in glucagon and fall in insulin are both prevented during exercise in humans by somatostatin infusion and these hormones replaced to basal levels, plasma glucose level falls by ~25–50 mg/dl over the course of an hour (4,7,8). Although changes in glucagon and insulin are individually very important, the interaction of these hormones is a component of the stimulus. The importance of this interaction is based on several observations (3). First, the ratio of glucagon to insulin is better correlated to glucose production than either glucagon or insulin alone. Second, the exercise-induced glucagon rise increases glucose production approximately fourfold when insulin is allowed to fall compared with when it is maintained at basal levels. Hence, during exercise, as is the case at rest, a fall in insulin sensitizes the liver to the effects of glucagon. Third, in the absence of biologically active glucagon, the exercise-induced fall in insulin does not stimulate hepatic glucose production. This suggests that the fall in insulin acts by potentiating the actions of glucagon. Factors involved in the regulation of glucose fluxes are described in Fig. 3.1.

In contrast to the importance of glucagon and insulin during moderate-intensity exercise, epinephrine plays only a minor role in regulating hepatic glucose production. The majority of the literature indicates that epinephrine is unimportant for the increase in hepatic glucose production, at least during moderate exercise of <120 min duration (3). Studies conducted in humans,

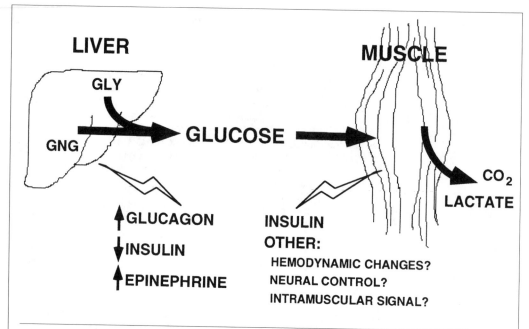

Figure 3.1. Regulation of exercise-induced increases in glucose fluxes. Hepatic glucose production is regulated primarily by the exercise-induced rise in glucagon and fall in insulin. During prolonged or heavy exercise or during exercise in IDDM, epinephrine may play an increased role in stimulating glucose production. In healthy subjects, most of the exercise-induced increase in muscle glucose uptake occurs because of an unknown stimulus that is independent of insulin. In the poorly controlled diabetic state, some insulin is needed during exercise to overcome the elevated NEFA and counterregulatory hormone levels.

adrenalectomized for treatment of Cushing's disease or bilateral pheochromocytoma, show that these patients have a normal increase in glucose production during 60 min of moderate exercise (9). Similarly, hepatic glucose production is equivalent in adrenalectomized dogs for the first 120 min of exercise regardless of whether they are receiving basal or exercise-simulated epinephrine replacement (10). The rise in epinephrine, however, controls a significant proportion of the increase in glucose output after 120 min of exercise. Since epinephrine stimulates glucose production during prolonged exercise when gluconeogenesis is high and it coincides with a diminished arterial lactate response, one can speculate that the effect of epinephrine is to facilitate gluconeogenic precursor mobilization from peripheral sites.

Sympathetic innervation of the liver has been proposed to be important in the stimulation of hepatic glucose production during exercise. This suggestion is based on two premises. First, increases in phosphorylase a activity and hepatic glycogenolysis occur with direct hepatic nerve stimulation (3). Second, the exercise-induced increase in glucose production is more rapid than changes in arterial glucagon, insulin, and epinephrine levels (2). Despite the circumstantial evidence that seems to implicate the sympathetic nerves, no role during exercise has been demonstrated. Combined α- and ß-adrenergic blockade does not attenuate glucose production in exercising humans (11), implying that sympathetic drive is unimportant to this process. Another study in humans showed that blocking sympathetic nerve activity to the liver and adrenal medulla with local anesthesia of the celiac ganglion while controlling the pancreatic hormone responses (somatostatin with insulin and glucagon replacement) does not impair the increase in glucose production during exercise (7). It is important to recognize that the effectiveness of the sympathetic receptor or nerve blockade was not determined in the studies cited above and may have been incomplete. Further supporting a lack of a role of hepatic innervation is the demonstration that human subjects who have had liver transplants have a normal increase in glucose production with exercise (12). Animal studies also suggest that hepatic innervation is unimportant for the increase in glucose production during exercise. Chemical sympathectomy with 6-OH dopamine does not affect hepatic glycogen breakdown (13), and surgical hepatic denervation has no effect on the increment in glucose production (14).

The role of glucocorticoids within a single bout of exercise has generally been considered to be small, because the effects of this hormone generally take hours to be manifested. Nevertheless, evidence suggests that they may play a role in the increase in intrahepatic gluconeogenic efficiency during prolonged exercise. Transgenic mice carrying a gene consisting of an intact phosphoenolpyruvate carboxykinase (PEPCK) promotor (including the glucocorticoid response element) linked to a reporter gene for bovine growth hormone (bGH) exhibit nearly a fivefold increase in hepatic bGH mRNA in response to exercise (15). However, transgenic mice with a deletion in the PEPCK gene glucocorticoid regulatory element show no change. This observation is supported by the finding that the exercise-induced increase in PEPCK mRNA is markedly attenuated in adrenalectomized mice and dexamethasone corrects the impairment (15).

The response of the liver to high-intensity exercise and the regulation of this response may be different than that outlined above for exercise of lesser intensities. The main identifiable difference in glucoregulation is that the increase in hepatic glucose production no longer matches but, in fact, exceeds the rise in glucose utilization. This results in an increase in arterial glucose levels that extends into the postexercise state. Since a single bout of high-intensity exercise can only be sustained for a short interval, it is likely that the added glucose released by the liver originates from liver glycogen. In a practical sense, activities such as basketball and soccer may consist of repeated bouts of high-intensity exertion that, if not preceded by caloric intake and if extended for a prolonged period, may draw on glucose that is derived from the gluconeogenic pathway. It has been hypothesized that during exercise of high intensity, the control of glucose production may shift away from the pancreatic hormones to the catecholamines (16). This is based on two observations. First, norepinephrine and epinephrine can increase by 10- to 20-fold, whereas the increase in the glucagon-to-insulin ratio is considerably less (16). Second, when high-intensity exercise is superimposed on a preexisting pancreatic clamp, hepatic glucose production increases normally even though the increase in glucagon is blunted and the fall in insulin is absent (17). Nevertheless, all studies that have assessed the role for catecholamines in stimulating hepatic glucose production during heavy exercise (>80% maximum O_2 uptake) have been negative (7,16,18).

Regulation of Fat Mobilization

Lipolysis, as assessed by the increase in arterial glycerol concentration and by isotopic techniques, increases with the onset of moderate exercise (19). Arterial NEFA levels, however, increase gradually. The slower time course for the rise in plasma NEFA levels reflects an increase in the clearance of this fuel by the working muscle (19). The ß-adrenergic effects of the catecholamines (20–22) and the fall in insulin (23) are the two most important regulators of NEFA mobilization during exercise. Circulating NEFAs are reduced during exercise by ß-adrenergic blockade (21,11). A parallel reduction in tracer-determined glycerol appearance indicates that this is due to a suppression of lipolysis (21). The exercise-induced increase in NEFA levels is retained in adrenalectomized (or adrenodemedullated) animals (10) and humans (9), suggesting that norepinephrine released from sympathetic nerves is the important stimulus. The mechanism by which catecholamines stimulate lipolysis is related not only to an increase in sympathetic nerve activity but also to an increased efficacy of ß-adrenergic stimulation (22). Adipocytes taken from human subjects after exercise have an increased lipolytic responsiveness to catecholamines that is mediated through ß-adrenergic mechanisms (22). This effect occurs without an increase in the binding of the ß-adrenergic receptor-specific catecholamine, ^{125}I-labeled cyanopindolol, suggesting that the effects of exercise are on a step distal to ligand binding. Prevention of the exercise-induced fall in insulin with an exogenous infusion of the hormone also attenuates the increase in arterial NEFA levels (4,23). Since this is accompanied by a diminished increase in circulating glycerol levels, it is likely that the fall in insulin increases NEFA levels, at least in part, by stimulating lipolysis (23). Nevertheless, the possibility of a decrease in reesterification resulting from the exercise-induced fall in insulin cannot be excluded.

In contrast to the importance of NEFA mobilization from adipose tissue during moderate-intensity exercise, its role during high-intensity exercise is considerably less. Despite the increased adrenergic drive that is present during high-intensity work, the arterial NEFA levels in plasma decrease. The contributions of a diminished lipolytic response and increased rate of reesterification to the diminished increase in NEFA mobilization have not been examined. It is notable, in this regard, that blood glycerol levels may still rise during heavy exercise. One explanation for this apparent discrepancy is that the increased blood glycerol levels are a result of glycerol release from triglycerides within the working muscle and that the NEFAs that are liberated in the process are oxidized locally, within the muscle.

Ketogenesis is increased with prolonged exercise because of elevated mobilization of NEFAs from adipose tissue and delivery to the liver, extraction of NEFAs by the liver, and conversion of NEFAs to ketone bodies within the liver (24). The rate that ketone bodies are released by the liver is unimportant as a direct fuel for the working muscle in healthy humans. The significance of hepatic ketogenesis is that it is a reflection of the energy state of the liver. It is a marker of fat oxidation, a key pathway in providing energy to fuel gluconeogenesis. Acute and chronic circumstances requiring accelerated gluconeogenic rates are characterized by high ketogenic rates. Inhibiting fat oxidation pharmacologically has been shown to reduce the exercise-induced increase in glucose production in depancreatized dogs that are heavily reliant on gluconeogenesis (25).

Few studies have assessed the role of potential hormonal and neural effectors in the control of ketogenesis during exercise. Any hormone or neurotransmitter that regulates hepatic NEFA delivery, hepatic NEFA extraction, or intrahepatic fat oxidation may play a role. Of these, hepatic NEFA delivery and ketone body output are particularly well correlated during rest and exercise (26). Therefore, factors that stimulate NEFA mobilization, such as a fall in insulin or the ß-adrenergic effects of the catecholamines, may stimulate ketogenesis. The exercise-induced rise in glucagon stimulates fat oxidation in the liver and is necessary for the full increase in ketogenesis observed during exercise (27). This stimulatory effect of glucagon occurs even though hepatic NEFA uptake is unaffected, indicating that glucagon is stimulating ketogenic processes with the liver.

Regulation of Muscle Glycogenolysis

Muscle glycogen is an important local fuel during the early stages of exercise.

As exercise duration progresses, glycogen stores decline in working muscle. With prolonged exercise, glycogenolysis is also stimulated in inactive muscle fibers. In these muscles, glycogen is metabolized to lactate, released from the muscle, and delivered to the liver, where it is used in the gluconeogenic pathway. The rate of glycogen breakdown in contracting muscle is accelerated by increasing work intensities. Studies using ß-adrenergic blockade indicate that the catecholamines play a major role in the mobilization of muscle glycogen during exercise (28). Studies in the isolated hindlimb indicate that in addition to epinephrine, contraction per se can stimulate muscle glycogenolysis even in the complete absence of catecholamines (29). Thus, it appears that catecholamines and some aspect of contraction, irrespective of neural and hormonal influence, control muscle glycogenolysis.

Regulation of Muscle Glucose Uptake

In contrast to muscle NEFA utilization, which is determined primarily by muscle NEFA availability, muscle glucose uptake is closely regulated by hormonal and nonhormonal mechanisms. Kinetic analyses of glucose uptake, conducted in vivo (30) and in vitro (31), generally indicate that the maximal velocity (V_{max}) for this process is increased by exercise without affecting the Michaelis-Menton constant (K_m). The K_m for glucose oxidation by the working limb is the same as that for glucose uptake, implying that both processes are characterized by the same rate-limiting step (30). The transport across the plasma membrane is probably rate-limiting, except perhaps at the onset of exercise or during heavy exercise, instances when intracellular glucose accumulates. Presuming that transport is limiting, the increases in V_{max} for glucose uptake and metabolism without a change in K_m suggest that exercise increases the number, turnover, and/or availability of active glucose transporters without a change in their affinity for glucose. This is con-

sistent with the demonstration that prior exercise increases transporter number and turnover in plasma membranes prepared from rat skeletal muscle (32,33). The increase in plasma membrane transporter number has been shown in some experiments to correspond to a decrease in transporter content in an intracellular microsomal fraction (33,34), indicating that, as during insulin stimulation, translocation of the glucose transporter is stimulated by muscle contraction. The results of other studies indicate, however, that exercise increases plasma glucose transporter number without a corresponding decrease in the intracellular glucose transporter pool mobilized by insulin (32). The conclusion drawn from these observations is that the glucose transporters recruited by muscle contraction are derived from a pool that is distinct from the glucose transporter source deployed by insulin and measured in the microsomal fraction.

Exercise is characterized by an increase in glucose utilization and a seemingly paradoxical fall in circulating insulin levels. Therefore, exercise must stimulate insulin-independent glucose uptake, increase insulin action, or both. Exercise does, in fact, appear to stimulate both insulin-independent glucose uptake and insulin action. Studies conducted in vitro show that contraction can stimulate glucose uptake in the complete absence of insulin (35). Studies conducted in vivo are somewhat less clear, because different model systems give different estimates of insulin-dependent and -independent mechanisms (3). In the insulin-deficient depancreatized dog, a model of poorly controlled diabetes, the exercise-induced increment in glucose metabolic clearance rate is very small, indicating that insulin-independent mechanisms are minimal. In contrast, in a model system characterized by insulin deficiency, but largely normal circulating NEFA and glucose levels (acute somatostatin-induced insulinopenia), the exercise-induced increase in glucose uptake and oxidation occurs primarily by insulin-independent processes. Finally, indirect estimates obtained by using multiple insulin clamps indicate that the glucose uptake and carbohydrate oxidation responses are insulin-independent. Taken together, it seems that in a physiological setting, the increase in glucose metabolism can occur to a large extent via insulin-independent processes. Under conditions characterized by the metabolic abnormalities present in diabetes (e.g., elevated NEFA levels), factors antagonistic to glucose uptake are present. Insulin becomes essential to glucose uptake during exercise in the insulin-deficient diabetic state to overcome this antagonism.

Muscle metabolism is sensitized to the actions of basal and elevated insulin levels (hyperinsulinemia). The mechanism(s) by which exercise en-hances insulin action may include 1) an increased blood flow to the working muscle, 2) increased transendothelial insulin transport, 3) indirect effects mediated by the insulin-induced suppression of NEFA levels, 4) potentiation by adenosine, and 5) an undefined insulin receptor or post-insulin receptor modification.

The potential importance of the muscle "metabolic state" in the regulation of glucose uptake is evident from the excessive increments in glucose uptake that occur under conditions in which oxygen availability is limited, such as during anemia, when breathing a hypoxic gas mixture, or during severe exercise (3). The high rates of glucose uptake during exercise when anemic or while breathing a hypoxic gas mixture occur even though insulin levels are no higher and catecholamine levels, which may be antagonistic to glucose uptake, are elevated. The mechanism of the link between muscle metabolism and glucose uptake remains to be identified. However, the energy state of the muscle, as determined by the muscle phosphocreatine level, correlates strongly to glucose uptake in the exercising limb (36). The ability of hypoxia and the muscle metabolic state to increase glucose uptake may be particularly important in individuals with diabetes and cardiovascular impairments.

Adaptations in the Postexercise State

The metabolic demands of exercise lead to adaptations that persist into the postexercise state. The more persistent metabolic effects during and after exercise are controlled, in large part, by glucoregulatory hormones. For this reason, individuals with IDDM may experience a derangement in metabolism long after the cessation of exercise. The hormone concentrations present during exercise are generally restored toward basal levels shortly after exercise (2). Exercise that results in significant changes in circulating glucose levels, however, will have more persistent effects on hormone levels. For example, the hyperglycemia that is associated with high-intensity exercise will result in postexercise hyperinsulinemia, and the fall in glucose that occurs during prolonged exercise can lead to a persistent elevation in counterregulatory hormone levels. Exercise, in many ways, simply accelerates the transition of the body into a more fasted state. Liver and muscle glycogen stores progressively deplete, and hepatic gluconeogenesis is accelerated. The extent of this effect depends on work intensity and duration. Muscle glycogen depletion is a potent stimulus for glycogen synthesis and facilitates the initial repletion of muscle stores in the postexercise state (37–39).

The repletion of muscle glycogen after exercise has been proposed to occur in two phases (37). In phase one, glucose uptake is elevated, glycogen synthase activity is elevated, and muscle glycogen is rapidly restored. This phase occurs immediately after the cessation of exercise and is notable in that it does not require insulin. In the second phase, muscle glycogen has returned to near-normal levels and glucose uptake requires insulin. Phase two is characterized by a marked and persistent increase in insulin action. This model for postexercise glycogen resynthesis is consistent with findings obtained using ^{13}C nuclear magnetic resonance spectroscopy following contraction of the human gastrocnemius muscle (39). These experiments showed that muscle glycogen synthesis is predominantly insulin-independent the first hour after the cessation of contraction, but it is insulin-dependent after this interval. An increase in insulin binding to muscle is not necessary for the increase in insulin action following exercise (37), indicating that postreceptor events are responsible. The added insulin-stimulated glucose disposal after exercise is solely due to an increase in nonoxidative glucose metabolism (37). The duration of these alterations in muscle glucose metabolism is probably longer after more extensive glycogen-depleting exercise and can be protracted by an absence of dietary carbohydrate (38). Glycogen repletion to preexercise levels requires ~24 h in humans maintained on a high-carbohydrate diet, but it may take as long as 8–10 days if carbohydrate is absent from the diet (38).

EXERCISE AND IDDM

It is apparent from the preceding discussion that the prevailing insulin level is an important determinant of the metabolic response to exercise. Nondiabetic subjects spontaneously regulate the release of insulin from the ß-cells of the pancreas in accordance with their metabolic needs. The inability of IDDM patients to regulate the delivery of insulin into the blood in a similar fashion can seriously compromise their ability to meet the requirements of exercise. Given current insulin treatment regimens, it is extremely difficult to duplicate the normal metabolic responses seen in nondiabetic individuals. Frequently, insulin delivery is mismatched to insulin needs, and the risk of hypoglycemia or exacerbated hyperglycemia can result. The following sections address the problems of over- and underinsulinization in IDDM. Table 3.2 summarizes the potential repercussions of too much or too little insulin.

Overinsulinization

The results of the Diabetes Control and Complications Trial (DCCT), an assessment of the effects of glucose control on the long-term complications of diabetes, demonstrate conclusively that tight glucose control prevents the advent and/or delays the progression of microvascular complications. While the DCCT findings provide a firm basis for advocating tight metabolic control in individuals with IDDM, the move toward more rigorous control creates an added risk of hypoglycemia. In the IDDM patient with excess circulating insulin, the increases in the release of glucose from the liver and NEFAs from adipose tissue that normally occur with exercise are inhibited. Since muscle glucose utilization increases with exercise, the attenuation of hepatic glucose

---

Table 3.2. Exercise and IDDM

Too little insulin
  Glucose production is accelerated
                                            → Blood glucose increases
  Glucose utilization is impaired

  Lipolysis is excessive   → Free fatty acids and ketone bodies
                                              are increased

Too much insulin
  Glucose production is impaired
                                            → Blood glucose decreases
  Glucose utilization is accelerated

  Lipolysis is reduced   → Free fatty acids and ketone bodies
                                              are lowered

production leads to a fall in circulating glucose. If the exercise period is sufficiently long, hypoglycemia will eventually result. Since exercise is one of the main causes of hypoglycemia in well-controlled IDDM, the implementation of treatment regimens designed to achieve tight control requires an understanding of the factors that can increase the risk of hypoglycemia during exercise. Three factors make patients with IDDM vulnerable to becoming overinsulinized and hypoglycemic during exercise.

■ The failure of plasma insulin to decrease as it does when people without diabetes exercise can lead to relative overinsulinization. As a result, a dose of insulin appropriate at rest may be excessive during exercise. Although the fall in insulin is essential to the metabolic response to exercise in nondiabetic subjects (4,5), this may not be uniformly true for individuals with IDDM receiving a peripheral infusion. In studies conducted in postabsorptive IDDM patients exercising during a constant basal infusion of insulin, glucose levels have been shown both to remain constant (40) and to fall (11). A reduction in premeal insulin dose may be more important for exercise conducted in the postprandial state (41).
■ The exercise-induced increase in insulin action may lead to a relative overinsulinization in IDDM patients if a compensatory decrease in insulin dosage is not made. Since the exercise-induced increase in insulin action can persist for many hours after exercise (42,37), IDDM patients who have not made appropriate adjustments in their insulin dosage risk becoming hypoglycemic long after the cessation of exercise.
■ The absorption of subcutaneously injected insulin can be accelerated by exercise (40). This effect can be minimized by injecting away from the site of contraction. The effect of exercise on insulin absorption can be increased even further if insulin is injected into the muscle as opposed to the subcutaneous region of the working limb (43). Thus, extra care must be given to avoid inadvertent injection into skeletal muscle. Even though precautions need to be made to minimize inappropriately rapid insulin absorption, it is important to realize that hypoglycemia can result even when insulin mobilization is not accelerated.

There are many possible ways to permute the timing and amount of insulin administration and food intake to best avoid hypoglycemia, and many different options have been studied. A reduction in insulin dose in anticipation of exercise clearly decreases the risk of hypoglycemia. This is particularly important in the postprandial state, because the extra insulin needed to minimize the glycemic excursion in response to feeding can create insulin levels that, while normal for meal ingestion, are excessive when exercise is added. In one study, IDDM patients maintained on intensive insulin therapy using either multiple subcutaneous injections or continuous subcutaneous insulin infusions (CSII) became hypoglycemic over the course of 45 min of moderate-intensity exercise conducted 2 h after an insulin injection and 90 min after a standard meal (44). Hypoglycemia was avoided in these individuals by reducing the insulin dose by 30–50%. This is consistent with the finding that insulin-infused subjects exercising 30 min after breakfast exhibit a rapid fall in circulating glucose if the insulin infusion rate is increased to simulate the normal insulin response (41). The fall in plasma glucose is avoided, however, if insulin is lowered by ~70% below the elevated postprandial insulin infusion rate. The results of one study indicate that it may not be necessary to reduce the amount of insulin injected subcutaneously in the postprandial state, provided that enough time is allowed following the injection for the insulin levels in the blood to be in a declining mode similar to that normally present during exercise (45).

More prolonged exercise may require a greater reduction in insulin dosage. Individuals with IDDM are able to exercise in the postabsorptive state for nearly 3 h without becoming hypoglycemic if the insulin dose is reduced by 80% compared with 90 min when the dosage is reduced by 50% (46). Furthermore, the glucose-lowering effect of insulin during heavy exercise is greater than that during moderate exercise of similar duration (47,48). Naturally, the magnitude of the glucose fall that can be tolerated by an individual before hypoglycemia ensues will depend on the glycemia at the onset of exercise. Nevertheless, if the primary objective of insulin therapy is tight glucose control, the margin of error in estimating an exercise insulin dose should be considered small.

Since exercise is often spontaneous, particularly in children, it is not always possible to anticipate the need to decrease the insulin dosage. In these instances, glucose ingestion takes on added importance as a means of preventing hypoglycemia. The effectiveness of an oral carbohydrate load will depend, in large part, on its intestinal absorption kinetics. Therefore, readily absorbable substrates are most suitable for ingestion during exercise or in the postexercise state if the individual is in immediate risk of developing hypoglycemia. On the other hand, it has been suggested that a slowly absorbed carbohydrate might be more useful in decreasing the risk of delayed-onset hypoglycemia, which can occur hours after the cessation of exercise (49). This is of particular importance if exercise is performed in the late afternoon or evening, since hypoglycemia may occur during sleep. A possible inhibitory effect of exercise on food absorption from the gut has been a concern. However, gastrointestinal glucose absorption does not appear to be a limitation, because the majority of [^{13}C]glucose contained in an oral glucose load consumed during prolonged moderate exercise can be accounted for by the $^{13}CO_2$ content of the expired air of nondiabetic subjects and well-controlled IDDM patients (50).

Selection of the ideal quantity of calories necessary to avoid hypo-glycemia will be determined by many of the factors summarized in Table 3.1. Of particular importance is the exercise intensity and duration. High-intensity exercise leads to a less efficient utilization of oral glucose compared with moderate- or light-intensity exercise, because the availability of oral glucose does not increase proportionally to metabolic demands (51). The amount of ingested glucose can be reduced if exercise is initiated under hyperglycemic conditions. Based on assumptions regarding the size of the body glucose pool, it can be estimated that a 70-kg individual requires ~5 g less of ingested glucose for every 50 mg/dl increment above the target blood glucose level.

Although ways to estimate the amount of added glucose needed during exercise have been suggested (52), it is impossible to identify precisely the amount needed for each individual. Variability exists not only between individuals but also for each individual, depending on the time that exercise is performed (53). The potential variability between and for individuals is illustrated by the results from one study, which showed that in a group of eight IDDM patients, three different types of responses to exercise following breakfast and lunch could be identified (53). In the majority of these patients, exercise reduced the glycemic excursion following both meals. In two patients, however, exercise lowered the glycemic response following lunch only, and in a third patient, exercise had no effect on glycemia at all. Considerable variation in the postexercise glycemic response is also observed (54). Making recommendations that are broadly applicable to the IDDM population on how to adjust insulin and diet for exercise is clearly not feasible. Recommendations for treatment modification need to be tailored to the specific exercise response for each individual. With the widespread use of self-monitoring of blood glucose (SMBG), however, an individual's specific exercise responses are very easy to obtain. Patients should be encouraged to document their responses to particular activities.

Underinsulinization

IDDM patients in poor control are hyperglycemic, hyperlipidemic, and may be ketotic. Although glucose fluxes may be normal or accelerated, the mechanisms responsible for the metabolic changes are different than in individuals with and without IDDM. A greater fraction of the glucose released by the liver is gluconeogenic in origin under insulin-deficient conditions (55). Muscle glucose utilization occurs even when insulin levels are deficient, since the mass action effect of the hyperglycemia overcomes the lack of insulin-stimulated glucose uptake (55). Nevertheless, a smaller percentage of the glucose that is used in poorly controlled IDDM is fully oxidized because of impaired pyruvate dehydrogenase activity. Elevated NEFA utilization compensates for the deficit in energy production that would otherwise occur as a result of impaired glucose oxidation. IDDM patients in poor control may also have diminished glycogen stores and increased lipid stores within the muscle. This may, in turn, result in a decrease and an increase, respectively, in the use of these intramuscular stores (56).

Exercise in the insulin-deficient state can result in a further deterioration of metabolic control. Exercise in IDDM patients deprived of insulin for 18–48 h results in an exacerbation of the hyperglycemia and ketosis already present in these individuals (57). The rise in blood glucose is due to an impairment in the exercise-induced increase in glucose utilization accompanied by a normal increase in hepatic glucose production. The added increase in hepatic ketone body output during exercise in poorly controlled IDDM is, in part, secondary to an unrestrained increase in lipolysis and possibly to an increase in intrahepatic ketogenic efficiency (24). In some instances, heavy exercise can be more deleterious to metabolic control than moderate exercise of the same duration. Even well-controlled IDDM patients receiving CSII may have an increase in blood glucose and NEFA levels following high-intensity exercise (58). This is probably due to a failure of insulin to rise as it normally would following heavy exercise in nondiabetic subjects.

In well-controlled IDDM patients who are free of autonomic neuropathies, the counterregulatory hormone response to exercise is similar to the response in nondiabetic subjects, provided that hypoglycemia does not occur. In the nondiabetic state, the counterregulatory system is sensitized to changes in glucose during exercise as both the counterregulatory hormone threshold and the magnitude of the counterregulatory hormone response are increased (1). Although this efficient counterregulation may be sustained in some patients with IDDM, it seems to be defective in others (59). In contrast to IDDM patients in good control, IDDM patients in poor control have increased counterregulatory hormone responses (57), all of which may contribute to the deleterious metabolic effect of exercise in these individuals. As is the case in the nondiabetic state, glucagon probably contributes to the increased hepatic glucose (60) and ketone body (26) outputs present in poorly controlled IDDM. The role of glucagon during exercise in IDDM is summarized with regard to metabolic control in Table 3.3. The β-adrenergic effects of the catecholamines play a minor role in controlling hepatic metabolism in nondiabetic control subjects, but may be of greater significance in IDDM (11). The potent effects of the catecholamines in stimulating fuel mobilization from muscle (glycogen) and adipose (triglycerides) and fuel delivery to the liver (in the form of lactate, alanine, glycerol, and NEFAs) is important in poorly controlled IDDM, because this process provides precursors for gluconeogenesis and ketogenesis to the liver. Recent work in humans suggests that the catecholamines may also be important during heavy exercise in IDDM, even though the probable source of the glucose released by the liver under these circumstances is hepatic glycogen (61). The increased role of the cate-

Table 3.3. Role of Glucagon During Exercise in IDDM

Too little insulin
    Glucagon response is exaggerated   → Increased hepatic glucose output
                                         → Increased ketogenesis
                                         → Worsened metabolic control

Too much insulin
    Glucagon response is reduced   → Decreased hepatic glucose output
                                    → Increased risk of hypoglycemia

cholamines is exemplified by the greater glucose lowering effect of propranolol in IDDM patients compared with nondiabetic subjects (11). The metabolic actions of the catecholamines during exercise in IDDM are summarized with respect to metabolic control in Table 3.4.

EXERCISE AND NIDDM

Although NIDDM is the predominant form of diabetes, the metabolic response to exercise in this population has not received a corresponding degree of attention. Insulin resistance may be a prominent feature of NIDDM and may be particularly important in the context of syndrome X (62). This syndrome is often characterized by obesity, hyperinsulinemia, and hypertension; treatment may consist of dietary prescriptions, oral hypoglycemic agents, lipid-lowering agents, and/or insulin. However, the use of exercise as a therapeutic modality may be particularly beneficial because it has a positive impact on insulin resistance, the fundamental abnormality of this metabolic state.

Obese NIDDM patients maintained on diet therapy alone or diet and sulfonylurea therapy with postabsorptive plasma glucose in excess of 200 mg/dl and normal basal insulin show a fall in glycemia of ~50 mg/dl during a 45-min exercise session (63). The fall in glucose under these conditions is due to an attenuated rise in hepatic glucose production coupled to a normal increase in glucose utilization. With regard to this increase in glucose utilization, note that rats made insulin-resistant by high-fat feeding still exhibit a normal exercise-induced increment in glucose metabolism (64). The reduced rise in glucose production could be due to the failure of insulin to fall as it does in control subjects and/or to the hepatic effects of hyperglycemia that are present in these subjects. Alternatively, a defect in a feedback mechanism that couples the

Table 3.4. Role of Catecholamines During Exercise in IDDM

Too little insulin
    Catecholamine response is exaggerated
                                    → Increased lipolysis
                                    → Increased free fatty acids and ketones
                                    → Impaired glucose utilization
                                    → Increase in glucose production?

Too much insulin
    In the absence of advanced autonomic neuropathy, catecholamine response is exaggerated if hypoglycemia ensues, leading to the above metabolic responses and prevention of more severe hypoglycemia.

increases in glucose production and utilization during exercise may exist in patients with NIDDM (65).

During 3 h of moderate-intensity exercise in NIDDM patients with moderate fasting hyperglycemia (140 mg/dl) and hyperinsulinemia (23 μU/ml), plasma glucose falls by ~40 mg/dl (66). Moreover, a decrease in the elevated insulin levels is also present. One recent study showed that a single session of glycogen-depleting exercise significantly increases insulin sensitivity at the liver and in muscle 12–16 h later in men with NIDDM (67). Prior exercise reduced basal hepatic glucose production and accentuated the suppressive effects of a low-dose insulin infusion on this variable. Peripheral insulin sensitivity was increased as reflected by an enhanced rate of nonoxidative glucose disposal and increased glycogen synthase activity. These studies that illustrate how exercise can lower circulating glucose levels and increase insulin sensitivity in NIDDM patients emphasize the potential importance of exercise as a therapy in this population.

NIDDM patients on diet therapy alone should be able to exercise with no more caution than the individual with normal glucose tolerance, provided there are no major vascular or neurological complications. When oral hypoglycemic agents (sulfonylureas) are used, there may be a tendency for hypoglycemia during prolonged exercise. When glyburide was given to normal subjects before exercise, insulin levels increased by about twofold and blood glucose fell to 50 mg/dl (68). Experimental use of the free fatty acid oxidation inhibitor methylpalmoxirate in the streptozotocin-induced diabetic rat has been shown to accelerate glucose oxidation in the liver and, to a lesser extent, in muscle, thereby depleting glycogen stores in these tissues (69). This drug has also been shown to impair total hepatic glucose production in exercising depancreatized dogs (25). If such compounds are to be used for therapeutic purposes, the tendency for hypoglycemia during exercise will be enhanced. In addition, chronic use of fatty acid oxidation inhibitors may lead to accumulation of esterified fat in the liver and to hypertrophy of the myocardium. Clearly, more work is necessary to fully understand the entire spectrum of the effects of fatty acid oxidation inhibitors. Regardless of the course of treatment, future studies should ascertain more precisely the metabolic response to exercise as a function of the therapeutic regimen.

For many patients with NIDDM, weight loss is an important aspect of their therapy. For this reason, these individuals may be maintained on a low-calorie diet in combination with exercise. Although calorie restriction is usually necessary to lose weight, it is also important that enough calories be provided for a subject to be able to exercise safely. Diets containing <400 kcal/day have been associated with cardiac arrhythmias and sudden death. An individual participating in an exercise program should probably be kept on a diet containing no less than 800 kcal/day. It seems that low-calorie diets can be used without affecting exercise tolerance, provided that they contain enough carbohydrate (at least 35% of the total calories) to maintain normal muscle glycogen levels.

Although many patients with NIDDM are reliant on exogenous insulin, all the data concerning the exercise response in patients receiving insulin have been derived from studies of patients with IDDM. Although there may be certain discrepancies, the practical considerations that apply when planning a therapeutic regimen for individuals with IDDM will probably apply to those with NIDDM who are receiving insulin.

PRACTICAL CONSIDERATIONS FOR ADAPTING THERAPY TO PHYSICAL ACTIVITY

As noted above, NIDDM individuals without extensive vascular or neurological complications can generally exercise with no more concern than nondiabetic individuals of equal cardiovascular fitness. However, IDDM patients should take several precautions. It is impossible to give precise guidelines for diet and insulin therapy that will be suitable for all patients with IDDM who wish to be physically active. Individuals will differ in their tolerance to exercise and insulin requirements. Moreover, the metabolic demands associated with exercise vary depending on the type of exercise. Nevertheless, some general strategies can be applied to help prevent the problems associated with exercise in IDDM. Regular SMBG should be conducted for two reasons. First, frequent SMBG before, during, and after exercise helps a patient identify when he or she is at an immediate risk of becoming hypoglycemic or hyperglycemic. In addition, SMBG provides feedback that forms the basis for implementing therapy for subsequent exercise. If blood glucose readings are <80 mg/dl before exercise, the risk of hypoglycemia is great, and exercise should not be initiated without the ingestion of glucose. If fasting blood glucose is >250–300 mg/dl and ketone bodies are present in the urine, it is generally advisable to administer more insulin and delay exercising. In addition to preexercise evaluation, SMBG should be done at regular intervals during and after exercise to minimize the risk of hypoglycemia. It is important to consider not only the absolute glycemic levels when monitoring blood glucose but also the rate at which any change in glycemia may occur. For example, a glucose level that is stable at 100 mg/dl may reflect a safe situation, but a glucose level of 100 mg/dl following a glucose level of 150 mg/dl is indicative of an imbalance between glucose production and utilization and may require further attention (i.e., glucose ingestion).

The need to reduce the insulin dose before exercise and avoid administrating insulin in the region of the working muscles was emphasized in a previous section. The precise size of any reduction in insulin is dependent on many variables that will vary from person to person and with different exercise parameters (i.e., work intensity and duration). Individuals maintained on inter-mediate- and short-acting insulin may decrease or omit the short-acting insulin, depending on the circumstances. Alternatively, the intermediate-acting dose could be reduced but supplemented with added short-acting insulin later in the day. People relying on CSII with the intention of exercising in the post-prandial state should reduce the pre-meal bolus. An advantage of using an insulin pump is that the pump eliminates much of the variability in circulating insulin levels that occurs because of exercise-induced changes in insulin absorption from subcutaneous depots. With a pump, the insulin store is in the device and not in a subcutaneous depot where it is subject to changes in the absorption profile. A disadvantage of insulin pumps is that they can be cumbersome and vulnerable to damage. Some pump users remove the devices before physical activity, administering a small bolus before removal. Of course, any added insulin must be given prudently and in conjunction with SMBG.

In addition to modifications in insulin delivery and glucose ingestion, the type, duration, and timing of exercise are necessary considerations when implementing exercise programs. Exercise that requires repetitive recruitment of large muscle groups (e.g., running or walking, cycling, or swimming) causes large and sustained increases in oxygen uptake and leads to long-term cardiovascular adaptations. A work intensity that causes an increase in the metabolic demand of ~50% of an individual's maximum oxygen uptake and an exercise duration of >20 min is sufficiently rigorous to obtain exercise-related adaptations. Exercise of extended duration, however, increases the risk of hypoglycemia and should be undertaken with appropriate precautions. Competitive sports frequently require high-intensity exertion. This type of exercise not only contributes to fitness but also is an important part of the socialization of children and young adults in particular. Because of the integral role of strenuous exercise in society, it is important to understand glucoregulation during this type of exercise. The time of day that one exercises should be considered. The risk of hypoglycemia from exercise appears to be lowest in the morning before the prebreakfast insulin dose (70). Insulin levels are usually lowest at this time. Late afternoon or early evening exercise can be hazardous if sufficient precautions are not taken to minimize the risk of hypoglycemia during sleep. Adapting insulin and diet therapy to regular exercise can be greatly facilitated if the time of day for exercise and the exercise parameters are consistent. While this may be a reasonable objective for some adults, the spontaneity with which children exercise and the variety of different sports in which they may participate make this goal difficult to obtain. Also, one of the chief obstacles patients face in undertaking and benefiting from an exercise program is compliance. Compliance to an exercise program will be highest if patients select a type of exercise they enjoy.

CONCLUSIONS

Exercise should be encouraged in people with diabetes for the same reasons that it should be encouraged in the general population. Regular exercise can decrease risk factors for cardiovascular disease and is believed by many to improve the general quality of life. Physical activity can improve metabolic control in NIDDM patients and even alleviate symptoms of the syndrome altogether. Evidence that the adaptations to regular exercise improve glucose control in IDDM is, however, lacking. While the benefits of regular physical activity in diabetic and nondiabetic populations are generally similar, patients with IDDM face a number of challenges before, during, and after each exercise session that are unique to diabetes. Exercise-induced changes in insulin and counterregulatory hormone levels control the mobilization of fuels from various storage sites. In people with IDDM, the normal endocrine response to exercise is lost, resulting in derangements in fuel metabolism. Exercise can lead to profound hypo-

glycemia if insulin levels are excessive or to an exacerbated diabetic state (e.g., hyperglycemia or ketosis) if insulin levels are deficient. A number of strategies must be considered to safely adapt insulin therapy and diet to accommodate daily exercise. Since the most serious and frequent metabolic problem is hypoglycemia during and after exercise, adjustments in therapy for IDDM patients involve a reduction in insulin dose in anticipation of exercise and/or the ingestion of readily absorbable carbohydrate. The value and appropriateness of an exercise program for the individual with IDDM is judged by the extent to which the beneficial adaptive effects of regular exercise exceed the risks of a single exercise session.

The results of the DCCT have emphasized the importance of tight glucose control in deterring the complications of diabetes and should lead to an increase in the number of individuals who make tight control an objective of their therapy. With this, the onus is on the patient and health-care providers to understand the factors that contribute to hypoglycemia during exercise and to develop strategies to avoid it. Research in the area of exercise and diabetes has progressed to the point where a knowledgeable patient can adjust therapy in anticipation of exercise of predetermined length and intensity and minimize the risk of hypoglycemia. Children, though, rarely set out with a precise agenda and frequently become involved in recreation after administration of insulin. Further research needs to be conducted to develop ways of minimizing the risk of hypoglycemia during spontaneous exercise when the option to reduce the insulin dose is no longer available. In addition, most of our understanding of exercise in individuals with diabetes is obtained from experiments designed to look at the effects of moderate exercise. Exercise is often conducted in high-intensity "bursts" (e.g., soccer, hockey, or basketball). More research needs to be focused on means to accommodate participation in competitive sports so that IDDM children and adults who wish to engage in them can do so safely.

REFERENCES

1. Wasserman DH, Zinman B: American Diabetes Association: Exercise in individuals with insulin-dependent diabetes mellitus (Technical Review). *Diabetes Care* 17:924–37, 1994
2. Galbo H: *Hormonal Adaptations to Exercise*. New York, Thieme-Stratton, 1983
3. Wasserman DH: Control of glucose fluxes during exercise in the postabsorptive state. In *Annual Review of Physiology*. Palo Alto, CA, Annual Reviews, 1995, p. 191–218
4. Hirsch IB, Marker JC, Smith J, Spina R, Parvin CA, Holloszy JO, Cryer PE: Insulin and glucagon in the prevention of hypoglycemia during exercise in humans. *Am J Physiol* 260:E695–704, 1991
5. Wasserman DH, Lacy DB, Goldstein RE, Williams PE, Cherrington AD: Exercise-induced fall in insulin and hepatic carbohydrate metabolism during exercise. *Am J Physiol* 256:E500–508, 1989
6. Wasserman DH, Spalding JS, Lacy DB, Colburn CA, Goldstein RE, Cherrington AD: Glucagon is a primary controller of the increments in hepatic glycogenolysis and gluconeogenesis during exercise. *Am J Physiol* 257:E108–17, 1989
7. Kjaer M, Engfred K, Fernandez A, Secher N, Galbo H: Regulation of hepatic glucose production during exercise in humans: role of sympathoadrenergic activity. *Am J Physiol* 265:E275–83, 1993
8. Wolfe RR, Nadel ER, Shaw JHF, Stephenson LA, Wolfe M: Role of changes in insulin and glucagon in glucose homeostasis in exercise. *J Clin Invest* 77:900–907, 1986
9. Hoelzer DR, Dalsky GP, Schwartz NS, Clutter WE, Shah SD, Holloszy JO, Cryer PE: Epinephrine is not critical to prevention of hypoglycemia during exercise in humans. *Am J Physiol* 251:E104–10, 1986
10. Moates JM, Lacy DB, Cherrington AD, Goldstein RE, Wasserman DH: The metabolic role of the exercise-induced increment in epinephrine. *Am J Physiol* 255:E428–36, 1988
11. Simonson DC, Koivisto VA, Sherwin RS, Ferrannini R, Hendler R, DeFronzo RA: Adrenergic blockade alters glucose kinetics during exercise in insulin-dependent diabetics. *J Clin Invest* 73:1648–58, 1984
12. Kjaer M, Engfred K, Galbo H, Sonne B, Rasmussen K, Keiding S: Hepatic glucose production during exercise in liver-transplanted subjects (Abstract). *Scand J Gastroenterol* 26 (Suppl.):46A, 1991
13. Richter EA, Galbo H, Holst JJ, Sonne B: Significance of glucagon for insulin secretion and hepatic glycogenolysis during exercise in rats. *Horm Metab Res* 13:323–26, 1981
14. Wasserman DH, Williams PE, Lacy DB, Bracy D, Cherrington AD: Hepatic nerves are not essential to the increase in hepatic glucose production during muscular work. *Am J Physiol* 259:E195–203, 1990
15. Friedman JE: Role of glucocorticoids in activation of hepatic PEPCK gene transcription during exercise. *Am J Physiol* 266:E560–66, 1994
16. Marliss EB, Purdon C, Halter JB, Sigal RJ, Vranic M: *Glucoregulation During and After Intense Exercise in Control and Diabetic Subjects*. London, Smith-Gordon, 1992
17. Sigal RJ, Fisher SF, Halter JB, Vranic M, Marliss EB: The roles of catecholamines in glucoregulation in intense exercise as defined by the islet cell clamp technique. *Diabetes*. Submitted
18. Sigal RJ, Purdon C, Bilinski D, Vranic M, Halter JB, Marliss EB: Glucoregulation during and after intense exercise: effects of beta-blockade. *J Clin Endocrinol Metab* 78:359–66, 1994
19. Wolfe RR, Klein S, Carraro F, Weber JM: Role of triglyceride-fatty acid cycle in controlling fat metabolism in humans during and after exercise. *Am J Physiol* 258:E382–89, 1990
20. Arner P, Kriegholm E, Engfeldt P, Bolinder J: Adrenergic regulation of lipolysis in situ at rest and during

exercise. *J Clin Invest* 85:893–98, 1990

21. Issekutz B: Role of beta-adrenergic receptors in mobilization of energy sources in exercising dogs. *J Appl Physiol* 44:869–76, 1978

22. Wahrenberg H, Engfeldt P, Bolinder J, Arner P: Acute adaptation in adrenergic control of lipolysis during physical exercise in humans. *Am J Physiol* 253:E383–90, 1987

23. Wasserman DH, Lacy DB, Goldstein RE, Williams PE, Cherrington AD: Exercise-induced fall in insulin and the increase in fat metabolism during prolonged exercise. *Diabetes* 38:484–90, 1989

24. Wahren J, Sato Y, Ostman J, Hagenfeldt L, Felig P: Turnover and splanchnic metabolism of free fatty acids and ketones in insulin-dependent diabetics during exercise. *J Clin Invest* 73:1367–76, 1984

25. Shi Z, Yamatani GAK, Fisher SJ, Lickley H, Vranic M: Effects of subbasal insulin infusion on resting and exercise-induced glucose turnover in depancreatized dogs. *Am J Physiol* 264:E334–41, 1993

26. Seftoft L, Trap-Jensen J, Lyngsoe J, Clausen JP, Holst JJ, Nielsen SL, Rehfeld JF, Muckadell OSD: Regulation of gluconeogenesis and ketogenesis during rest and exercise in diabetic subjects and normal men. *Clin Sci Mol Med* 53:411–18, 1977

27. Wasserman DH, Spalding JS, Bracy DP, Lacy DB, Cherrington AD: Exercise-induced rise in glucagon and the increase in ketogenesis during prolonged muscular work. *Diabetes* 38:799–807, 1989

28. Chasiostis D, Sahlin K, Hultman E: Regulation of glycogenolysis in human muscle at rest and during exercise. *J Appl Physiol* 53:708–15, 1982

29. Richter EA, Ruderman NB, Gavras H, Belur E, Galbo H: Muscle glycogenolysis during exercise: dual control by epinephrine and contractions. *Am J Physiol* 242:E25–32, 1982

30. Zinker BA, Bracy D, Lacy DB, Jacobs J, Wasserman DH: Regulation of glucose uptake and metabolism during exercise: an in vivo analysis. *Diabetes* 42:956–65, 1993

31. Nesher R, Karl I, Kipnis D: Dissociation of effects of insulin and contraction on glucose transport in rat epitrochlearis muscle. *Am J Physiol* 249:C226–32, 1985

32. Douen AG, Ramlal R, Cartee GD, Klip A: Exercise-induced increase in glucose transporters of plasma membranes of rat skeletal muscle. *Endocrinology* 124:449–54, 1989

33. Fushiki T, Wells JA, Tapscott EB, Dohm GL: Changes in glucose transporters in muscle in response to exercise. *Am J Physiol* 256:E580–87, 1989

34. Goodyear LJ, Hirshman MF, Horton ES: Exercise-induced translocation of skeletal muscle glucose transporters. *Am J Physiol* 261:E795–99, 1991

35. Ploug T, Galbo H, Richter EA: Increased muscle glucose uptake during contractions: no need for insulin. *Am J Physiol* 247:E726–31, 1984

36. Katz A, Broberg S, Sahlin K, Wahren J: Leg glucose uptake during maximal dynamic exercise in humans. *Am J Physiol* 251:E65–70, 1986

37. Garetto LP, Richter EA, Goodman MN, Ruderman NB: Enhanced muscle glucose metabolism after exercise in the rat: the two phases. *Am J Physiol* 246:E471–75, 1984

38. Hultman E, Bergstrom J, Roch-Norland AE: Glycogen storage in human skeletal muscle. In *Muscle Metabolism During Exercise.* Pernow BSB, Ed. New York, Plenum, 1971, p. 273–88

39. Price TB, Rothman DL, Taylor R, Avison MJ, Shulman GI, Shulman RG: Human muscle glycogen resynthesis after exercise: insulin-dependent and -independent phases. *J Appl Physiol* 76:104–11, 1994

40. Zinman B, Murray FT, Vranic M, Albisser AM, Leibel BS, McClean PA, Marliss EB: Glucoregulation during moderate exercise in insulin-treated diabetics. *J Clin Endocrinol Metab* 45:641–52, 1977

41. Nelson JD, Poussier P, Marliss EB, Albisser AM, Zinman B: Metabolic response of normal man and insulin-infused diabetics to post-prandial exercise in type I diabetics. *Am J Physiol* 242:E309–16, 1982

42. Bogardus C, Thuillez P, Ravnussin E, Vasquez B, Narimiga M, Azhar S: Effect of muscle glycogen depletion on in vivo insulin action in man. *J Clin Invest* 72:1605–10, 1983

43. Frid A, Ostman J, Linde B: Hypoglycemia risk during exercise after intramuscular injection of insulin in thigh in IDDM. *Diabetes Care* 13:473–77, 1990

44. Schiffrin A, Parikh S: Accommodating planned exercise in type I diabetic patients on intensive treatment. *Diabetes Care* 8:337–43, 1985

45. Trovati M, Anfossi G, Vitali S, Mularoni E, Massucco P, Facis RD, Carta Q: Postprandial exercise in type I diabetic patients on multiple daily insulin injection regimen. *Diabetes Care* 11:107–10, 1988

46. Kemmer FW, Berger M: Therapy and better quality of life: the dichotomous role of exercise in diabetes mellitus. *Diabetes Metab Rev* 2:53–68, 1986

47. Hubinger A, Ridderskamp I, Lehmann E: Metabolic response to different forms of physical exercise in type I diabetics and the duration of the glucose lowering effect. *Eur J Clin Invest* 15:197–205, 1985

48. Zander E, Bruns W, Wulfert P, Besch W, Lubs D, Chlup R, Schulz B: Muscular exercise in type I diabetics: different metabolic reactions during heavy muscular work: independence on actual insulin availability. *Exp Clin Endocrinol* 82:78–90, 1983

49. Nathan DM, Madnek SF, Delahanty L: Programming pre-exercise snacks to prevent post-exercise hypoglycemia in intensively treated insulin-dependent diabetics. *Ann Intern Med* 102:483–86, 1985

50. Krzentowski G, Pirnay F, Pallikarakis N, Luyckx AS, Lacroix M, Mosora F, Lefebvre PJ: Glucose utilization during exercise in normal and diabetic subjects: the role of insulin. *Diabetes* 30:983–89, 1981

51. Pirnay F, Crielaard JM, Pallikarakis N, Lacroix M, Mosora F, Luyckx A, Lefebvre PJ: Fate of exogenous glucose during exercise of different intensities in humans. *J Appl Physiol* 43:258–61, 1982

52. Horton ES: Role and management of exercise in diabetes mellitus. *Diabetes Care* 11:201–11, 1988

53. Caron D, Poussier P, Marliss EB, Zinman B: The effect of postprandial exercise on meal-related glucose intolerance in insulin-dependent diabetic individuals. *Diabetes Care* 5:364–69, 1982

54. Campaigne BN, Wallberg-Henricksson H, Gunnarsson R: Glucose and insulin responses in relation to insulin dose and caloric intake 12 h after physical exercise in men with IDDM. *Diabetes Care* 10:716–21, 1987

55. Wahren J, Hagenfeldt L, Felig P: Splanchnic and leg exchange of glucose, amino acids, and free fatty acids during exercise in diabetes mellitus. *J Clin Invest* 55:1303–14, 1975

56. Standl E, Lotz N, Dexel TH, Janka H, Kolb H: Muscle triglycerides in diabetic subjects. *Diabetologia* 18:463–69, 1980

57. Berger M, Berchtold P, Kuppers HJ, Drost H, Kley HK, Muller WA, Wiegelmann W, Zimmerman-Telschow H, Gries FA, Kruskemper HL, Zimmerman H: Metabolic and hormonal effects of muscular exercise in juvenile type diabetics. *Diabetologia* 13:355–65, 1977

58. Mitchell RH, Abraham G, Schiffrin A, Leiter A, Marliss EB: Hyperglycemia after intense exercise in IDDM subjects during continuous subcutaneous insulin infusion. *Diabetes Care* 11:311–17, 1988

59. Schneider SH, Vitug A, Ananthakrishnan R, Khachadurian AK: Impaired adrenergic response to prolonged exercise in type I diabetes. *Metabolism* 40:1219–25, 1991

60. Wasserman DH, Lickley HLA, Vranic M: Important role of glucagon during exercise in diabetic dogs. *J Appl Physiol* 59:1272–81, 1985

61. Purdon C, Brusson M, Nyreen SL, Miles PDG, Halter J, Vranic M, Marliss EB: The roles of insulin and catecholamines in the glucoregulatory response during intense exercise and early recovery in insulin-dependent diabetic and control subjects. *J Clin Endocrinol Metab* 76: 566–73, 1993

62. Reaven GM: Role of insulin resistance in human disease. *Diabetes* 37:1595–1607, 1988

63. Minuk HL, Vranik M, Hanna AK, Albisser AM, Zinman B: Glucoregulatory and metabolic response to exercise in obese non-insulin-dependent diabetes. *Am J Physiol* 240:E458–64, 1981

64. Kusunoki M, Storlien LH, Macdessi J, Oakes ND, Kennedy C, Chisholm DJ, Kraegen EW: Muscle glucose uptake during and after exercise is normal in insulin-resistant rats. *Am J Physiol* 264:E167–72, 1993

65. Jenkins AB, Furler SM, Bruce DG, Chisholm DJ: Regulation of hepatic glucose output during moderate exercise in non-insulin-dependent diabetes. *Metabolism* 37:966–72, 1988

66. Koivisto V, DeFronzo RA: Exercise in the treatment of type II diabetes. *Acta Endocrinol* 262 (Suppl.):107–16, 1984

67. Devlin JT, Hirshman M, Horton ED, Horton ES: Enhanced peripheral and splanchnic insulin sensitivity in NIDDM men after single bout of exercise. *Diabetes* 36:434–39, 1987

68. Kemmer FW, Tacken M, Berger M: Mechanism of exercise-induced hypoglycemia during sulfonylurea treatment. *Diabetes* 36:1178–82, 1987

69. Young JC, Treadway JL, Fader EI, Caslin R: Effects of oral hypoglycemic agent methylpalmoxirate on exercise capacity of streptozotocin diabetic rats. *Diabetes* 35: 744–48, 1986

70. Ruegemer JJ, Squires RW, Marsh HM, Haymond MW, Cryer PE, Rizza RA, Miles JM: Differences between prebreakfast and late afternoon glycemic responses to exercise in IDDM. *Diabetes Care* 13: 104–10, 1990

4. Reduction in Risk of Coronary Heart Disease and Diabetes

Highlights
Reduction in Risk of Coronary
Heart Disease and Diabetes

Reduction in Risk of Coronary Heart Disease (CHD)

■ Increased physical activity improves the cardiovascular risk factor profile; its effects include, reducing adiposity, blood pressure, dyslipidemia, and platelet adhesiveness, as well as enhancing fibrinolysis.

■ Increased physical activity may also reduce CHD risk independently of favorable alterations in traditional coronary risk factors.

■ The estimated reduction in the risk of myocardial infarction with the maintenance of an active, compared with a sedentary, lifestyle is estimated to be 35–55%.

Reduction in Risk of Non-Insulin-Dependent Diabetes Mellitus (NIDDM)

■ Physical activity improves insulin sensitivity and glycemic control among nondiabetic individuals, as well as among those with impaired glucose tolerance or overt NIDDM.

■ The addition of exercise to caloric restriction facilitates loss of adipose tissue, assists in maintenance of reduced body weight, and may independently improve insulin sensitivity.

■ The potential reduction in the risk of NIDDM associated with an active, compared with a sedentary, lifestyle is 30–50%.

Reduction in Risk of Coronary Heart Disease and Diabetes

JOANN E. MANSON, MD, DrPH, AND ANGELA SPELSBERG, MD, SM

INTRODUCTION

A sedentary lifestyle should be considered an important modifiable risk factor for both cardiovascular disease (CVD) and diabetes in the general population (1). Based on national survey data, 56% of men and 61% of women in the U.S. either never or irregularly engage in physical activity (2). Physical activity favorably influences a variety of known cardiovascular risk factors, including obesity, hypertension, dyslipidemia, fibrinolysis, and platelet adhesiveness. In addition, physical activity improves insulin sensitivity and glycemic control among nondiabetic individuals as well as among those with impaired glucose tolerance (IGT) or overt non-insulin-dependent diabetes mellitus (NIDDM).

Individuals with mild to moderate diabetes (fasting plasma glucose <200 mg/dl) appear to benefit more than those with severe hyperglycemia (3); the pronounced hyperinsulinemia in the former appears to be reduced effectively by physical training (4). Among patients with diabetes, atherosclerotic disease (including coronary heart disease [CHD], stroke, hypertension, and peripheral vascular disease) is a major cause of morbidity and mortality (3). Therefore, increased physical activity among individuals with diabetes or at increased risk of glucose intolerance may be of particular importance.

In this chapter, a summary of the currently available evidence concerning the role of increased physical activity in the primary prevention of CHD and diabetes is presented. Because insulin-dependent diabetes mellitus (IDDM) and NIDDM have different etiologies and because exercise is unlikely to be relevant to the primary prevention of IDDM, this chapter will focus primarily on NIDDM.

REDUCTION IN RISK OF CHD

Epidemiological Evidence

The available observational epidemiological literature on exercise and CHD consistently demonstrates risk reductions among more physically active individuals compared with their more sedentary peers (5). A recent meta-analysis of 27 prospective cohort studies in which the association between physical activity and CHD was assessed revealed a 90% elevated risk of CHD for people with sedentary compared with more active occupations (95% confidence interval [CI] 1.6–2.2) and a relative risk (RR) of 1.6 (95% CI 1.2–2.2) among more sedentary compared with more recreationally active individuals (6).

Differences in the magnitude of the association across studies were found to depend on the methodological features of the analyzed studies. Those studies with high quality scores (i.e., those without major apparent biases, including misclassification of activity levels, use of surrogate indicators of exercise, or inadequate control for potential confounding by dietary and other factors) tended to demonstrate a stronger benefit of physical activity than methodologically weaker studies. In a separate review paper, the estimated reduction in the risk of myocardial infarction with the maintenance of an active, compared with a sedentary, lifestyle was estimated to be 35–55% (1).

Because of the high prevalence of physical inactivity, the proportion of CHD deaths in the U.S. due to a sedentary lifestyle has been estimated to be 34.6% (Table 4.1). The attributable risk, i.e., the excess rate of CHD deaths that can be related to physical inactivity, is higher than for any other coronary risk factor except high serum cholesterol. Based on a cost-effectiveness analysis to estimate the health and economic implications of a physical activity program in the prevention of CHD, the cost per quality-adjusted life-year was found to be lower than for any other coronary risk factor intervention (Table 4.1).

Because previous epidemiological studies have been predominantly observational in design, the possibility that unmeasured or unknown factors influencing the selection and participation of study subjects (selection bias), as well as unmeasured or unknown third factors (confounding bias), cannot be excluded in interpreting the inverse association observed between physical activity and CHD. However, the consistency of the results across the studies, as well as the biological plausibility due to the known salutary effects of increased physical activity levels on the coronary risk factor profile, including obesity (7,8), dyslipidemia (9), hypertension (10), platelet adhesiveness, and fibrinolysis (11), support a causal association.

Physical activity may also confer protection from CHD by other mechanisms, including improvement in functional work capacity and myocardial oxygen demand (12), as well as reduction in the adrenergic response to stress (13). Benefits of exercise in relation to CHD are also supported by animal studies. Primates fed an atherogenic diet over an 18-month period showed a substantial reduction in the severity of atherosclerosis with moderate conditioning exercise compared with primates without exercise (14). This inverse association could not be explained by alterations in plasma lipids, glucose, or blood pressure, suggesting an independent antiatherogenic effect of physical activity. For a summary of the potential beneficial effects of physical activity on coronary risk factors and atherosclerosis, see Fig. 24.1 in chapter 24.

Sparse data are available concerning the benefits of physical activity in preventing CHD among diabetic individuals. Physical activity improves insulin sensitivity and glycemic control among lean nondiabetic individuals as well as among obese individuals and patients with NIDDM. In IDDM, exercise also increases skeletal muscle sensitivity to insulin and reduces insulin requirements; glycemic control does not appear to be favorably altered (15,16), perhaps because of associated increases in caloric intake (17). The effects of long-term exercise among IDDM patients remain inconclusive. The sparse available follow-up data suggest that IDDM patients who participate in physical activity early in life

Table 4.1. Selected Risk Factors for CHD, by Prevalence, Population Attributable Risk, and Cost-Effectiveness: United States

RISK FACTOR	PREVALENCE (%)	ATTRIBUTABLE RISK (%)	COST-EFFECTIVENESS
Physical inactivity	58.0	34.6	$11,313 per QALY
Hypertension	18.0	28.9	$25,000 per QALY
Smoking	25.5	25.0	$21,947 total lifetime benefits of quitting
Obesity	23.0	32.1	Not available
Elevated serum cholesterol (≥200 mg/dl)	37.0	42.7	$28,000 per QALY

Percentages for attributable risk cannot be summed because they are calculated independently for each risk factor. QALY denotes quality-adjusted life-years. Cost-effectiveness data for physical inactivity and hypertension are from Hatziandreu EI, Koplan JP, Weinstein MC, Caspersen CJ, Warner KE: A cost-effectiveness analysis of exercise as a health-promotion activity. *Am J Public Health* 78: 1417–21, 1988. Cost-effectiveness data for smoking are from Weinstein MC, Stanson WB: Cost-effectiveness of interventions to prevent or treat coronary heart disease. *Annu Rev Public Health* 6:41–63, 1985. Cost-effectiveness data for elevated serum cholesterol are from Oster G, Colditz GA, Kelly NL: The economic costs of smoking and benefits of quitting for individual smokers. *Prev Med* 13:377–89, 1984.

Modified from CDC: Public health focus: physical activity and the prevention of coronary heart disease. *Morb Mortal Wkly Rep* 42:669–72, 1993 may experience fewer macrovascular complications, as well as less nephropathy and neuropathy, compared with nonparticipants (18,19). Studies in patients with mild NIDDM have demonstrated a benefit of exercise in increasing insulin sensitivity and glucose tolerance, as well as inducing favorable changes in blood lipids (20–22). Exercise as an adjunct to diet regimens produces greater weight loss and higher maintenance rates in obese nondiabetic individuals (23,24) and NIDDM patients (25). In combination with weight-loss programs, exercise potentially counteracts the decrease in resting energy expenditure observed with dietary treatment, producing greater overall weight reductions and a greater percentage of fat loss (26–29). Benefits of exercise, when added to weight loss, have not been consistently reported in all studies, however (30,31). Methodological differences between the studies, such as the intensity of the applied exercise regimens, compliance, and differing degrees of control of food intake, may explain the observed inconsistencies (25). No randomized clinical trials have been conducted to assess reductions in clinical CHD events induced by increased physical activity in NIDDM patients. Based on the available evidence, however, physical activity may play an important role in the reduction of CHD among diabetic as well as nondiabetic individuals (32).

REDUCTION IN RISK OF NIDDM

Epidemiological Evidence

The potential beneficial effects of physical activity on the development of NIDDM have been investigated in only a few epidemiological studies (33). Support for benefits of exercise in relation to NIDDM risk is provided by descriptive comparisons of active rural versus more sedentary urban high-risk Pacific populations (34,35), as well as cross-sectional (36–39), retrospective cohort (40), and prospective studies of active compared with sedentary individuals (29,41,42).

Cross-Sectional and Retrospective Cohort Studies

In Melanesian and Indian Fijian men, the age-standardized prevalence of NIDDM among men classified as sedentary was more than twice the rate in those classified as exercising moderately to heavily (36). The same association was observed among migrant Asian Muslim and Hindu Indian men, African Creole men, and Hindu Indian women, but not among Chinese Mauritians of both sexes (37), after control for potential confounders, such as body mass index (BMI), central adiposity, age, and family history of diabetes. Not all cross-sectional studies, however, have demonstrated a significant association between glucose tolerance and physical activity (38,39). RR estimates in cross-sectional studies comparing most sedentary individuals with most active people range from no association to a 2.7-fold increased risk of NIDDM among the most sedentary. In a retrospective cohort study of 5,398 female college alumnae (ages 20–70), those women who did not engage in vigorous athletic activities during their college years had a 3.4-fold increased risk of developing NIDDM compared with women who trained regularly (40).

Prospective Cohort Studies

The prospective observational, nonrandomized studies that have assessed the relationship between physical activity and risk of NIDDM have consistently shown a marked reduction in NIDDM risk among physically active individuals compared with their sedentary peers (Table 4.2) (29,41,42). In a prospective study of 5,990 male alumni of the University of Pennsylvania during 14 years of follow-up, leisure-time activity was inversely associated with the risk of NIDDM; for every 500-kcal increment of energy expenditure, a 6% reduction in diabetes risk was observed after adjustment for age, BMI, and other variables (P, trend = 0.01) (41). The strongest protective effect was observed among those at highest risk

Table 4.2. Association Between Physical Activity and Risk of NIDDM: Prospective Epidemiology Studies

PROSPECTIVE COHORT STUDIES	AGE (YEARS)	SEX	YEAR(S) OF STUDY	COMPARISON GROUPS	RR ASSOCIATION: MOST ACTIVE/ MOST SEDENTARY	POTENTIAL CONFOUNDING FACTORS CONTROLLED IN ANALYSIS
University of Pennsylvania alumni (36)	39–68	M	1962–1976	Each 500 kcal/week increase in physical activity index	0.94	Age, BMI, history of hypertension, parental history of diabetes
		M	1962–1976	Moderate and/or vigorous exercise vs. sedentary	0.65	Age
U.S. nurses (37)	34–59	F	1980–1988	Vigorous exercise ≥weekly vs.<weekly	0.67	Age
				Vigorous exercise ≥weekly vs.<weekly	0.84	Age, BMI, family history of diabetes, smoking, alcohol, hypertension, high serum cholesterol
U.S. physicians (24)	40–84	M	1980–1988	Vigorous exercise ≥weekly vs.<weekly	0.64	Age
				Vigorous exercise ≥weekly vs.<weekly	0.70	Age, BMI, smoking, alcohol, hypertension, high serum cholesterol

RR, adjusted for variables in the right column, is the ratio of the incidence of NIDDM in those who are most active divided by the incidence of NIDDM in those most sedentary. Participants in each of the prospective cohort studies were predominantly white. Median length of follow-up was 5 years.

for NIDDM (men with high BMI, history of hypertension, or family history of diabetes). Men with regular moderate and/or vigorous exercise (measured by a weekly physical activity index) were found to have a 35% lower risk of NIDDM than their sedentary counterparts.

Risk reductions with physical activity were also found among 87,253 women in the Nurses' Health Study. During 8 years of follow-up, women who exercised vigorously (long enough to produce a sweat) at least once a week had an age-adjusted RR of NIDDM of 0.67 (95% CI 0.60–0.75; $P < 0.001$) compared with women exercising less than once a week; a significant 16% reduction in NIDDM risk persisted after additional adjustment for BMI, family history of diabetes, and other variables (42).

Finally, in a study of 21,271 U.S. male physicians, the age-adjusted RR of NIDDM was again found to decrease with increasing frequency of exercise (29). Compared with men exercising vigorously less than once a week, the age-adjusted RR was 0.77 for vigorous exercise once a week, 0.67 for 2–4 times/week, and 0.58 for 5 times/week (P, trend = 0.0002). The reduction in risk of NIDDM remained significant after adjustment for age, BMI, smoking, hypertension, and high serum cholesterol (RR = 0.70; 95% CI 0.5–0.92) for an exercise frequency of at least once a week compared with less than once a week. Risk reductions were particularly pronounced among obese men (BMI >26.4 kg/m^2) (29).

Intervention Studies

A recently published nonrandomized intervention study among Swedish men, ages 47–49 at baseline, compared a diet and exercise regimen to no intervention among individuals with newly diagnosed NIDDM, IGT, and healthy individuals in relation to magnitude of weight loss, CVD risk profiles, and clinical outcome (43). Only 10.6% of participants with IGT assigned to the intervention group developed NIDDM within 5 years compared with 28.6% with IGT assigned to the control group. This result suggests that sustained modification of lifestyle factors directed at weight loss, including dietary changes and increase in physical activity, are feasible and may help to prevent, or at least postpone, the onset of NIDDM.

To assess the independent effect of physical activity on the risk of NIDDM, control for BMI is important. All of the prospective studies were able to control for age, BMI, and several other potential confounding variables. Furthermore, the prospective studies were conducted in populations relatively homogeneous in educational attainment and socioeconomic status, thereby minimizing selection and confounding biases. The consistently observed reductions in risk of NIDDM among physically active compared with sedentary individuals in all the prospective studies and most of the cross-sectional investigations support the hypothesis that physical inactivity is an important determinant of NIDDM and that regular moderate and/or vigorous exercise may reduce the incidence of NIDDM.

However, at present, data are limited with respect to the intensity, frequency, and duration of exercise that will be most effective in reducing the occurrence of NIDDM. According to the estimates derived from the prospective studies, the potential reduction in the risk of NIDDM associated with regular moderate and/or vigorous exercise, compared with a sedentary lifestyle, is 30–50% (44).

Biological Mechanisms

A benefit of physical activity in the prevention of NIDDM is biologically plausible and could be explained by several mechanisms. First, exercise is associated with lower BMI, and studies among nondiabetic individuals suggest that the addition of exercise to caloric restriction will facilitate loss of adipose tissue and assist in maintenance of reduced body weight (45). Obesity, in particular central adiposity, has been linked to glucose intolerance, hyperinsulinemia, and hypertension; insulin resistance has been identified as the mediating factor (46,47). In addition, exercise appears to have independent effects on insulin sensitivity and glucose metabolism (48-55). These mechanisms are discussed in detail in Chapters 3 and 6.

SUMMARY

The currently available epidemiological evidence indicates a substantial reduction in the risk of CHD and NIDDM with the maintenance of an active, compared with a sedentary, lifestyle. The estimated risk reductions are 35–55% for CHD and 30–50% for NIDDM, respectively. Clinician counseling and prescription of regular physical activity should represent a major goal in the primary prevention of CHD and NIDDM. This responsibility is of paramount importance, particularly in light of the high prevalence of physical inactivity and the high incidence of atherosclerotic diseases and diabetes in the U.S. and throughout the world.

REFERENCES

1. Manson JE, Tosteson H, Ridker PM, Satterfield S, Hebert P, O'Connor GT, Buring JE, Hennekens CH: The primary prevention of myocardial infarction. *N Engl J Med* 326:1406–16, 1992
2. Public Health Focus: Physical activity and the prevention of coronary heart disease. *MMWR* 42:669–72, 1993
3. Ruderman NB, Schneider SH: Diabetes, exercise, and atherosclerosis. *Diabetes Care* 15 (Suppl. 4):1787–93, 1992
4. Holloszy JO, Schultz J, Kusnierkiewicz J, Hagberg JM, Ehsani AA: Effects of exercise on glucose tolerance and insulin resistance. *Acta Med Scand* (Suppl. 711):55–65, 1986
5. Powell KE, Thompson PD, Caspersen CJ, Kendrick JS: Physical activity and the incidence of coronary heart disease. *Annu Rev Public Health* 8:253–87, 1987
6. Berlin JA, Colditz GA: A meta-analysis of physical activity in the prevention of coronary heart disease. *Am J Epidemiol* 132:612–26, 1990
7. Wood PD, Stefanick ML, Williams PT, Haskell WL: The effects on plasma lipoproteins of a prudent weight-reducing diet with or without exercise, in overweight men and women. *N Engl J Med* 325:461–66, 1991
8. Gwinnup G: Weight loss without dietary restriction: efficacy of different forms of aerobic exercise. *Am J Sports Med* 15:275–79, 1987
9. Wood PD, Haskell WL: The effect of exercise on plasma high-density lipoproteins. *Lipids* 14:417–27, 1979
10. Seals DR, Hagberg JM: The effect of exercise training on human hypertension: a review. *Med Sci Sports Exercise* 16:207–15, 1984
11. Oberman A: Rehabilitation of patients with coronary artery disease. In *Heart Disease: A Textbook of Cardiovascular Medicine.* 3rd ed. Braunwald E, Ed. Philadelphia, Saunders, 1988, p. 1395–1409
12. Maskin CS: Aerobic exercise training in cardiopulmonary disease. In *Cardiopulmonary Exercise Testing: Physiologic Principles and Clinical Applications.* Weber KT, Janicki JS, Eds. Philadelphia, Saunders, 1986, p. 317–32
13. Cooksey JD, Reilly P, Brown S, Bomze H, Cryer PE: Exercise training and plasma catecholamines in patients with ischemic heart disease. *Am J Cardiol* 42:372–76, 1978
14. Kramsch DM, Aspen AJ, Abramowitz BM, Kriemendahl T, Hood WB: Reduction of coronary atherosclerosis by moderate conditioning exercise in monkeys on an atherogenic diet. *N Engl J Med* 305:1483–89, 1981
15. Wallberg-Henriksson H, Gunnarsson R, Henriksson J, DeFronzo R, Felig P, Östmann J, Wahren J: Increased peripheral insulin sensitivity and muscle mitochondrial

enzymes but unchanged blood glucose control in type I diabetes after physical training. *Diabetes* 31: 1044–50, 1982

16. Zinman B, Zuniga–Guajardo S, Kelly D: Comparison of the acute and long-term effects of physical training on glucose control in type I diabetes. *Diabetes Care* 7:515–19, 1984

17. Devlin JT: Effects of exercise on insulin sensitivity in humans. *Diabetes Care* 15 (Suppl. 4):1690–93, 1992

18. LaPorte RE, Dorman JS, Tajima N, Cruickshanks KJ, Orchard TJ, Cavender DE, Becker DJ, Drash AL: Pittsburgh Insulin-Dependent Diabetes Mellitus Morbidity and Mortality Study: physical activity and diabetic complications. *Pediatrics* 78:1027–33, 1986

19. Kriska AM, LaPorte RE, Patrick SL, Kuller LH, Orchard TJ: The association of physical activity and diabetic complications in individuals with insulin-dependent diabetes mellitus: The Epidemiology of Diabetes Complications Study VII. *J Clin Epidemiol* 44:1207–14, 1991

20. Ruderman NB, Ganda OP, Johansen K: The effect of physical training on glucose tolerance and plasma lipids in maturity-onset diabetes. *Diabetes* 28 (Suppl. 1):89–94, 1979

21. Saltin B, Lindgärde F, Houston M, Hörlin R, Nygaard E, Gad P: Physical training and glucose tolerance in middle-aged men with chemical diabetes. *Diabetes* 28 (Suppl. 1):30–37, 1979

22. Ruderman NB, Apelian AZ, Schneider SH: Exercise in therapy and prevention of type II diabetes: implication for blacks. *Diabetes Care* 13 (Suppl. 4):1163–68, 1990

23. Pavlou KN, Krey S, Steffee WP: Exercise as an adjunct to weight loss and maintenance in moderately obese subjects. *Am J Clin Nutr* 49:1115–23, 1989

24. Pavlou KN, Whatley JE, Jannace PW, DiBartolomeo JJ, Burrows BA, Duthie EA, Lerman RH: Physical activity as a supplement to weight-loss regimen. *Am J Clin Nutr* 49:1110–14, 1989

25. Wing RR, Epstein LH, Paternostro-Bayles M, Kriska A, Nowalk MP, Gooding W: Exercise in a behavioral weight control programme for obese patients with type 2 (non-insulin-dependent) diabetes. *Diabetologia* 31:902–909, 1988

26. Kenrick M, Ball FM, Canary JJ: Exercise and weight reduction in obesity. *Arch Phys Med Rehab* 53:232–37, 1972

27. Donahue RP, Lin DH, Kirschenbaum DS, Keesey RE: Metabolic consequences of dieting and exercise in the treatment of obesity. *J Consult Clin Psychol* 5:827–36, 1984

28. Pavlou KN, Steffee WP, Lerman RH, Burrows BA: Effects of dieting and exercise on lean body mass, oxygen uptake, and strength. *Med Sci Sports Exercise* 17:466–71, 1985

29. Manson JE, Nathan DM, Krolewski AS, Stampfer MJ, Willett WC, Hennekens CH: A prospective study of exercise and incidence of diabetes among U.S. male physicians. *JAMA* 268:63–67, 1992

30. Van Dale D, Saris WHM, Schoffelen PFM, Ten Hoor F: Does exercise give an additional effect in weight reduction regimens? *Int J Obes* 11:367–75, 1987

31. Phinney SD, LaGrange BM, O'-Connell M, Danforth E: Effects of aerobic exercise on energy expenditure and nitrogen balance during very low calorie dieting. *Metabolism* 37:758–65, 1988

32. Schneider SH, Vitug A, Ruderman NB: Atherosclerosis and physical activity. *Diabetes Metab Rev* 1: 445–81, 1986

33. Jarrett RJ: Epidemiology and public health aspects of non-insulin-dependent diabetes mellitus. *Epidemiol Rev* 11:151–71, 1989

34. Zimmet P, Dowse G, Finch C, Serjeantson S, King H: The epidemiology and natural history of NIDDM: lessons from the South Pacific. *Diabetes Metab Rev* 6: 91–124, 1990

35. King H, Zimmet P, Raper LR, Balkau B: Risk factors for diabetes in three Pacific populations. *Am J Epidemiol* 119:396–409, 1984

36. Taylor R, Ram P, Zimmet P, Raper LR, Ringrose H: Physical activity and prevalence of diabetes in Melanesian and Indian men in Fiji. *Diabetologia* 27:578–82, 1984

37. Dowse GK, Zimmet PZ, Gareboo H, Alberti KGMM, Tuomilehto J, Finch CF, Chitson P, Tulsidas H: Abdominal obesity and physical activity as risk factors for NIDDM and impaired glucose tolerance in Indian, Creole, and Chinese Mauritians. *Diabetes Care* 14:271–82, 1991

38. King H, Taylor R, Koteka G, Nemaia H, Zimmet PZ, Bennett PH, Raper LR: Glucose tolerance in Polynesia: population-based surveys in Rarotonga and Niue. *Med J Aust* 145:505–10, 1986

39. Jarrett RJ, Shipley MJ, Hunt R: Physical activity, glucose tolerance and diabetes mellitus: The Whitehall Study. *Diabetic Med* 3:549–51, 1986

40. Frisch RE, Wyshak G, Albright TE, Albright NL, Schiff I: Lower prevalence of diabetes in female former college athletes compared with nonathletes. *Diabetes* 35:1101–105, 1986

41. Helmrich SP, Ragland DR, Leung RW, Pfaffenbarger RS: Physical activity and reduced occurrence of non-insulin-dependent diabetes mellitus. *N Engl J Med* 325:147–52, 1991

42. Manson JE, Rimm EB, Stampfer MJ, Colditz GA, Willett WC, Krolewski AS, Rosner B, Hennekens CH, Speizer FE: Physical activity and incidence of non-insulin-dependent diabetes mellitus in women. *Lancet* 338:774–78, 1991

43. Eriksson KE, Lingärde F: Prevention of type 2 (non-insulin-dependent) diabetes mellitus and physical exercise: the 6-year Malmö feasibility study. *Diabetologia* 34:891–98, 1991

44. Manson JE, Spelsberg A: Primary prevention of non-insulin-dependent diabetes mellitus. *Am J Prev Med* 10:172–84, 1994

45. Stern JS, Titchenal CA, Johnson PR: Does exercise make a difference? In *Recent Advances in Obesity Research*. London, Libbey, 1987, p. 337–49

46. Kaplan NM: The deadly quartet: upper body obesity, glucose intolerance, hypertriglyceridemia, and hypertension. *Arch Intern Med* 149:1514–20, 1989

47. Reaven GM: Role of insulin resistance in human disease (Banting Lecture 1988). *Diabetes* 37:1595–1607, 1988

48. DeFronzo RA, Bonadonna RC, Ferrannini E: Pathogenesis of NIDDM: a balanced overview. *Diabetes Care* 15:318–68, 1992

49. Mondon CE, Dolkas CB, Reaven GM: Site of enhanced insulin sensitivity in exercise-trained rats. *Am J Physiol* 239:E169–77, 1980

50. Dohm GL, Sinha MK, Caro JF: Insulin receptor bindings and protein kinase activity in muscles of trained rats. *Am J Physiol* 252:E170–75, 1987

51. Schneider SH, Amorosa LF, Khachadurian AK, Ruderman NB: Studies on the mechanism of improved glucose control during regular exercise in type 2 (non-insulin-dependent) diabetes. *Diabetologia* 26:355–60, 1984

52. Koivisto VA, Yki-Jarvinen H, DeFronzo RA: Physical training and insulin sensitivity. *Diabetes Metab Rev* 1:445–81, 1986

53. Burstein R, Polychronakos C, Toews CJ, MacDougall JD, Guyda HJ, Posner BI: Acute reversal of the enhanced insulin action in trained athletes: association with insulin receptor changes. *Diabetes* 34:756–60, 1985

54. Bjorntorp P, DeJounge K, Sjostrom L, Sullivan L: The effect of physical training on insulin production in obesity. *Metabolism* 19:631–38, 1970

55. Soman VR, Koivisto VA, Deibert D, Felig P, DeFronzo RA: Increased insulin sensitivity and insulin binding to monocytes after physical training. *N Engl J Med* 301:1200–204, 1979

5. Psychological Benefits of Exercise

Highlights
Psychological Benefits of Exercise

- Exercise can have important effects on mental health for individuals with and without psychiatric disorders.
- Regular exercise can have an antidepressant effect in patients with mild depressive disorders.
- Aerobic exercise can reduce anxiety levels acutely, and regular exercise may have a role in chronically reducing anxiety in individuals with anxiety disorders.
- Emotionally healthy individuals who exercise regularly report improved mood, sense of well-being, and self-esteem.
- Rarely, exercise may have negative psychological effects, such as exercise addiction.
- It is not known how often or for how long individuals should exercise in order to achieve optimal psychological benefit.
- Adherence to exercise regimens is problematic; 50% of those beginning an exercise program will drop out.
- Patients with diabetes, like healthy individuals, can benefit emotionally as well as physically from regular exercise.

Psychological Benefits of Exercise

S. TZIPORAH COHEN, BA, AND ALAN M. JACOBSON, MD

INTRODUCTION

While the physical benefits of regular exercise are well-known, important psychological effects need to be considered. These include possible benefits for *1)* individuals with psychiatric disorders, *2)* emotionally healthy individuals, and *3)* individuals who may be at risk for future psychiatric disorders.

Initial interest in the effects of exercise on mental health was spurred by the finding of an inverse relationship between an individual's level of physical fitness and the presence of psychopathology; more physically fit individuals generally showed lower degrees of psychopathology (1). Although only a cross-sectional association, subsequent studies examined whether exercise was effective in actually lowering the degree of psychopathology in affected individuals.

Several studies have examined the effects of exercise on psychological functioning, looking for effects on anxiety, depression, self-esteem and self-concept, and general sense of well-being. Most of these studies have looked at aerobic exercise, such as running or aerobics classes, and have involved nonclinical as well as clinical populations. A few have looked at non-aerobic exercise, such as weight training or yoga. In this chapter, we briefly summarize some of these findings and address some important clinical issues in the use of exercise in the treatment of emotional distress. Although these studies were not done in diabetic populations, their findings are likely to be useful for and applicable to individuals with diabetes.

EFFECTS OF EXERCISE ON INDIVIDUALS WITH PSYCHIATRIC DISORDERS

The effects of exercise on mood and anxiety disorders have been fairly well established. Regular exercise has an antidepressant effect in patients with mild to moderate unipolar depressive disorders (2). This effect is seen with both aerobic and nonaerobic forms of exercise and thus seems to be independent of any change in aerobic fitness. Preliminary evidence shows that exercise may be as effective as some psychotherapies in treating depression (3,4). Another study showed positive effects of exercise on hospitalized depressed patients, with regular aerobic exercise having an antidepressant effect (5). A meta-analysis of 15 studies examining depressed patients found a statistically significant decrease in depression scores in exercisers versus nonexercisers (6). Importantly, however, exercise has not been evaluated in severely depressed patients, e.g., those with severe psychomotor retardation or psychotic symptoms. In the studies cited above, patients were excluded if they were psychotic or thought to have a high suicide risk. *There is no evidence that exercise alone is adequate to treat severe depression, and exercise should not be used in place of traditional therapies, but rather as an adjunct.*

Aerobic exercise apparently has an anxiolytic effect as well. Studies measuring anxiety generally focus on either *trait* anxiety (the general predisposition of an individual to respond across many situations with high levels of anxiety) or *state* anxiety (the more specific measure of an individual's anxiety at a particular moment) (7). In studies that measured state anxiety, aerobic exercise of 20–40 min duration resulted in decreased anxiety for up to 4 h after exercise (7,8). At least two meta-analyses examining the effect of aerobic exercise on anxiety found a significant decrease in state and trait anxiety in the exercisers, although the effects were limited to men (6,9). As in the depression studies, this decrease in anxiety has been shown to be independent of any increase in aerobic fitness (10).

EFFECTS OF EXERCISE ON EMOTIONALLY HEALTHY INDIVIDUALS

A few studies suggest that exercise may reduce normal feelings of depression and anxiety among individuals without a history of psychiatric illness. In one study of healthy adults without psychiatric disorders, 10 weeks of regular aerobic exercise (walking or running for 1 h, 3 times/week) decreased state and trait anxiety, tension, depressive feelings, and fatigue in exercisers compared with a control group (11). A more recent study comparing similar aerobic exercise to yoga and a wait-list control group showed aerobic exercise to be associated with reduced depression and anxiety. In addition, the subjects in the exercise and yoga groups reported improved mood, self-confidence and life satisfaction, and better family relations and sex lives (12). In a study of college students, regular exercise was associated with decreased anger, fatigue, hostility, and inertia, as well as improved sleep (13). Even in studies where no objective difference was seen, the majority of subjects reported "feeling better" and experiencing feelings of "exhilaration" following exercise, evidence of a possible effect that is not picked up by traditional measures (14). In general, however, exercise has less of a psychological effect on emotionally healthy individuals than on individuals with psychiatric disorders like depression or anxiety (6). It is important to remember that exercise does not make psychologically normal people supernormal, much as antidepressants do not make nondepressed individuals euphoric.

In addition to having beneficial effects on specific symptoms of anxiety and depression, research indicates that exercise is associated with an improved sense of well-being, self-esteem, and self-efficacy (15,16). A meta-analysis of 37 studies of the effect of exercise on self-concept (defined as how one sees oneself, including variables such as self-esteem, self-image, self-awareness, and self-ideal) found a significant increase in self-concept scores of exercisers versus nonexercisers (6).

If exercise improves well-being in healthy individuals and reduces symptoms in patients with psychiatric disorders, could exercise prevent or slow the onset of psychiatric disorders? One theory suggests that the acute decrease in depression and anxiety following exercise might prevent the development of chronic depression or anxiety (17). Unfortunately, no studies have examined this intriguing hypothesis.

NEGATIVE EFFECTS OF EXERCISE

Exercise may have negative psychological consequences in some individuals. A small subgroup of individuals may begin to exercise compulsively, becoming, in effect, addicted to exercise. Morgan describes such an addiction as "present if the person feels compelled to exercise daily and feels unable to live without it and when deprived of exercise, experiences withdrawal symptoms including anxiety, irritability, and depression" (18). Such individuals may continue to exercise despite serious injury or interference with social and occupational activities (19).

Exercise compulsion is often seen in individuals with eating disorders, especially anorexia nervosa. Exercise may begin as a way to decrease hunger and increase weight loss and may progress to an addiction in its own right. These individuals become "obligate exercisers." Some researchers have proposed that obligatory exercise is actually a variant of anorexia nervosa, and they have reported that many of these individuals, even if they do not have the hallmark weight loss and fear of fatness, share many of the obsessive characteristics, as well as character, style, and background, of anorexic patients (20).

A few studies have tried to identify personality traits that would predict individuals at risk for becoming addicted to exercise, but only one was able to find any correlation (21). This study found that weight preoccupation in men and women and obsessive-compulsiveness in men were strongly related to excessive exercising. Because this is only one study, more research needs to be done to determine which individuals are at risk for developing an exercise addiction, although individuals who are excessively weight conscious may be one group at risk.

Another negative effect of exercise is the "staleness syndrome," characterized by mood and sleep disturbances and often resembling depression (17). Because this is almost exclusively seen in serious athletes in intensive training, it will not be discussed here.

Despite these occasional detrimental effects, exercise is still a safe, low-risk activity, even for individuals with symptoms of depression or anxiety. Among patients with bulimic or anorexic symptoms, however, there is a theoretical risk that exercise prescriptions may promote obligate and dangerous regimens. Table 5.1 summarizes the psychological benefits and potential side effects of exercise.

CLINICAL ISSUES

Does exercise have a therapeutic index or a dose-response curve in terms of psychological benefit? Some of the transient benefits of exercise, such as a decrease in state anxiety or an improvement in well-being, may be seen after just a single exercise session. In most studies, subjects exercised 3 times/week, but no studies have examined exactly how many exercise sessions per week are necessary for long-lasting psychological benefit. Also, as the number of exercise sessions per week increases, so might the rates of injury, an important factor in prescribing an exercise regimen.

Adherence is an issue when prescribing any medical or psychiatric treatment, and exercise is no exception. While some of the symptoms of depression (fatigue, anhedonia, psychomotor retardation) may make it difficult for patients to initiate and maintain an exercise regimen, adherence rates to exercise programs are similar between psychiatric and nonpsychiatric populations (2). Approximately 50% of patients continue to exercise regularly after the end of a formal training program (2). To state this differently, *half* of the individuals beginning an exercise program will drop out, usually after only a few weeks. This is a major detriment in

Table 5.1. Potential Psychological Benefits and Side Effects of Exercise

BENEFITS	SIDE EFFECTS
Antidepressant effect	Compulsive exercising
Antianxiolytic effect	Exercise addiction
Increased sense of well-being	"Staleness syndrome"
Enhanced self-esteem	

using exercise as a treatment for any benefit, whether physical or psychological.

Whether adherence to exercise programs is more problematic in patients with diabetes is not clear. Given the regimen complexities posed by taking insulin and the weight-related issues for obese patients, adherence may be more difficult in these individuals than among those without a concomitant illness. There is also no research to indicate whether exercise promotes or impedes adherence to other elements of the diabetic treatment program.

Exercise, in general, is not contraindicated in patients on psychiatric medications, although certain issues must be taken into account. Patients on antipsychotic medications, such as haloperidol or chlorpromazine, can safely exercise; however, the sedation and Parkinsonian-like side effects of these medications can interfere with motivation to exercise and with coordination (22). Antidepressants are commonly prescribed for moderate to severe depression, and again, patients taking these drugs can safely exercise. However, orthostatic hypotension secondary to the use of certain antidepressants can make exercise dangerous and thus should be monitored. This is an especially important problem among the elderly and among diabetic patients with signs of autonomic neuropathy. It is generally recommended that only light exercise be attempted during adjustment to a new medication and during the initial titration to therapeutic dosage (2). Once patients are on full doses and are not experiencing certain side effects (orthostatic hypotension, hypertension), they can participate in a full-intensity exercise program appropriate for their level of physical fitness.

Table 5.2. Clinical Recommendations

- Include regular exercise (30–60 min, 3 times/week) as part of the treatment plan for mild to moderately depressed or anxious patients if no contraindications are present.
- For patients on psychotropic medications, defer regular exercise until adjustment to medication is complete and no serious side effects are present.
- Recognizing that adherence is a long-term issue in maintaining regular exercise routines, refer patients to organized exercise programs/classes and provide active follow-up and encouragement.

SUMMARY

In summary, the majority of studies have found beneficial effects of exercise on psychosocial functioning. Exercise can help reduce depression and anxiety, as well as give individuals an improved sense of well-being. Although negative effects of exercise, such as exercise addiction, can occur, exercise is generally a safe method for improving psychological health. Table 2 summarizes our clinical recommendations for prescribing exercise to patients as part of a mental health treatment plan.

ACKNOWLEDGMENTS

This research was supported by National Institutes of Health Grants DK–27845 and DK–42315 and a donation from Herbert Graetz.

REFERENCES

1. Morgan WP: Physical fitness and emotional health: a review. *Am Corrective Ther J* 23:124–27, 1969
2. Martinsen EW: Benefits of exercise for the treatment of depression. *Sports Med* 9:380–89, 1990
3. Klein MH, Greist JH, Gurman AS, Neimeyer RA, Lesser DP, Bushnell NJ, Smith RE: A comparative outcome study of group psychotherapy vs. exercise treatments for depression. *Int J Ment Health* 13:148–77, 1985
4. Greist JH, Klein MH, Eischens RR, Faris J, Gurman AS, Morgan WP: Running as treatment for depression. *Comp Psychiatry* 20:41–54, 1979
5. Martinsen EW, Medhus A, Sandvik L: Effects of aerobic exercise on depression: a controlled study. *Br Med J* 291:109, 1985
6. McDonald DG, Hodgdon JA: *Psychological Effects of Aerobic Fitness Training: Research and Theory.* New York, Springer-Verlag, 1991
7. Landers DM, Petruzzello SJ: Physical activity, fitness and anxiety. In *Physical Activity, Fitness, and Health: International Proceedings and Consensus Statement.* Bouchard C, Shepard RG, Stephens T, Eds. Champaign, IL, Human Kinetics Publishers, 1994, p. 868–82
8. Morgan WP: Reduction of state anxiety following acute physical activity. In *Exercise and Mental Health.* Morgan WP, Goldston SE, Eds. Washington, Hemisphere Publishing, 1987, p. 105–109
9. Petruzzello SJ, Landers DM, Hatfield BD, Kubitz KA, Salazar W: A meta-analysis on the anxiety-reducing effects of acute and chronic exercise. *Sports Med* 11:143–82, 1991
10. Martinsen EW, Hoffart A, Solberg Y: Aerobic and non-aerobic forms of exercise in the treatment of anxiety disorders. *Stress Med* 5:115–20, 1989
11. Blumenthal JA, Williams RS, Needels TL, Wallace AG: Psychological changes accompany aerobic exercise in healthy middle-aged adults. *Psychosom Med* 44:529–36, 1982
12. Blumenthal JA, Emery CF, Madden DJ, George LK, Coleman RE, Riddle MW, McKee DC, Reasoner J, Williams RS: Cardiovascular and behavioral effects of aerobic exercise training in healthy older men

and women. *J Gerontol* 44:M147–57, 1989

13. Brown RS: Exercise as an adjunct to the treatment of mental disorders. In *Exercise and Mental Health*. Morgan WP, Goldston SE, Eds. Washington, Hemisphere Publishing, 1987, p. 131–37

14. Ismail AH: Psychological effects of exercise in the middle years. In *Exercise and Mental Health*. Morgan WP, Goldston SE, Eds. Washington, Hemisphere Publishing, 1987, p. 111–16

15. McAuley E: Physical activity and psychosocial outcomes. In *Physical Activity, Fitness, and Health: International Proceedings and Consensus Statement*. Bouchard C, Shepard RG, Stephens T, Eds. Champaign, IL, Human Kinetics Publishers, 1994, p. 551–68

16. Sonstroem RJ, Morgan WP: Exercise and self-esteem: rationale and model. *Med Sci Sports Exercise* 21:329–37, 1989

17. Raglin JS: Exercise and mental health: beneficial and detrimental effects. *Sports Med* 9:323–29, 1990

18. Morgan WP: Negative addiction in runners. *Physical Sports Med* 7:57–70, 1979

19. Polivy J: Physical activity, fitness, and compulsive behaviors. In *Physical Activity, Fitness, and Health: International Proceedings and Consensus Statement*. Bouchard C, Shepard RG, Stephens T, Eds. Champaign, IL, Human Kinetics Publishers, 1994, p. 883–96

20. Yates A, Leehey K, Shisslak CM: Running—an analogue of anorexia? *N Engl J Med* 308:251–55, 1983

21. Davis C, Brewer H, Ratusny D: Behavioral frequency and psychological commitment: necessary concepts in the study of excessive exercising. *J Behav Med* 16:611–27, 1993

22. Martinsen EW: Exercise and medications in the psychiatric patient. In *Exercise and Mental Health*. Morgan WP, Goldston SE, Eds. Washington, Hemisphere Publishing, 1987

II. The Treatment Plan

6. The Exercise Prescription

Highlights
The Exercise Prescription

- To optimize the likelihood of a safe and effective response, the exercise prescription should take into consideration safety aspects as well as the mode, frequency, duration, intensity, rate of progression, and timing of physical activity.
- The foremost priority in compiling the exercise prescription is to minimize the potential adverse effects of exercise via appropriate screening, program design, monitoring, and patient education.
- Before embarking on an exercise program, all people with diabetes should undergo a complete medical history and physical examination aimed at the identification of macrovascular, microvascular, and neurological complications. A continuing-care plan with follow-up medical evaluations is also necessary.
- An exercise electrocardiogram should be performed on *1)* people with known or suspected coronary artery disease and *2)* people who have had insulin-dependent diabetes mellitus (IDDM) for >15 years, have IDDM and are >30 years old,

or have non-insulin-dependent diabetes mellitus (NIDDM) and are >35 years old.
- The type, frequency, duration, and intensity of exercise training should be modulated to achieve an energy expenditure of 700–2,000 calories/week.
- Generally, to accomplish the desired weekly energy expenditure, aerobic exercise should be performed for 20–60 min, 3–5 days/week, at an intensity corresponding to 50–74% of maximal aerobic capacity.
- Exercise training should begin at a comfortable intensity and gradually progress in accordance with baseline cardiorespiratory fitness level, age, weight, health status, personal preferences, and individual goals.
- Appropriately designed resistance training programs may be safe and effective for select patients.
- Exercise participation should be timed so that it does not coincide with periods of peak insulin absorption.
- Specific steps should be taken to enhance compliance with exercise training.

The Exercise Prescription

NEIL F. GORDON, MD, PhD, MPH

INTRODUCTION

Exercise prescription is the process whereby a person's physical activity regimen is formulated in a systematic and individualized manner. Recent advances in basic and clinical exercise physiology have facilitated a more precise approach to exercise prescription for healthy people and those with chronic medical conditions. However, the existing body of scientific information is not so extensive as to warrant its application in a highly rigid fashion. In this respect, it must be emphasized that while the principles for exercise prescription outlined in this chapter are based on a solid foundation of scientific knowledge, they should not be construed as being theorems or laws. Rather, the recommended procedures should be viewed as guidelines that may be applied to a given person in a flexible manner. Health professionals who compile exercise prescriptions should recognize that the process is an art as well as a science (1).

To optimize the likelihood of a safe and effective response, the exercise prescription should take into consideration safety aspects as well as the mode, frequency, duration, intensity, rate of progression, and timing of physical activity. These fundamental components are interrelated and partly dependent on the purposes for which exercise is prescribed in a given person. The purposes will vary depending on the individual's interests, needs, background, and health status.

For people with diabetes, the major potential benefits of a physically active lifestyle include increased physical fitness, improved glycemic control, reduced risk for cardiovascular disease, decreased adiposity, and enhanced psychological well-being (2,3). From a health-promotion perspective, the various components of the exercise prescription therefore should be modulated with these purposes in mind. However, the purposes need not carry equal or consistent weight in all people with diabetes. In some instances, for example, in an overweight person with non-insulin-dependent diabetes mellitus (NIDDM), decreased adiposity and improved insulin sensitivity may be the central concerns. In other instances, for example, in a young person with insulin-dependent diabetes mellitus (IDDM), enhancement of physical fitness and psychological well-being may be the primary goals. Thus, the exercise prescription should focus on achieving the potential health-related benefits of exercise while at the same time reflecting the specific outcomes that are sought by a particular person with diabetes.

SAFETY: THE PREEXERCISE EVALUATION

Exercise is a normal human function that can be undertaken with a high level of safety by most people, including those with diabetes. However, exercise is not without risks, and the recommendation that people with diabetes participate in an exercise program is based on the premise that the benefits outweigh these risks. Therefore, the foremost priority in compiling the exercise prescription is to pay careful attention to minimizing the potential adverse effects of exercise via appropriate screening, program design, monitoring, and patient education (Table 6.1).

As is the case for the general population, the major potential health hazards of exercise for people with diabetes include musculoskeletal injury and sudden cardiac death. Other potential adverse effects that apply specifically to people with diabetes are listed in Table 6.2. Health professionals who counsel patients on exercise should be familiar with these adverse effects and how to prevent them.

Specific safety precautions for people with diabetes who participate in exercise are addressed in detail later (see Chapters 13–25). Depending on the severity of diabetes complications and other coexisting medical conditions, certain patients may need to participate in a medically supervised exercise program. However, before embarking on an exercise program, it is recommended that all people with diabetes undergo a

Table 6.1. Summary of Exercise Recommendations for Patients With Diabetes

Screening
- Search for vascular and neurological complications, including silent ischemia
- Exercise ECG in patients with known or suspected CAD, >30 years of age with IDDM, with IDDM for >15 years, or >35 years of age with NIDDM

Exercise program
- Type: Aerobic
- Frequency: 3–5 times/week
- Duration: 20–60 min
- Intensity: 50–74% of maximal aerobic capacity
- Energy expenditure: Modulate type, frequency, duration, and intensity to attain an energy expenditure of 700–2,000 calories/week
- Timing: Time participation so that it does not coincide with peak insulin absorption

Avoid complications
- Warm up and cool down
- Careful selection of exercise type and intensity
- Patient education
- Proper footwear
- Avoid exercise in extreme heat or cold
- Inspect feet daily and after exercise
- Avoid exercise when metabolic control is poor
- Maintain adequate hydration
- Monitor blood glucose if taking insulin or oral hypoglycemic agents, and follow guidelines to prevent hypoglycemia

Compliance
- Make exercise enjoyable
- Convenient location
- Positive feedback from involved medical personnel and family

Adapted in part from the American Diabetes Association (3).

complete medical history (Table 6.3), usually the most important part of the preexercise evaluation, and physical examination (Table 6.4) aimed at the identification of macrovascular, microvascular, and neurological complications as well as other medical conditions that constitute a contraindication to exercise or require special consideration (Table 6.5) (3). Because diabetes is potentially a progressive chronic disease, a continuing-care plan with follow-up medical evaluations is also necessary. Follow-up evaluations may be integrated into the patient's regular office visits, which should be scheduled at least quarterly for insulin-treated patients and at least semi-annually for other patients. The precise frequency and nature of follow-up physician visits, of course, will also depend on other factors, such as degree of blood glucose control and presence of complications or other medical conditions (4).

From a preexercise evaluation perspective, it must be emphasized that the most serious complication of exercise participation is sudden cardiac death. Although habitual physical activity is associated with an overall reduction in the risk of sudden cardiac death in the general adult population, and the chances of sustaining a fatal cardiac event during exercise training

Table 6.2. Potential Adverse Effects of Exercise in Patients With Diabetes

Cardiovascular
- Cardiac dysfunction and arrhythmias due to ischemic heart disease (often silent)
- Excessive increments in blood pressure during exercise
- Postexercise orthostatic hypotension

Microvascular
- Retinal hemorrhage
- Increased proteinuria
- Acceleration of microvascular lesions

Metabolic
- Worsening of hyperglycemia and ketosis
- Hypoglycemia in patients on insulin or sulfonylurea therapy

Musculoskeletal and traumatic
- Foot ulcers (especially in presence of neuropathy)
- Orthopedic injury related to neuropathy
- Accelerated degenerative joint disease
- Eye injuries and retinal hemorrhage

Adapted with permission from the American Diabetes Association (3).

are extremely small, it is well established that exercise can precipitate sudden cardiac death (5–7). Moreover, several studies have now shown that in adults the transiently increased risk of cardiac arrest that occurs during exercise results primarily from the presence of preexisting coronary artery disease (CAD) (8,9). In view of this, and because diabetes increases the risk for CAD by about threefold in men and possibly even more in women and is associated with a high prevalence of silent ischemia (3), it is recommended that the following individuals perform a graded exercise test with electrocardiogram (ECG) monitoring as part of a medical evaluation before beginning an exercise program: *1*) irrespective of their age, all people with known or suspected (on the basis of symptoms) CAD and *2*) asymptomatic people who have had IDDM for >15 years, have IDDM and are >30 years old, or have NIDDM and are >35 years old. Graded exercise testing in these individuals should be conducted in accordance with traditional guidelines that are outlined in detail elsewhere (1).

FITNESS VERSUS HEALTH BENEFITS OF EXERCISE: IMPLICATIONS FOR EXERCISE PRESCRIPTION

Much is known about the physiological adaptations that result from regular exercise. In particular, the exercise stimuli that are needed to improve maximal oxygen uptake, the most widely accepted index of cardiorespiratory fitness, have been well documented. Based on existing research in this area, guidelines for the quality and quantity of exercise required to promote cardiorespiratory fitness have been formulated (10).

Because cardiorespiratory fitness and health are frequently considered synonymous, such guidelines are often extrapolated to the prescription of exercise for the purpose of disease prevention and rehabilitation (11). In reality, however, changes in clinical status and health do not necessarily parallel increases in maximal oxygen uptake. Interestingly, recent epidemiological studies strongly suggest that regular participation in light-to-moderate inten-

Table 6.3. Major Components of the Preexercise Medical History

Individuals should be questioned about a past or present history of the following:

- Heart attack, coronary angioplasty, bypass surgery, other cardiac surgery
- Pain or discomfort in the chest or surrounding areas that may be ischemic in nature
- Light-headedness or syncope, particularly with exercise
- Unaccustomed shortness of breath or shortness of breath with mild exertion
- Palpitations or tachycardia
- Symptoms of congestive heart failure
- Heart murmurs, clicks, or other unusual cardiac findings
- Hypertension
- Stroke or transient ischemic attacks
- Phlebitis, emboli
- Symptoms and laboratory test results related to diabetes
- Current treatment of diabetes, including medications, diet, and results of glucose monitoring
- Frequency, severity, and cause of acute diabetes complications, such as ketoacidosis and hypoglycemia
- Symptoms and treatment of chronic complications associated with diabetes (eye, heart, kidney, nerve, peripheral vascular, and cerebral vascular)
- Pulmonary disease, including asthma, emphysema, and bronchitis
- Abnormal serum lipids and lipoproteins
- Anemia
- Emotional disorders
- Recent illness, hospitalization, or surgical procedure
- Pregnancy and breast-feeding
- Medications of all types
- Drug allergies
- Musculoskeletal disorders and injuries
- Family history, in particular, coronary heart disease and sudden death
- Habits, such as tobacco use, alcohol use, caffeine use, and eating disorders
- Exercise history with information on available resources, personal preferences, environmental considerations, and exercise type, frequency, duration, and intensity
- Psychosocial and economic factors that might influence the precise nature of the exercise prescription

Adapted with permission from the American College of Sports Medicine (1) and from the American Diabetes Association (4).

sity physical activities, which are unlikely to exert an optimal effect on maximal oxygen uptake, may be beneficial for the prevention of several diseases, including CAD, hypertension, and NIDDM (5,12,13). Furthermore, these studies suggest that strenuous exercise may not offer substantially more benefit from a health standpoint. Similarly, moderate levels of cardiorespiratory fitness, which probably are attainable by most adults without resorting to particularly strenuous exercise, have been shown to be partially protective against premature mortality (14). In addition, longitudinal training studies indicate that exercising at intensities that do not have an optimal effect on maximal oxygen uptake may produce equally favorable changes in CAD risk factors, including serum lipids and lipoproteins, blood pressure, and adiposity (12,15). Unlike improvements in maximal oxygen uptake, which are closely coupled to the volume and intensity of exercise training, the effectiveness of exercise in the possible prevention of CAD appears to be dependent primarily on the total energy expenditure (16). Thus, provided the frequency and duration are modulated appropriately, even physical activity

Table 6.4. Major Components of the Preexercise Physical Examination, Including Laboratory Testing

The physical examination should specifically assess the following:

- Height, weight, waist-to-hip ratio, and if possible, percent body fat
- Ophthalmoscopic examination
- Pulse rate and regularity
- Blood pressure determination, with orthostatic measurements
- Chest auscultation
- Cardiac examination
- Palpation and auscultation of carotid, abdominal, and femoral arteries
- Palpation and inspection of lower extremities for edema and presence of arterial pulses
- Foot examination
- Neurological examination
- Absence or presence of xanthoma and xanthelasma
- Orthopedic or other medical conditions that would limit exercise or require special consideration
- Laboratory tests (if not recently performed and clinically indicated), including fasting blood glucose, glycosylated hemoglobin, fasting serum lipids and lipoproteins, serum creatinine, urinalysis, thyroid function tests, resting ECG, exercise ECG, pulmonary studies, and review of results of previous pertinent tests (e.g., coronary angiography, echocardiographic studies, nuclear medicine studies)

Adapted with permission from the American College of Sports Medicine (1) and from the American Diabetes Association (4).

performed at an intensity below the critical threshold above which significant improvements in maximal oxygen uptake occur may be beneficial (11).

How can such knowledge be used to help promote physical activity participation among people with diabetes? Many individuals dislike strenuous exercise. Therefore, one approach is to reassure these individuals that they will derive important health benefits from less strenuous exercise training, place no emphasis on the intensity component of their exercise prescription (with the exception of ensuring that they do not exercise at too high an intensity), and focus on attainment of the desired level of energy expenditure (11). A potential disadvantage to this approach is that the efficacy of such low-intensity exercise in enhancing insulin sensitivity is unknown at present. Another disadvantage is that although any increase in physical activity may increase a sedentary person's maximal oxygen uptake, clinically relevant changes would be unlikely to result. Because important goals of exercise training for people with diabetes include enhancement of

insulin sensitivity and physical fitness, a somewhat modified version of this approach may be preferable. Rather than completely ignoring the intensity component, a middle ground may be reached. This can be accomplished by encouraging people to achieve the desired energy expenditure level while exercising at intensities of their choice that are above the minimal threshold needed to significantly increase maximal oxygen uptake but below that which may elicit undesirable physiological responses or clinical consequences (such as hypoglycemia, hyperglycemia, ketosis, myocardial ischemia, arrhythmia, exacerbation of proliferative retinopathy, and orthopedic injury) (11).

MODE OF EXERCISE

A key goal of the exercise prescription is caloric energy expenditure (1,16). To accomplish this, activities that use large muscle groups, that can be maintained for a prolonged period, and that are rhythmic and aerobic in nature are preferred. Typical examples include walking, jogging, swimming, cycling, cross-

Table 6.5. Contraindications to Exercise Participation

Absolute contraindications

- Recent significant change in the resting ECG that has not been adequately investigated and managed
- Recent complicated myocardial infarction
- Unstable angina pectoris
- Uncontrolled ventricular dysrhythmia
- Uncontrolled atrial dysrhythmia that compromises cardiac function
- Third-degree A-V block
- Acute or inadequately controlled heart failure
- Severe aortic stenosis or hypertrophic cardiomyopathy
- Suspected or known dissecting aneurysm
- Active or suspected myocarditis or pericarditis
- Acute thrombophlebitis or intracardiac thrombi
- Recent systemic or pulmonary embolus
- Untreated high-risk proliferative retinopathy
- Recent significant retinal hemorrhage
- Acute or inadequately controlled renal failure
- Acute infection or fever
- Significant emotional distress (psychosis)

Relative contraindications

- Blood glucose >300 mg/dl or >240 mg/dl with urinary ketone bodies
- Uncontrolled hypertension with resting systolic blood pressure >180 mmHg or diastolic blood pressure >105 mmHg
- Severe autonomic neuropathy with exertional hypotension
- Moderate valvular heart disease
- Cardiomyopathy
- Frequent or complex ventricular ectopy
- Ventricular aneurysm
- Resting heart rate >120 beats/min
- Recent fall in systolic blood pressure of more than 20 mmHg that was not caused by medication
- Known electrolyte abnormalities (e.g., hypokalemia, hypomagnesemia)
- Uncontrolled metabolic disease (e.g., thyrotoxicosis, myxedema)
- Chronic infectious disease (e.g., hepatitis, AIDS)
- Neuromuscular, musculoskeletal, or rheumatoid disorders that are exacerbated by exercise
- Complicated pregnancy.

Adapted with permission from the American College of Sports Medicine (1) and Gordon NF: *Diabetes: Your Complete Exercise Guide.* Champaign, IL, Human Kinetics Publishers, 1993.

country skiing, rowing, dancing, skating, rope skipping, stair climbing, and various endurance game activities. For a given level of energy expenditure, the health-related benefits of exercise appear to be independent of the mode of aerobic activity. Therefore, provided no contraindications exist, the types of aerobic exercise a patient performs are a matter of personal preference.

Aerobic activities that require running and jumping are considered high-impact types of exercise. Generally, these activities are associated with a higher incidence of musculoskeletal injuries in beginning as well as long-term exercisers than are low-impact and non-weight-bearing type activities (1). This increased risk for musculoskeletal injury is particularly evident in the elderly. Such activities are also more likely to traumatize the feet in patients with peripheral neuropathy (3). Thus, these factors must be considered when the exercise modality is prescribed.

When precise control of exercise intensity is needed, as in the early stages of an exercise program for patients with diabetes complications, preferred activities are those that can be readily maintained at a constant intensity and for which interindividual variability in energy expenditure is relatively low (1). Such activities include walking and stationary cycling.

Although aerobic exercise is of primary importance, a persuasive body of scientific evidence indicates that resistance training sufficient to develop and maintain strength should also be an integral component of an adult physical activity program. Based on existing research, both the American College of Sports Medicine and the American Association of Cardiovascular and Pulmonary Rehabilitation have added resistance training guidelines to their exercise recommendations for healthy adults and low-risk cardiac patients (10,17). Recent studies suggest that appropriately designed resistance training programs may be safe and effective for patients with diabetes, provided they do not have contraindications to such exercise (18,19) (see Chapter 7).

FREQUENCY, INTENSITY, DURATION, RATE OF PROGRESSION, AND TIMING OF EXERCISE

According to the American Heart Association, leisure-time activity for minimum physical conditioning and health benefits should consume at least 700 calories/week (16). They further recommend that individuals be encouraged to engage in activities requiring up to 2,000 calories/week for maximum health benefits (16). There is little convincing evidence of substantially greater health benefit at more than 2,000 calories/week (16).

In addition to the mode of exercise, weekly energy expenditure during training is dependent on the frequency, intensity, and duration of physical activity. Therefore, these factors should be modulated in accordance with the patient's clinical status and personal preferences to achieve the desired weekly energy expenditure.

Frequency

The frequency at which exercise should be performed depends, in part, on the duration and intensity of each exercise session. Existing research indicates that a frequency of <2 days/week generally does not evoke a meaningful change in maximal oxygen uptake (10). In contrast, the magnitude of improvement in maximal oxygen uptake tends to plateau when the frequency of training is increased above 3 days/week, with little additional benefit with training more than 5 days/week (10). Available evidence further suggests that the duration of glycemic improvement after the last bout of exercise in patients with diabetes is >12 but <72 h (20). In view of the above, it is recommended that exercise be performed on at least 3 nonconsecutive days each week and ideally on 5 days/week. Patients on insulin who experience difficulty in balancing their daily insulin and caloric needs may find it preferable to exercise daily. Similarly, obese patients may need to exercise more frequently (that is, 6–7 days/week) to optimize weight loss.

Multiple shorter bouts of exercise spread throughout the day may produce improvements in exercise capacity similar to a single longer session (21). Although more comprehensive scientific inquiry is needed, note that multiple short bouts of exercise closely resemble the physical activity that typically has been measured in epidemiological studies (22). In these studies, the accumulation of energy expenditure has been found to be inversely related to the risk for CAD and the development of NIDDM. Therefore, while no confirmatory data currently exist, it is thought that if the total daily energy expenditure is the same, comparable health benefits should accrue with multiple versus single bouts of exercise.

Intensity

The prescription of the appropriate exercise intensity is the most difficult problem in designing exercise programs. According to the American College of Sports Medicine, the minimum training intensity threshold for improvement in maximal oxygen uptake is 60% of the maximal heart rate (HR_{max}) (10). This corresponds to 50% of maximal oxygen uptake (VO_{2max}) or HR_{max} reserve and a perceived exertion rating (RPE) of 12 on the Borg 6–20 scale (Table 6.6).

Higher intensity exercise is associated with greater cardiovascular risk, greater chance for musculoskeletal injury, and lower compliance to training than lower intensity exercise. Therefore, programs emphasizing low-to-moderate intensity exercise are preferable for people with diabetes. If the complications of diabetes permit, it is recommended that exercise be prescribed at an intensity corresponding to 60–79% HR_{max}, 50–74% of maximal oxygen uptake or HR_{max} reserve, or an RPE of 12–13.

As indicated above, various techniques can be used to prescribe and monitor exercise intensity. These include heart rate, percent maximal oxygen uptake, and RPE (1). Patients usually find the concept of heart rate and RPE easier to understand than the concept of maximal oxygen uptake, and these two methods are generally preferred (23). Generally for people with diabetes complications, both heart rate and RPE should be used. Although the use of heart rate as an estimate of intensity of exercise is the recommended approach, for those without diabetes complications or coexisting medical conditions that may be worsened by exercise, RPE may be used on its own.

The heart-rate method of exercise prescription is based on the linear relationship that exists between heart rate and exercise intensity. Ideally, target heart rates should be prescribed using the individual's HR_{max} determined during graded exercise testing. This is particularly important for patients with cardiovascular complications or autonomic neuropathy or those receiving medications, such as ß-blockers, that may alter the heart-rate response to exercise. When the true HR_{max} is unknown, it can be estimated by the equation $HR_{max} = 220 -$ the patient's age.

The two most commonly used ways of prescribing target heart rates are the percent HR_{max} method and the percent HR_{max} reserve method (1,3,23). The percent HR_{max} method simply involves multiplying HR_{max} by 0.6 and 0.79, respectively, to determine the lower and upper limits of the target heart-rate range. The percent HR_{max} reserve method differs from this in that the individual's true resting heart rate, determined before arising in the morning, is also taken into consideration, as follows:

Lower limit
$$= 0.5(HR_{max} - HR_{rest}) + HR_{rest}$$

Upper limit
$$= 0.74(HR_{max} - HR_{rest}) + HR_{rest}$$

The use of RPE has become a valid method for monitoring and prescribing exercise intensity. It is generally regarded as an adjunct to heart-rate monitoring, but it can be used in place of heart rate in patients in whom a precise knowledge of heart rate is not clinically indicated. It should be kept in mind, however, that about 10% of participants tend to select unrealistic RPE scores. In these individuals, the RPE method for exercise prescription is inappropriate. The commonly used Borg 6–20 scale is shown in Table 6.7.

Irrespective of the precise manner of exercise intensity prescription, importance should be placed on an adequate warm-up and cooldown. Patients should warm up with low-intensity aerobic exercise for at least 5 min. The most practical way to accomplish this is to perform the prescribed aerobic activity at a lower intensity. Ideally, the aerobic warm-up should raise the heart rate to within at least 20 beats/min of the lower limit of the prescribed target heart-rate range. On completion of the aerobic phase of the exercise session, it is also important to keep exercising at a reduced intensity for at least 5 min before stopping completely. This cooldown helps ensure the gradual return of heart rate and blood pressure to near-resting

Table 6.6. Classification of Intensity of Exercise Based on 20–60 min of Aerobic Exercise Training

Relative Intensity (%)		RATING OF PERCEIVED EXERTION	CLASSIFICATION OF INTENSITY
HR_{max}	VO_{2max} OR HR_{max} RESERVE		
< 35	< 30	< 10	Very light
35 – 59	30 – 49	10 – 11	Light
60 – 79	50 – 74	12 – 13	Moderate (somewhat hard)
80 – 89	75 – 84	14 – 16	Heavy
≥ 90	≥ 85	> 16	Very heavy

Published with permission from Pollock ML, Wilmore JH: *Exercise in Health and Disease: Evaluation and Prescription for Prevention and Rehabilitation.* 2nd ed. Philadelphia, Saunders, 1990.

levels and reduces the potential for post-exercise hypotension together with its adverse clinical sequelae. The importance of an adequate aerobic warm-up and cooldown is emphasized by the observation in one study that of 61 cardiac complications during the exercise training of CAD patients, 44 occurred at the beginning or end of an exercise session (24).

To help prevent musculoskeletal injuries, stretching exercises may also be included in the warm-up and/or cooldown. However, they must be done without holding the breath, which can result in large increases in systolic

Table 6.7. Borg 6–20 Perceived Exertion Scale

RATING OF PERCEIVED EXERTION OR RPE	VERBAL DESCRIPTION OF RPE
6	
7	Very, very light
8	
9	Very light
10	
11	Fairly light
12	
13	Somewhat hard
14	
15	Hard
16	
17	Very hard
18	
19	Very, very hard
20	

From Borg GA: Psychophysical bases of perceived exertion. *Med Sci Sports Exercise* 14:377–87, 1982.

blood pressure due to a Valsalva effect. For patients with microvascular or coronary disease, such increases in systolic blood pressure are potentially detrimental (3).

Duration

The appropriate duration of each exercise session is inversely related to the intensity at which the exercise is performed. Thus, lower intensity physical activity should be conducted over a longer period of time than higher intensity exercise. When performed 3–5 days/week at 50–74% of maximal oxygen uptake, exercise sessions will typically need to last 20–60 min to achieve the desired weekly energy expenditure. Shorter exercise sessions will need to be performed several times during the day. Longer exercise sessions may result in a higher incidence of musculoskeletal injury and difficulty with compliance.

Rate of Progression

The rate of progression in the exercise training program is dependent on several factors. These include baseline cardiorespiratory fitness level, age, weight, health status, personal preferences, and individual goals. It is usually best initially to alter the duration of exercise rather than the intensity of effort. Generally, exercise training should begin at a comfortable intensity that is well within the individual's current capacity. Exercise sessions initially should be no more than 10–15 min in duration and should be gradually increased in accordance with the individual's capabilities. Once a desired duration is reached, exercise intensity may likewise be gradually increased. To prevent musculoskeletal injury and untoward physiological responses, beginning exercisers should be advised to progress gradually and cautioned against attempting to perform too much exercise too soon (1).

Timing of Exercise

Ideally, exercise training should be performed at the time of day that is most convenient for the participant. However, because exercise can potentiate the effects of insulin, hypoglycemia during or after exercise is a definite risk for individuals receiving treatment with insulin (and, to a lesser degree, oral hypoglycemic agents). While details of hypoglycemia prevention are presented elsewhere (see Chapter 11), it is important when prescribing exercise to time participation so that it does not coincide with periods of peak insulin absorption. Initially, in order to enhance blood glucose control, it may be preferable for patients on insulin to exercise at a similar time each day. However, this is not absolutely necessary, especially once the patient gains adequate experience with hypoglycemia prevention.

COMPLIANCE

Research on adherence to exercise training reveals that 50% of participants drop out within 1 year (1). Specific steps can be taken to enhance exercise compliance. These are discussed in detail elsewhere (1,3) and include 1) ensuring that the person has reasonable expectations at the start of the program, 2) having the new participant make a firm commitment to adhere to the program via a written contract, 3) starting the exercise program at a comfortable level and progressing gradually, 4) choosing enjoyable activities that can be performed at a convenient time and location, 5) setting realistic goals to ensure a gradual progression of exercise training, 6) reviewing the person's performance on a regular basis and giving them feedback about their progress, 7) reinforcing positive changes in behavior via appropriate rewards, 8) using stimulus control strategies (e.g., write exercise time in appointment books, set watch alarms for exercise time, lay out clothes the night before) and cognitive strategies (e.g., have participants systematically consider the pros and cons of exercise), 9) optimizing social support from friends and relatives, and 10) training in relapse prevention.

THE ROLE OF PHYSICIANS AND OTHER HEALTH-CARE PROFESSIONALS IN THE EXERCISE PRESCRIPTION

Physicians have both the opportunity and responsibility to promote regular exercise to their patients with diabetes. If the physician does not have the time or does not feel knowledgeable enough to personally prescribe and supervise an exercise program, he or she may delegate the task to other appropriately qualified members of the health-care team. In this respect, the services of nurses, exercise physiologists, physical therapists, and other health-care professionals may be extremely useful. However, the physician must set the agenda, because staff members under a physician's supervision cannot deliver preventive and rehabilitative services, such as the exercise prescription, unless the physician defines the services as medically appropriate (5).

REFERENCES

1. American College of Sports Medicine: *Guidelines for Exercise Testing and Prescription.* Philadelphia, Lea & Febiger, 1991
2. American Diabetes Association: Diabetes mellitus and exercise (Position Statement). *Diabetes Care* 16 (Suppl. 2):37, 1993
3. American Diabetes Association: Exercise and NIDDM (Technical Review). *Diabetes Care* 16 (Suppl. 2):54–58, 1993
4. American Diabetes Association: Standards of medical care for patients with diabetes mellitus (Position Statement). *Diabetes Care* 16 (Suppl. 2):10–13, 1993
5. Fletcher GF, Blair SN, Blumenthal J, Caspersen C, Chaitman B, Epstein S, Falls H, Sivarajan Froelicher ES, Froelicher VF, Pina IL: Benefits and recommendations for physical activity programs for all Americans (Statement on Exercise). *Circulation* 86:340–44, 1992
6. Thompson PD, Funk EJ, Carleton RA, Sturner WQ: Incidence of death during jogging in Rhode Island from 1975 through 1980. *JAMA* 247: 2535–38, 1982
7. Siscovick DS, Weiss NS, Fletcher RH, Lasky T: The incidence of primary cardiac arrest during vigorous exercise. *N Engl J Med* 311: 874–77, 1984
8. Kohl HW, Gordon NF, Powell KE, Blair SN, Paffenbarger RS: Physical activity, physical fitness and sudden cardiac death. *Epidemiol Rev* 14: 37–58, 1992
9. Thompson PD, Klocke FJ, Levine BD, Van Camp SP: Task force 5: coronary artery disease. *Med Sci Sports Exercise* 26:S271–75, 1994
10. American College of Sports Medicine: The recommended quantity and quality of exercise for developing and maintaining cardiorespiratory and muscular fitness in healthy adults (Position Stand). *Med Sci Sports Exercise* 22:265–74, 1990
11. Gordon NF, Kohl HW, Blair SN: Lifestyle exercise: a new strategy to promote physical activity for adults. *J Cardiopulm Rehab* 13:161–63, 1993
12. American College of Sports Medicine: Physical activity, physical fitness, and hypertension (Position Stand). *Med Sci Sports Exercise* 25:i-x, 1993
13. Helmrich SP, Ragland DR, Leung RW, Paffenbarger RS: Physical activity and reduced occurrence of non-insulin-dependent diabetes mellitus. *N Engl J Med* 325:147–52, 1991
14. Blair SN, Kohl HW III, Paffenbarger RS Jr, Clark DG, Cooper KH, Gibbons LW: Physical fitness and all-cause mortality: a prospective study of healthy men and women. *JAMA* 262:2395–401, 1989
15. Duncan JJ, Gordon NF, Scott CB: Women walking for health and fitness: how much is enough? *JAMA* 266:3295–99, 1991
16. Fletcher GF, Froelicher VF, Hartley LH, Haskell WL, Pollock ML: A statement for health professionals from the American Heart Association (Exercise Standards). *Circulation* 82:2286–322, 1990
17. American Association of Cardiovascular and Pulmonary Rehabili-

tation: *Guidelines for Cardiac Rehabilitation Programs.* Champaign, IL, Human Kinetics Books, 1994

18. Miller WJ, Sherman WM, Ivy JL: Effect of strength training on glucose tolerance and post-glucose insulin response. *Med Sci Sports Exercise* 16:539–43, 1984

19. Durak EP, Jovanovic-Peterson L, Peterson CM: Randomized crossover study of effect of resistance training on glycemic control, muscular strength, and cholesterol in type I diabetic men. *Diabetes Care* 13:1039–43, 1990

20. Vranic M, Wasserman D: Exercise, fitness, and diabetes. In *Exercise, Fitness, and Health.* Bouchard C, Shephard RJ, Stephens T, Sutton J, McPherson B, Eds. Champaign, IL, Human Kinetics Books, 1990, p. 467–90

21. De Busk RF, Stenestrand U, Sheehan M, Haskell WL: Training effects of long versus short bouts of exercise in healthy subjects. *Am J Cardiol* 65:1010–13, 1990

22. De Busk RF, Haskell WL: Do multiple short bouts of exercise really produce the same benefits as single long bouts? (Letter). *Am J Cardiol* 67:326, 1991

23. Campaigne BN, Lampman RM: *Exercise in the Clinical Management of Diabetes.* Champaign, IL, Human Kinetics Books, 1994

24. Haskell WL: Cardiovascular complications during exercise training of cardiac patients. *Circulation* 57: 920–24, 1978

7. Resistance Training

Highlights
Resistance Training

- Properly designed resistance training programs may provide important benefits for patients with diabetes.
- Patients should be carefully screened before beginning resistance training and should receive proper supervision and monitoring.
- Intense resistive exercise often produces an acute hyperglycemic effect. Patients on insulin or oral hypoglycemic agents may develop hypoglycemia in the hours following resistance training.
- Proper technique should be taught for all of the exercises used in the program. Patients should be instructed to perform lifting movements through a full range of motion while breathing freely and rhythmically.
- Exercise prescriptions for resistance training must be developed on an individual basis after consideration of the patient's goals and limitations, as well as selection of the appropriate modality, choice of exercise, intensity, volume, and frequency of training.

Resistance Training

W. GUYTON HORNSBY, Jr, PhD, CDE

INTRODUCTION

Resistance training refers to forms of exercise that use muscular strength to move a weight or work against a resistive load. Resistance training may provide substantial benefits to patients with diabetes. As with any form of exercise, benefits must outweigh risks. Resistance training has previously been regarded as unsafe for many patients with cardiovascular disease or for those with microvascular or neurological complications. With thorough preexercise screening, proper supervision and monitoring, and appropriate attention to modifications of the training regimen, resistance training may allow many patients to safely improve muscular strength and endurance, enhance flexibility, improve insulin sensitivity and glucose tolerance, enhance body composition, and decrease risk factors for cardiovascular disease (1-4).

CARDIOVASCULAR AND METABOLIC EFFECTS

Chronic resistance training has been associated with a number of favorable metabolic and cardiovascular effects in nondiabetic study groups. Improvements in oral glucose tolerance and insulin sensitivity, similar to those produced by aerobic training, have been reported following resistance training (5). Miller et al. (6) demonstrated lower fasting plasma insulin following resistance training that was correlated with increased lean body mass. Ullrich et al. (7) found resistance training improved plasma lipids and enhanced cardiovascular function. Improvements in glycemic control have been reported in subjects with insulin-dependent diabetes mellitus (IDDM) when resistance training has been combined with aerobic exercise (8) and when resistance training has been used exclusively (9). Effects of chronic resistance training have not been reported in subjects with non-insulin-dependent diabetes mellitus (NIDDM).

Little is known about the acute effects of resistance exercise in diabetes. An informal survey of members of the International Diabetic Athletes Association suggests that resistance exercise is often associated with hyperglycemia during and shortly after acute training sessions. This anecdotal evidence is consistent with findings of hyperglycemic responses to intense (>80% VO_{2max}) aerobic exercise in subjects with IDDM (10) and NIDDM (11). Glucoregulation with intense exercise has been reviewed by Marliss et al. (12). Short-term increases in blood glucose with resistance exercise are frequently followed by hypoglycemia, which may appear many hours after the exercise has ended. This postexercise hypoglycemia is likely due to restoration of muscle glycogen (13).

Acute resistance exercise has been associated with extreme elevations in both systolic and diastolic blood pressure in healthy subjects performing high-intensity exhaustive exercise (14). Increased arterial pressure and heart rate increase the work of the heart and myocardial requirements for oxygen. Holding the breath during maximal tension exercise may cause reductions in venous return and can lead to inadequate blood flow to the heart and brain. Increases in blood pressure are most pronounced during Valsalva maneuvers with sustained isometric contractions. There is a fear that inappropriate hemodynamic responses may place an excessive burden on patients with diabetes. Caution should be observed in patients with advanced retinal and cardiovascular complications (see Chapters 14 and 15).

SAFETY

The safety of resistance training has been well documented in geriatric patients (15) (see Chapter 22), as well as in patients with cardiac disease (16) and diabetes (9). Attention to modifications in training, such as lowering the intensity of lifting, eliminating exercise to the point of exhaustion, and limiting the amount of sustained gripping or isometric contractions may be useful in reducing exercise-induced blood pressure elevations. Patients should be instructed to perform lifting movements while breathing freely and rhythmically, without holding the breath. Exhalation should occur during the lifting phase of the movement and inhalation should be done while lowering the weight. If patients are unable to perform this breathing pattern, telling them to "breathe regularly and do not hold your breath" usually is adequate to help them avoid the Valsalva maneuver.

While intense resistance exercises are expected to produce a short-term hyperglycemic effect, it is important to instruct patients that responses can vary. Hypoglycemic responses following resistance exercise have been reported (9) and should always be considered a possible consequence. Any patient on insulin or an oral hypoglycemic agent should be advised to monitor blood glucose before, during, and after exercise and should be instructed to take appropriate actions in response to undesirable glycemic effects.

To reduce the risk of injury, proper technique should be learned for each exercise. Whenever possible, exercises should be done through a full range of motion. Adequate warm-up and cooldown periods should always be performed. A 5- to 10-min general warm-up period consisting of light aerobic activity and stretching should be done before resistance training. If moderate or intense lifting is to be performed, this should be preceded by low resistance movements. Light aerobic activity and stretching should be done for 5-10 min in the cooldown period.

All patients should have a thorough medical examination before beginning a resistive training program to detect the presence of macrovascular, microvascular, or neurological complications, as well as to determine any orthopedic limitations. The evaluation should include a symptom-limited graded exercise test with electrocardiographic and blood pressure monitoring for all patients with known or suspected coronary artery disease, people who

have had IDDM >15 years, have IDDM and are >30 years of age, or have NIDDM and are >35 years of age. Heart rate, blood pressure, and rating of perceived exertion should be determined during lifting movements (see Chapters 6, 15, and 18).

TYPES OF RESISTANCE TRAINING

Modalities for resistance training include calisthenic activities using body weight for resistance; various types of springs, rubber bands, or elastic tubing; free weights, such as barbells or dumbbells; and weight machines that provide resistance by pulleys, chains, hydraulic cylinders, or electromagnets. The resistance that is applied may be described as *1*) constant, if the load remains the same throughout the exercise or *2*) variable, if the resistance is altered during the exercise by special pulleys or cams. Muscular contractions are classified as *1*) isometric or static, with force being applied without movement, *2*) isotonic or dynamic, with force being applied to produce movement, or *3*) isokinetic, with variable force being applied to move a resistance at a constant speed.

THE RESISTIVE EXERCISE PRESCRIPTION

Once properly screened, various techniques can be used to establish initial resistance training loads. One of the safest methods is to begin with the lightest weight that can be set for each exercise and monitor patient responses for 6-10 repetitions. Heart rate and blood pressure should be within individual limits established by exercise testing, and the rating of perceived exertion should be no greater than 13 (somewhat hard). If the patient tolerates this weight well, he or she can increase repetitions to 10-15 and then 15-20 every 1-2 weeks. After patients are comfortable with the movements and have demonstrated good technique, the number of sets can be increased to 2-3, and heavier weight can be added. Typically, 2-5 pounds for upper body exercises and 5-10 pounds for lower body exercises will be appropriate.

Alternatively, the maximal weight lifted in one full range of motion (the one repetition maximum or 1 RM) or the maximal weight that can be lifted for 10 (10 RM) or 15 (15 RM) repetitions can be determined, and initial training loads can be set as percentages of these values. Generally, resistive loads are classified as light (40-60% 1 RM), moderate (60-80% 1 RM), or heavy (80-100% 1 RM). While 1 RM testing is the standard for determining initial loads in most research studies, the previously described technique of starting with the lightest weight is more practical in clinical settings. This method puts less initial stress on patients, allows for better patient orientation, and may allow for a more accurate exercise prescription.

The volume of resistance training depends on the number of complete movements or repetitions that are performed for a given exercise. Repetitions are typically performed in groups or sets, depending on the intensity of training and the goals of the program. Rest between sets should be adequate to allow successful completion of the next set. For low-intensity training, rest periods are as brief as 15 s to 1 min. Moderate-intensity training usually requires 1-2 min of rest, and high-intensity exercise may require 2-5 min, for adequate recovery.

Exercises should be selected for each major muscle group including *1)* the hip and legs (gluteal, quadriceps, and hamstring groups), *2)* the chest (pectoral group), *3)* the shoulders (deltoid and trapezius groups), *4)* the back (latissimus dorsi, rhomboid, and teres and erector spinae groups), *5)* the arms (biceps, triceps, and wrist flexor and extensor groups), *6)* and the abdominal muscle groups. For each muscle group, at least 48 h recovery should be allowed between training sessions. Two resistance training sessions per week appear to be the minimum number required to produce positive physiological effects. Concepts involved in prescribing resistance training have been described by Fleck and Kraemer (17,18).

THE NATIONAL STRENGTH AND CONDITIONING ASSOCIATION

The National Strength and Conditioning Association certifies exercise professionals who demonstrate fundamental competencies to plan and supervise resistance training programs. This organization may be helpful in providing physicians and health-care professionals with a list of Certified Strength and Conditioning Specialists who can work with the health-care team to instruct patients on proper exercise technique and training. National Strength and Conditioning Association, P.O. Box 38909, Colorado Springs, CO 80934. Tel: 719-632-6367.

REFERENCES

1. Poehlman ET, Gardner AW, Ades PA, Katzman-Rooks SM, Montgomery SM, Atlas OK, Ballor DL, Tyzbir RS: Resting metabolism and cardiovascular disease risk in resistance-trained and aerobically trained males. *Metabolism* 41: 1351–60, 1992
2. Smutok MA, Kokkinos PF, Farmer C, Dawson P, Shulman R, DeVane-Bell J, Patterson J, Charabogos C, Goldberg AP, Hurley BF: Aerobic versus strength training for risk factors intervention in middle-aged men at high risk for coronary heart disease. *Metabolism* 42:177–84, 1993
3. Soukup JT, Kovaleski JE: A review of the effects of resistance training for individuals with diabetes mellitus. *Diabetes Educator* 19:307–12, 1993
4. Stone MH, Fleck SJ, Triplett NT, Kraemer WJ: Health- and performance-related potential of resistance training. *Sports Med* 11:210–31, 1991
5. Hurley BF, Seals DR, Ehsani AA, Carter L-J, Dalsky GP, Hagberg JM, Holloszy JO: Effects of high-intensity strength training on cardiovascular function. *Med Sci Sports Exercise* 16:483–88, 1984
6. Miller WJ, Sherman WM, Ivy JL: Effect of strength training on glu-

cose tolerance and post-glucose insulin response. *Med Sci Sports Exercise* 16:539–43, 1984

7. Ullrich IH, Reid CM, Yeater RA: Increased HDL-cholesterol levels with a weight lifting program. *Southern Med J* 80:328–31, 1987

8. Peterson CM, Jones RL, DuPuis A, Levine BS, Bernstein R, O'Shea ML: Feasibility of improved blood glucose control in patients with insulin-dependent diabetes mellitus. *Diabetes Care* 2:329–35, 1979

9. Durak EP, Jovanovic-Peterson L, Peterson CM: Randomized crossover study of effect of resistance training on glycemic control, muscular strength, and cholesterol in type I diabetic men. *Diabetes Care* 13:1039–43, 1990

10. Mitchell TH, Abraham G, Schiffrin A, Leiter LA, Marliss EB: Hyperglycemia following intense exercise in insulin-dependent diabetic subjects during continuous subcutaneous insulin infusion. *Diabetes Care* 11:311–17, 1988

11. Kjaer M, Hollenbeck CB, Frey-Hewitt B, Galbo H, Haskell W, Reaven GM: Glucoregulation and hormonal responses to maximal exercise in non-insulin-dependent diabetes. *J Appl Physiol* 68:2067–74, 1990

12. Marliss EB, Purdon C, Miles PDG, Halter JB, Sigal RJ, Vranic M: Glucoregulation during and after intense exercise in control and diabetic subjects. In *Diabetes Mellitus and Exercise.* Devlin JT, Horton ES, Vranic M, Eds. London, Smith-Gordon, 1992, p. 173–90

13. Ivy JL: Resynthesis of muscle glycogen after exercise. In *Diabetes Mellitus and Exercise.* Devlin JT, Horton ES, Vranic M, Eds. London, Smith-Gordon, 1992, p. 153–64

14. MacDougall JD, Tuxen D, Sale DG, Moroz JR, Sutton JR: Arterial blood pressure response to heavy resistance exercise. *J Appl Physiol* 58:785–90, 1985

15. Fiatarone MA, Marks EC, Ryan ND, Meredith CN, Lipsitz LA, Evans WJ: High-intensity strength training in nonagenarians. *JAMA* 263:3029–34, 1990

16. Ghilarducci LE, Holly RG, Amsterdam EA: Effects of high resistance training in coronary artery disease. *Am J Cardiol* 64:866–70, 1989

17. Fleck SJ, Kraemer WJ: Resistance training—basic principles (part 1 of 4). *Physician Sportsmed* 16(3):160–71, 1988

18. Fleck SJ, Kraemer WJ: Resistance training—exercise prescription (part 4 of 4). *Physician Sportsmed* 16(6):69–81, 1988

SUGGESTED READING

1. National Strength and Conditioning Association: *Essentials of Strength Training and Conditioning.* Baechle TR, Ed. Champaign, IL, Human Kinetics Publishers, 1994

8. Nutritional Strategies to Optimize Athletic Performance

Highlights

Fuel Use During Endurance Exercise

Does the Availability of Fat Limit Endurance Performance?

Does the Availability of Protein Limit Endurance Performance?

Does the Availability of Carbohydrate Limit Endurance Performance?

Nutritional Strategies to Optimize Body Carbohydrate Stores

Nutritional Strategies for the Endurance Athlete

Nutritional Strategies During Daily Heavy Training
Nutritional Strategies the Week Before an Important Event
Nutritional Strategies During the Hours Before Competition
Nutritional Strategies During Competition
Nutritional Strategies During the 4–6 h After Training or Competition
Nutritional Strategies During the 24 h After Training or Competition

Nutritional Strategies for Recreational Athletes

Highlights
Nutritional Strategies to
Optimize Athletic Performance

- The primary substrate that is oxidized during moderate-intensity exercise (65–75% VO_{2max} lasting 90–120 min) is carbohydrate.
- The body's stores of carbohydrate are limited; thus, it is important to consume adequate dietary carbohydrate during all phases of endurance training and performance.
- Endurance athletes should concentrate on consuming 8–10 g carbohydrate/kg body wt/day, at least 1.2 g protein/kg body wt/day, and the balance of energy from fat.

- Recreational athletes, however, should concentrate on consuming a healthy diet that contains <0.4 g fat/kg body wt/day (<30 g/day for a 70-kg person), at least 0.8 g protein/kg body wt/day, and the balance of energy from carbohydrate.
- Both endurance and recreational athletes should consume fluids during exercise to match the fluid lost from sweating.

Nutritional Strategies to Optimize Athletic Performance

W. MICHAEL SHERMAN, PhD, CYNTHIA FERRARA, PhD, AND
BARBARA SCHNEIDER, MS

FUEL USE DURING ENDURANCE EXERCISE

The bodily fuel reserves, protein, fat, and/or carbohydrate, are metabolized to provide the energy necessary for muscular contraction during endurance exercise. Protein metabolism may make a small contribution to energy expenditure but only when bodily carbohydrate stores are low or when the exercise is of a very long duration. Of the other fuel reserves, fat and carbohydrate are the primary substrates that are metabolized to produce energy for muscle contraction. The duration, intensity, and mode of exercise influence the relative proportion of fat and carbohydrate that are metabolized to provide the energy required for muscle contraction during endurance exercise.

DOES THE AVAILABILITY OF FAT LIMIT ENDURANCE PERFORMANCE?

During low-intensity long-duration exercise such as walking, the primary fuel that is metabolized to produce energy for muscle contraction is fat. Fat circulates in the blood as a fatty acid–albumin complex, or fat is stored in muscle or adipose tissues as triglyceride. After 60 min of exercise at 40% VO_{2max} (walking), fat contributes 40% of the total energy expenditure, whereas after 240 min of exercise at this walking intensity, fat contributes 70% of the total energy expenditure (1). However, because the body's fat stores are so large, the depletion of bodily fat stores has not been identified as a factor that limits performance (i.e., depletion of bodily fat stores or available fat energy almost never occurs and thus does not contribute to fatigue during endurance exercise).

DOES THE AVAILABILITY OF PROTEIN LIMIT ENDURANCE PERFORMANCE?

Metabolism of protein during exercise may provide a relatively small proportion of the total energy expenditure, depending on nutritional status and the duration of exercise. During exercise at 60% VO_{2max} for longer than 1 h, protein oxidation may contribute up to 5% of the total energy expenditure (2). If muscle glycogen stores are low, the contribution of protein oxidation may increase to 10–15% of the total energy expenditure. These findings indicate that metabolism of protein contributes an increasing proportion of the energy expenditure as the duration of exercise increases and the bodily carbohydrate stores decrease (3,4). However, there is no association between the onset of fatigue and a low content of muscle protein or the rate of protein breakdown during endurance exercise. This seems reasonable because the body protects this critical tissue to preserve the essential elements for muscle contraction and bodily structure. Therefore, it is unlikely that protein oxidation is a limiting factor during prolonged exercise (i.e., depletion of bodily protein reserves or available protein energy almost never occurs and thus does not contribute to fatigue during endurance exercise).

DOES THE AVAILABILITY OF CARBOHYDRATE LIMIT ENDURANCE PERFORMANCE?

During moderate-intensity exercise, a large proportion of the energy for muscle contraction is provided by the metabolism of the body's carbohydrate stores (5,6). Moderate-intensity exercise is between 65 and 75% VO_{2max}: within this range of exercise intensities, it would be slightly to extremely difficult to carry on a normal conversation during the exercise session. The bodily stores of carbohydrate include muscle and liver glycogen and blood glucose. Because bodily carbohydrate stores are limited, a significant reduction in or depletion of the bodily carbohydrate stores can limit the ability of the muscle to continue producing force at the required rate (i.e., a lowering of the muscle glycogen or blood glucose concentrations or muscle glycogen depletion causes fatigue during endurance exercise).

Stored carbohydrate energy in a 70-kg person is 5 MJ (2,7). This carbohydrate energy is found in muscle (79%) and liver (14%) as glycogen and in the blood (7%) as glucose (2). These carbohydrate stores can sustain moderate-intensity exercise for only about 120 min if carbohydrates are the only fuels metabolized to produce energy for muscular contraction during endurance exercise (2).

The rate of muscle glycogen degradation (glycogenolysis) increases with increasing exercise intensity (6). At exercise intensities between 65 and 85% VO_{2max}, fatigue appears to be related to a low muscle glycogen concentration. Furthermore, the preexercise muscle glycogen concentration is directly proportional to the endurance time to fatigue (5,8,9). For exercise at <60% VO_{2max}, fatigue likely occurs as a result of boredom, dehydration, hyperthermia, or orthopedic injury. For exercise at >90% VO_{2max}, fatigue is probably related to the increased lactic acid concentration in the blood and muscle.

Blood glucose is also metabolized to provide energy for muscle contraction. A lowering of the blood glucose concentration or a low blood glucose concentration (i.e., hypoglycemia) during exercise may impair endurance performance (1,10,11). These blood glucose responses can occur during moderate-intensity exercise that lasts for longer than 90–120 min (11,12). Therefore, it is extremely important to maintain a blood glucose concentration in the normal range during prolonged moderate-intensity endurance exercise.

The blood glucose concentration during exercise is dependent on the rate of muscle glucose uptake and the rate of glucose released from the splanchnic areas (1). The liver degrades glycogen to glucose (glycogenolysis) and releases the glucose into the blood to maintain the blood glucose concentration. In a 70-kg person exercising at 75% VO_{2max}, the blood glucose concentration remains at about 5 mmol/l for 90–120 min. The blood glucose concentration is maintained because the rate of splanchnic glucose release equals the rate of glucose uptake by the contracting muscles. If exercise continues at a moderate intensity for longer than 90–120 min, glucose uptake by the contracting muscle remains constant, but splanchnic glucose release declines because of the depletion of liver glycogen (11,13). Formation of glucose by glucose precursors (gluconeogenesis) cannot completely compensate for the decreased splanchnic glucose release that is due to liver glycogen depletion, and consequently, the blood glucose concentration declines. For 70% of the population, a lowering of the blood glucose concentration causes fatigue (11).

In conclusion, carbohydrate, fat, and protein may be metabolized and contribute by varying degrees to the total energy expenditure during prolonged moderate-intensity exercise. The major energy sources for exercise at intensities appropriate for improving cardiovascular endurance (between 65 and 75% VO_{2max}) are the bodily carbohydrate stores (e.g., muscle and liver glycogen and blood glucose) (2). When exercise is undertaken at these intensities for longer than 90–120 min, a reduction of these carbohydrate reserves can limit exercise performance (e.g., a lowering or depletion of muscle and liver glycogen and/or blood glucose causes fatigue).

NUTRITIONAL STRATEGIES TO OPTIMIZE BODY CARBOHYDRATE STORES

Normally active, untrained individuals have an energy expenditure between

2,000 and 2,500 kcal/day, whereas an athlete undertaking strenuous, prolonged exercise training may have an energy expenditure that is 1.5–3 times higher (2,7). The typical American diet contains 40–45% of the total energy from carbohydrate, 40% of the total energy from fat, and 10–15% of the total energy from protein. The recommended amounts of these nutrients in the diet for active people should probably be based on body weight (14). Thus, physically active people should consume at least 5–6 g carbohydrate/kg body wt/day, 0.8 g protein/kg body wt/day, and no more than 0.4 g fat/kg body wt/day (or 30% of the total calories from fat or 30 g of fat/day).

The endurance athlete should choose foods during training that will maintain bodily carbohydrate stores to optimize training and performance capabilities. Because carbohydrates are the primary source of fuel for exercising muscle, the carbohydrate intake must be carefully monitored (2,15).

Athletes undertaking intense daily exercise should consume additional energy equal to the energy expenditure of exercise to maintain a constant body weight. The percent of energy consumed as fat should not exceed 30% of the total energy intake in most people. Additionally, the endurance athlete should probably increase protein intake to 1.2 g/kg body wt/day, with the balance of energy intake derived primarily from dietary carbohydrate. Based on these recommendations, an endurance athlete may consume as much as 8–10 g carbohydrate/kg body wt/day (2,14,16). This high carbohydrate intake should maintain or increase glycogen stores in the muscle and liver. It appears that muscle glycogen may be normalized within 24 h following intermittent exercise if only 5–6 g carbohydrate/kg body wt/day is consumed, although this perspective has not been extensively studied (2). It is possible that some athletes participating in strength or endurance activities, or those athletes subjecting their muscles to recurring muscle trauma or sudden increases in training load, may require a slightly higher protein intake (17).

However, it is likely that the increased protein requirement for these conditions will be adequately met by the increased food intake to meet the energy expenditure associated with exercise.

NUTRITIONAL STRATEGIES FOR THE ENDURANCE ATHLETE

For the endurance athlete, nutritional strategies to optimize carbohydrate stores in muscle and liver are essential to optimize training and performance capabilities. These nutritional strategies should be used in every phase of the endurance athlete's training regimen, including daily training, the week before a competition, the hours before competition, during competition, and the 4–6 h and 24 h after competition or training. The application of these recommendations to the endurance and recreational athlete are summarized in Table 8.1.

Nutritional Strategies During Daily Heavy Training

Intense daily training will acutely reduce the bodily stores of carbohydrate. If inadequate dietary carbohydrate is consumed on a daily basis, there may be a suboptimal level of bodily carbohydrate that may impair daily training capabilities. Consuming 10 g carbohydrate/kg body wt/day during twice-daily intense rowing training for 28 days produced higher muscle glycogen and significantly better training/performance responses than consuming 5 g carbohydrate/kg body wt/day (18). Thus, adequate dietary carbohydrate intake on a daily basis has the potential to facilitate a more "optimal" training adaptation.

Nutritional Strategies the Week Before an Important Event

Because of the direct relationship between a low muscle glycogen concentration and fatigue, it has been hypothesized that starting exercise with a supra-elevated muscle glycogen

Table 8.1. Synopsis of Nutritional Strategies and Phases of Training/Competition for Endurance and Recreational Athletes

PHASE OF TRAINING	ENDURANCE ATHLETE	RECREATIONAL ATHLETE
■ During daily training	Consume <0.4 g fat/kg body wt/day; 0.8–1.2 g protein/kg body wt/day; 8–10 g CHO/kg body wt/day	Consume <30% total daily energy from fat; 10–12% total daily energy from protein; balance of energy from CHO
■ Week before event (CHO loading; note cautions in text for IDDM)	Do 90, 40, 40, 20, 20, and 0 min of exercise at moderate intensity; Consume 5 g CHO/kg body wt/day during first 3 days followed by 8–10 g CHO/kg body wt/day during second 3 days	Probably not applicable
■ Hours before event (see cautions in text for those who might be sensitive to an early lowering of blood glucose)	Consume 4–5 g liquid CHO/kg body wt 3–4 h before event, or consume 1–2 g liquid CHO/kg body wt 1 h before event, or solids may be used as tolerated; test individual responsiveness to recommendation	Exercise need not be undertaken on an empty stomach, although the work-enhancing effect of a preexercise CHO meal for the recreational athlete is doubtful
■ During the event	Consume fluids at a rate equal to sweat loss, or at minimum, consume 250 ml every 20 min during exercise; do not wait until thirst develops to begin consuming fluids; desirable fluids are CHO/electrolyte beverages (6–10% wt/vol); consume at a rate to provide 40–65 g CHO/h. If CHO consumption is delayed, consume 200 g of liquid CHO before completing 2 h of exercise and then consume 40–65 g CHO/h	Consume fluids at a rate equal to sweat loss, or at minimum, consume 250 ml every 20 min during exercise to produce moderate to heavy sweating; do not wait until thirst develops to begin consuming fluids; fluids may be CHO/electrolyte beverages, water, or other fluids according to individual preference
■ 4–6 h after event	Consume 0.7–3.0 g CHO/kg body wt immediately after and every 2 h thereafter for 4 h; if tolerated, 0.4 g CHO/kg body wt every 15 min after exercise for 4 h	Probably not applicable
■ 24 h after event	Consume 8–10 g CHO/kg body wt/day; mixed CHO foods can be consumed; high-glycemic index foods probably promote glycogen synthesis	See daily training recommendation

Individual tolerances to these recommendations may vary. Before individuals with diabetes undertake these nutritional strategies, they should consult a physician or diabetes educator about appropriate activity level. CHO, carbohydrate.

concentration (supercompensation) may extend, in time, the point at which fatigue occurs during endurance exercise.

An accepted glycogen supercompensation regimen reported by Sherman et al. (19) incorporates dietary manipulation with a tapering of the duration of exercise during the 6 days before an important endurance competition. Exercise is undertaken during these days at a moderate intensity for 90, 40, 40, 20, 20, and 0 min, respectively. During the first 3 days, the diet should contain 5 g carbohydrate/kg body wt/day, and during the next 3 days, the diet should contain 8–10 g carbohydrate/kg body wt/day. The protein intake should be 0.8–1.2 g/kg body wt/day over the 6-day period. This regimen increases muscle glycogen to more than 210 mmol/kg wet wt: 1.6-fold above the "normal" glycogen concentration of 130 mmol/ kg wet wt that is found in trained athletes consuming a diet containing 5 g carbohydrate/kg body wt/day (20).

The supercompensation or carbohydrate-loading regimen must be used with caution in people with diabetes. Specifically among those with insulin-dependent diabetes mellitus, careful manipulation of the insulin regimen and doses guided by frequent blood glucose monitoring will be needed to maintain glucose control while achieving the goals of the regimen.

Nutritional Strategies During the Hours Before Competition

Many endurance athletes train or compete after an overnight fast. An overnight fast will reduce the liver glycogen concentration, and this may produce a premature lowering of the blood glucose concentration and premature fatigue during endurance exercise. Thus, endurance athletes should consider consuming a preexercise carbohydrate meal during the hours before training and/or competition in endurance events.

Wright et al. (21) reported an 18% increase in total work and a 36-min increase in endurance time to exhaustion in well-trained cyclists who consumed 5 g of liquid carbohydrate/kg body wt compared with a placebo solution 3 h before exercise. Additionally, consuming either 1.1 or 2.2 g liquid carbohydrate/kg body wt 1 h before endurance exercise also produced a significant 12% increase in cycling time-trial performance in moderately trained cyclists (22).

If blood insulin is elevated at the start of exercise as a result of a preexercise carbohydrate feeding, there may be an initial lowering of the blood glucose concentration by as much as 1 mmol/l during the first 15–20 min of exercise (15). Thus, preexercise carbohydrate feedings may cause fatigue in those individuals who may be sensitive to this lowering of blood glucose. Thus, adoption of this strategy to improve endurance performance should be evaluated by the athlete in advance and not for the first time during an important competition.

Nutritional Strategies During Competition

During endurance performance, it is imperative to maintain the body's fluid balance and available carbohydrate energy.

The body's heat content increases during exercise. The body attempts to minimize the increase in body temperature primarily by sweating. As sweat evaporates, heat is lost from the body. The heat that is dissipated by sweating is especially critical for minimizing the increase in body temperature during exercise in a warm or hot environment.

Sweating reduces the amount of fluid in the body. The loss of body water and electrolytes during exercise may lead to heat cramps, heat exhaustion, and even heat stroke, which can cause death (2). When sweating occurs during exercise, the primary objective is to consume as much water as is lost. The sweat rate may range from 0.75 to 1.0 liter/h; thus, at least 250 ml fluid should be consumed every 20 min during exercise (2). Because the sensation of thirst occurs after there is already a significant body fluid deficit, the consumption of fluid should begin within the first 20 min of exercise.

Carbohydrate consumption during moderate-intensity exercise lasting longer than 90–120 min will delay the onset of fatigue during endurance exercise. Endurance time until exhaustion may be extended by as much as 60 min with carbohydrate feeding during exercise (11,16,23). The preservation of exercise tolerance is attributed largely to the maintenance of a high rate of carbohydrate oxidation during the later stages of exercise that is facilitated by maintaining the availability of blood glucose (11,23). Based on many studies of carbohydrate feedings during endurance exercise, it appears that the endurance athlete should ingest 40–65 g of carbohydrate/h consumed as a 6–10% (wt/vol) solution (10–12,16,23).

Under certain circumstances, it may not be practical or possible to consume carbohydrate in liquids during the early stages of an endurance event. However, for carbohydrate ingestion to positively affect endurance performance under this circumstance, the carbohydrates must be consumed before the blood glucose concentration begins to decline (24). If carbohydrate consumption must be delayed during endurance exercise, 200 g of liquid carbohydrate should be consumed before completing 2 h of moderate-intensity exercise. Thereafter, carbohydrate should be consumed at a rate to provide 40–65 g carbohydrate/h (16,24). Carbohydrate feedings during intermittent exercise also improve performance; however, the mechanism for the enhanced performance appears to be the result of a slowing of the degradation of muscle glycogen (25).

Nutritional Strategies During the 4–6 h After Training or Competition

The rate of glycogen synthesis is linear during the first 6 h after exercise. When muscle glycogen has been depleted, muscle glycogen synthesis occurs at a rate of 6 mmol/kg wet wt/h if 0.7–3.0 g of carbohydrate/kg is consumed immediately after exercise and at 2-h intervals thereafter for 6 h (15,26,27). However, if carbohydrate ingestion is delayed for 2 h after stopping exercise, the rate of muscle glycogen synthesis will be 50% slower (i.e., only 3 mmol/kg wet wt/h). It may be possible to double the rate of muscle glycogen synthesis (10–12 mmol/kg wet wt/h) after exercise by ingesting small amounts of carbohydrate (0.4 g carbohydrate/kg body wt) at 15-min intervals for 4 h after endurance exercise (28). Ingestion of carbohydrates immediately after glycogen-depleting exercise may be especially important if multiple glycogen-depleting sports events are to be undertaken in a given day (16).

Nutritional Strategies During the 24 h After Training or Competition

Muscle glycogen synthesis during the 24–48 h after exercise is largely dependent on the amount of carbohydrate ingested. Muscle glycogen can be replenished in 24 h if more than 525 g carbohydrate or 8 g carbohydrate/kg body wt/day is consumed (2,29). One study suggested that consuming complex carbohydrate produced a greater muscle glycogen storage during the second 24-h period after exercise; however, this study has not been replicated (2). More recently, it has been demonstrated that a high glycemic index carbohydrate diet (10 g/kg body wt/day) results in more muscle glycogen storage than consuming a low glycemic index carbohydrate diet (30). Exercise that significantly depletes muscle glycogen also often impairs muscle function. While most studies focus on the ideal methods to "normalize" muscle glycogen, few studies have determined if muscle function is also normal when a "normal" muscle glycogen concentration has been achieved.

NUTRITIONAL STRATEGIES FOR RECREATIONAL ATHLETES

Because most recreational athletes will not undertake exercise lasting longer than 90–120 min at a moderate intensity for more than 3 or 4 days/week, it is unlikely that the nutritional strategies outlined above will have a direct benefit for them. Most likely, adequate body carbohydrate stores will be maintained by consuming a "healthy" diet that matches caloric expenditure and maintains body weight. Thus, most recreational athletes should consume a diet that contains <30% of total energy from fat, roughly 10–12% of energy as protein, and the balance of energy from carbohydrate. Probably the most significant threat to the endurance capabilities of the recreational athlete are the negative consequences of dehydration due to sweating. Thus, the primary emphasis for the recreational athlete should be to consume fluids at a rate that is equal to the loss of body water from sweating. Normal body weight should be attained between exercise sessions that produce significant sweating to eliminate the consequences of chronic dehydration. Because thirst is increased after significant sweating has already occurred, fluid consumption should begin before the onset of the sensation of thirst during exercise.

REFERENCES

1. Ahlborg B, Bergstrom J, Brohult J, Eklund LG, Hultman E, Maschio G: Human muscle glycogen content and capacity for prolonged exercise after different diets. *Foersvarsmedicin* 3:85–99, 1967
2. Ahlborg G, Felig P, Hagenfeldt L, Hendler R, Wahren J: Substrate turnover during prolonged exercise in man: splanchnic and leg metabolism of glucose, free fatty acids, and amino acids. *J Clin Invest* 53:1080–90, 1976
3. Ahlborg G, Felig P: Lactate and glucose exchange across the forearm, legs, and splanchnic bed during and after prolonged leg exercise. *J Clin Invest* 69:45–54, 1982
4. Bergstrom J, Hermansen L, Saltin B: Diet, muscle glycogen, and physical performance. *Acta Physiol Scand* 75:140–50, 1967
5. Blom PCS, Hostmark AT, Vaage O, Kardel KR, Maehlum S: Effect of different post-exercise sugar diets on the rate of muscle glycogen synthesis. *Med Sci Sports Exercise* 19:491–96, 1987
6. Brotherhood JR: Nutrition and sports performance. *Sports Med* 1:350–89, 1984
7. Burke LM, Collier GR, Hargreaves M: Muscle glycogen storage after prolonged exercise: effect of the glycemic index of carbohydrate feedings. *J Appl Physiol* 75:1019–23, 1993
8. Coggan AR, Swanson SC: Nutritional manipulations before and during endurance exercise: effects on performance. *Med Sci Sports Exercise* 24:S331–35, 1992
9. Coggan AR, Coyle EF: Reversal of fatigue during prolonged exercise by carbohydrate infusion or ingestion. *J Appl Physiol* 63:2388–95, 1987
10. Coggan AR, Coyle EF: Metabolism and performance following carbohydrate ingestion late in exercise. *Med Sci Sports Exercise* 21:59–65, 1989
11. Costill DL, Sherman WM, Fink WJ, Maresh C, Whitten M, Miller JM: The role of dietary carbohydrates in muscle glycogen resynthesis after strenuous running. *Am J Clin Nutr* 34:1831–36, 1981
12. Coyle EF: Timing and method of increased carbohydrate intake to cope with heavy training, competition, and recovery. *J Sports Sci* 9:29–52, 1993
13. Coyle EF, Coggan AR, Hemmert MK, Ivy JL: Muscle glycogen utilization during prolonged strenuous exercise when fed carbohydrate. *J Appl Physiol* 61:165–72, 1986
14. Coyle EF, Coggan AR: Effectiveness of carbohydrate feeding in delaying fatigue during prolonged exercise. *Sports Med* 1:446–58, 1984
15. Doyle JA, Sherman WM, Strauss RL: Effects of eccentric and concentric exercise on muscle glycogen replenishment. *J Appl Physiol* 74:1848–55, 1993

16. Hermansen L, Hultman E, Saltin B: Muscle glycogen during prolonged severe exercise. *Acta Physiol Scand* 71:129–39, 1967

17. Ivy JL, Lee MC, Brozinick JT, Reed MJ: Muscle glycogen storage after different amounts of carbohydrate ingestion. *J Appl Physiol* 65:2018–23, 1988

18. Lemon PWR, Yarasheski KE, Dolony DG: The importance of protein for athletes. *Sports Med* 1:474–84, 1984

19. Lemon PWR, Mullin JP: Effect of initial muscle glycogen levels on protein catabolism during exercise. *J Appl Physiol* 48:624–29, 1980

20. McArdle WD, Katch FI, Katch VL: *Exercise Physiology: Energy, Nutrition, and Human Performance.* Lea & Febiger, Malvern, PA, 1991

21. Saltin B, Karlsson J: Muscle glycogen utilization during work of different intensities. In *Muscle Metabolism During Exercise.* Pernow B, Saltin B, Eds. New York, Plenum, 1971, p. 289–300

22. Sherman WM: Carbohydrate feedings before and after exercise. In *Perspectives in Exercise Science and Sports Medicine: Ergogenics: Enhancement of Performance and Exercise in Sport.* Vol. 4. Lamb DR, Williams MH, Eds. Indianapolis, IN, Benchmark, 1991, p. 1–34

23. Sherman WM, Wimer GS: Insufficient dietary carbohydrate: does it impair athletic performance? *Int J Sports Nutr* 1:28–44, 1991

24. Sherman WM, Brodowicz G, Wright DA, Allen WK, Simonsen J, Dernbach A: Effects of 4 h pre-exercise carbohydrate feedings on cycling performance. *Med Sci Sports Exercise* 21:598–604, 1989

25. Sherman WM, Lamb DR: Nutrition and prolonged exercise. In *Perspectives in Exercise Science and Sports Medicine: Prolonged Exercise.* Vol. 1. Lamb DR, Murray R, Eds. Indianapolis, IN, Benchmark, 1988, p. 213–80

26. Sherman WM: Carbohydrate, muscle glycogen and muscle glycogen supercompensation. In *Ergogenic Aids in Sport.* Williams MH, Ed. Champaign, IL, Human Kinetics Books, 1983, p. 3–26

27. Sherman WM, Costill DL, Fink WJ, Miller JM: The effect of exercise and diet manipulation on muscle glycogen and its subsequent use during performance. *Int J Sports Med* 2:114–18, 1981

28. Simonsen JC, Sherman WM, Lamb DR, Dernbach AR, Doyle JA, Strauss R: Dietary carbohydrate, muscle glycogen, and power output during rowing training. *J Appl Physiol* 70:1500–505, 1990

29. Wright DA, Sherman WM, Dernbach AR: Carbohydrate feedings before, during, or in combination improve cycling endurance performance. *J Appl Physiol* 71:1082–88, 1991

30. Yaspelkis BB III, Patterson JG, Anderla PA, Ding Z, Ivy JL: Carbohydrate supplementation spares muscle glycogen during variable intensity exercise. *J Appl Physiol* 75:1477–85, 1993

9. Nutrition, Exercise, and Diabetes

Highlights
Nutrition, Exercise, and Diabetes

■ An adequate caloric intake should be planned for the person with diabetes who participates in regular exercise. A nutrition assessment of usual food intake followed by monitoring of weight, height (if pertinent), and appetite (hunger) is the best way to judge adequacy of caloric intake. However, if glucose control is inadequate, eating additional calories is futile.

■ Carbohydrate feedings before, during, and after exercise can be especially important for the exerciser with diabetes.

■ A higher carbohydrate intake (60% of daily calories) during training with adequate blood glucose control can maintain maximal liver and muscle glycogen stores.

■ Eating a meal containing carbohydrate 3–4 h before activities or consuming a carbohydrate feeding within the hour before exercise can improve performance. For the exerciser with diabetes, this may also facilitate glucose control.

■ During exercise, blood glucose levels decline gradually beginning at 90–180 min. Ingesting a carbohydrate feeding during prolonged exercise can improve performance by maintaining the availability and oxidation of blood glucose. For the exerciser with diabetes whose blood glucose level may drop sooner and lower, ingesting carbohydrate after 60 min of exercise is important and may also assist in preventing hypoglycemia.

■ Consuming carbohydrate immediately after exercise optimizes repletion of muscle and liver glycogen. This takes on added importance for the exerciser with diabetes who is also at increased risk for late-onset hypoglycemia.

■ Fluids are important for all exercisers. For the first 60–90 min, water is the preferred beverage. After 60–90 min, fluids containing 8% carbohydrate are recommended. These beverages can also help prevent hypoglycemia in the exerciser with diabetes.

Nutrition, Exercise, and Diabetes

MARION J. FRANZ, MS, RD, CDE

INTRODUCTION

Adequate and appropriate nutrition is important for any person engaging in physical activity or fitness programs. For the person with diabetes, however, it takes on added importance. Not only can adequate nutrition help with physical performance, but nutrition also plays a pivotal role in the regulation of blood glucose levels before, during, and after physical activities.

Fatigue that causes anyone, with or without diabetes, to stop exercising can result from deficiencies of oxygen, fluid, or fuel. These shortages can occur separately or in combination. The ability to take in and process an adequate supply of oxygen is related to physical training, while fluid and fuel status and utilization are primarily related to nutrition. Dehydration leads progressively to fatigue, heat cramps, heat exhaustion, and heat stroke. However, for exercise to continue, muscles must also have a source of fuel. Although all athletes will eventually need fuel replacements to continue exercising, individuals with diabetes may need replenishment of fuel, especially carbohydrates, sooner (1).

Total energy requirements, the source and amount of energy, and fluid intake are important considerations for the person with diabetes.

ENERGY NEEDS

People participating in regular physical activity programs usually have higher energy needs compared with sedentary individuals. Total daily caloric requirements for individuals engaged in physical training programs vary and may range from 2,000 kcal (i.e., a gymnast) to 6,000 kcal or more (i.e., a football player or body builder) (2). The lower caloric density of the recommended high-carbohydrate/low-fat diet often makes it difficult to provide sufficient food to meet high energy requirements. High-carbohydrate food choices in a pattern of more frequent eating, with planned snacks, are often necessary. Nutritional beverages (liquid meal supplements) or energy bars may be helpful for the athlete wanting to gain weight or maintain a high weight, because they provide a high-carbohydrate beverage/snack in ready-to-consume concentrated form (2) (Table 9.1).

Men may require up to 50 kcal/kg body wt or more during periods of regular heavy physical activity. This is in contrast to 40 kcal/kg body wt for more moderate physical activity and 30 kcal/kg body wt for very light physical activity. Women may require 44 kcal/kg body wt for regular heavy physical activity compared with 37 kcal/kg body wt for more moderate activity and 30 kcal/kg body wt for very light physical activity (3). However, there is considerable person-to-person variation in calorie needs. In general, these values, along with the individual's weight, growth (if pertinent), and hunger, can be used to evaluate adequacy of caloric intake (Tables 9.2 and 9.3).

Without sufficient energy intake, both fat stores and body proteins are used to fuel daily activities. As a consequence, circulating levels of protein by-products increase as lean tissue is degraded, and water and electrolytes are lost in the excretion of these by-products. Because active people do not want to lose muscle mass, matching individual intake with energy expenditure is critical.

For exercisers with diabetes, the best way to determine caloric needs is to begin with a detailed nutrition history. Compare current intake with estimated caloric needs and develop a meal plan based on the nutrition assessment. Weight and appetite should be monitored and used to evaluate caloric adequacy.

CARBOHYDRATE

In general, it is recommended that 60% of total energy for exercisers should come from carbohydrate (2). An

Table 9.1. Nutritive Analysis of Nutritional Beverages and Energy Bars

	SERVING SIZE	CALORIES	CARBO-HYDRATE g (% total calories)	PROTEIN g (% total calories)	FAT g (% total calories)
■ Beverages					
Ensure	8 fl oz	250	34 (54)	9 (14)	9 (32)
GatoPro	8 fl oz	360	58 (65)	16 (18)	7 (17)
Sport Shake	8 fl oz	310	45 (58)	11 (13)	10 (29)
Sustacal	8 fl oz	240	33 (55)	14.5 (24)	5.5 (21)
■ Bars					
Exceed Sports Bar	1 bar (2.8 oz)	280	53 (76)	12 (17)	2 (7)
Power Bar	1 bar (2.25 oz)	225	42 (75)	10 (16)	2.5 (9)
Tiger Sport Ultimate Performance Bar	1 bar (2.3 oz)	230	40 (69)	11 (19)	3 (12)

adequate intake of carbohydrate is necessary to maintain maximal muscle and liver glycogen stores in endurance athletes (4). Chronic low intake of carbohydrate leads to progressive depletion in glycogen stores. If liver and muscle glycogen is not replenished on a daily basis, chronic fatigue is the result.

For the athlete with diabetes, blood glucose control is also essential. Consuming additional carbohydrate and/or calories and then losing it through glycosuria is futile. Therefore, coordination of insulin doses with food intake is essential to assure both glucose control and desirable muscle and liver glycogen stores.

Carbohydrate for Daily Training

For individuals training 1 h/day, 5–6 g of carbohydrate/kg body wt/day is needed to replenish muscle glycogen stores on a regular basis. For most individuals this is 60% of total daily calories. For individuals training ≥2 h/day, 8 g of carbohydrate/kg body wt/day or 65–70% of the total daily calories may be needed. For endurance activities this may be increased up to 10 g of carbohydrate/kg body wt/day (4) (Table 9.3). Because average intake is generally 4–5 g of carbohydrate/kg body wt/day (46% of calories), increasing carbohydrate requires effort and concentration on the part of the exerciser.

Despite the increase in glucose uptake by muscles during moderate-intensity exercise, glucose levels change very little in individuals without diabetes. Hepatic glycogenolysis and gluconeogenesis closely match the increase in glucose uptake. Muscular work causes a fall in plasma insulin and a rise in glucagon (5,6). This balance is the major determinant of hepatic glucose production, underscoring the need for insulin adjustments along with adequate carbohydrate intake during training for people with diabetes.

Carbohydrate Feedings Before Exercise

Recommendations to athletes to not eat during the 3 h before exercise or to avoid sugar 30–45 min before exercise no longer apply. Preexercise carbohydrate feedings do not impair athletic performance and may, in fact, improve performance. Consuming 200–350 g of carbohydrate 3–6 h before exercise appears to consistently improve performance (7,8), supporting the concept that active individuals should eat before exercise. As a result, the recommended pre-event carbohydrate intake is 1 g/kg body wt within the hour before exercise and up to 4 g/kg body wt in an easily digested meal within 3–4 h before activities (9,10). Intakes in the range of 1.1 g of carbohydrate/kg body wt 1 h before exercise have been reported to lead to carbohydrate oxidation and adequate beginning blood glucose levels (11).

For example, 1 g of carbohydrate/kg body wt 1 h before an event might be toast, jam, or juice; 4 g of carbohydrate/kg body wt 3–4 h before an event might be pancakes or potatoes, bread, and fruit. For an event early in the morning, athletes can eat an hour before exercise. This will enhance performance compared with exercising in a fasting state. Exercising or competing in the early morning after an overnight fast may cause liver and muscle glycogen to be low at the start of exercise and may contribute to fatigue and poor performance.

For events later in the day, a small meal may be eaten 3–4 hours before the event. The meal should contain mostly carbohydrate and some protein, but a minimal amount of fat. The menu could include lean meat (fish or poultry without skin), potatoes without gravy, vegetables, bread with no butter, salad without dressing, fruit, and skim milk. Three to four cups of fluid should be included with the meal and continued up to the time of the event.

For the athlete with diabetes, additional carbohydrate may be needed about 20 min before an event. Nathan et al. (12) reported that a simple pre-exercise snack, eaten 15–30 min before

exercise of short duration (<45 min), prevented postexercise hypoglycemia; 13 g of carbohydrate was an adequate amount. Low-fat carbohydrate foods (such as crackers, muffins, yogurt, or soups), rather than sugary sweets, are good choices. Other nutritious snacks include peanut butter and crackers, fig bars, oatmeal-raisin cookies, dried fruit, bread sticks, and granola bars. Fruit juices and fruits such as apples, peaches, plums, and pears not only have natural sugars, vitamins, and minerals but also are 85% water (1).

However, several studies (13,14) have reported that people with type I diabetes tend to overeat rather than undereat with exercise. Guidelines for increasing carbohydrate intake and decreasing insulin doses should be based on blood glucose levels before and after exercise, how close to scheduled meals and snacks exercise

Table 9.2. Approximate Calorie Requirements for Different Activity Levels

ACTIVITY LEVEL	MEN (kcal/kg body wt)	WOMEN (kcal/kg body wt)
■ Heavy	50	44
■ Moderate	40	37
■ Light	30	30

Table 9.3. Examples of Estimated Daily Nutrient Needs for Typical Athletes

WEIGHT	CALORIES	CARBO-HYDRATE	PROTEIN
70–kg man	50 kcal/kg 3,500 kcal	8 g/kg 560 g (64%) 6 g/kg 420 g (48%)	1.2 g/kg 84 g (10%)
55–kg woman	44 kcal/kg 2,420 kcal	8 g/kg 440 g (73%) 6 g/kg 330 g (55%)	1.2 g/kg 66 g (11%)

will occur, and how often the person exercises. The more regular the exercise, the more the body adapts. As a result, not as much extra carbohydrate is required. If exercise is done on a regular basis, the snacks should be part of the usual meal plan. Furthermore, with regular exercise, usual insulin doses can be adjusted. Self-monitoring of blood glucose can provide valuable information to document and maximize the benefits of nutrition. This will give the athlete the information needed to modify food choices and portions and to adjust insulin for best results for both performance and blood glucose control.

Moderate-intensity exercise (<50% maximum oxygen uptake) is reported to increase muscle glucose uptake and utilization by 2–3 mg/kg body wt/min above usual daily requirements. When exercising, a 70-kg person would need an added 140–210 mg of glucose for every minute of moderate exercise, or an added 8.4–12.6 g for every hour. During high-intensity exercise (80–100% maximum oxygen uptake), glucose uptake may increase by 5–6 mg/kg body wt/min above usual needs. As a result, 350–420 mg of glucose is used every minute. Despite the increased rate of glucose use, the demand on glucose stores and the risk of hypoglycemia is less, because exercise of this intensity cannot be sustained for long intervals (15).

Therefore, it may be prudent for exercisers with diabetes to eat a carbohydrate snack before or after a short period (about 1 h) of moderate-intensity exercise, although care must be taken not to overeat; 15 g of carbohydrate (60 kcal) may be enough to prevent hypoglycemia while not adding excessive calories.

Reduction in the dose of insulin before exercise (and possibly after) may also be required. Several guidelines are available for decreasing insulin. A reduction of the short-acting insulin of 30–50% has been reported to decrease the risk of hypoglycemia (16). Another method is to decrease the insulin acting during the time of exercise by 10% of the total daily insulin dose (1).

Carbohydrate loading is a technique used to increase glycogen stores by athletes doing events of long duration (9) (see Chapter 8 for additional information on carbohydrate loading). Individuals with diabetes who carbohydrate load must monitor blood glucose levels carefully and adjust insulin doses appropriately, both to preserve glucose control and to accomplish the goals of the carbohydrate-loading process.

Carbohydrate Intake During Exercise

Carbohydrate is needed to maintain carbohydrate oxidation for fuel utilization during exercise of a long duration. As muscle glycogen becomes depleted, blood glucose supplies the carbohydrate oxidation fuel source and is responsible for 75–90% of the total carbohydrate consumed during the first 40 min of exercise. Beyond 40 min, the rate of glucose use by contracting muscles increases progressively to a peak at 90–180 min, after which it declines in parallel with a gradual fall in the blood glucose level (17). Ingesting carbohydrate during prolonged moderate- to high-intensity exercise can improve performance by maintaining the availability and oxidation of blood glucose late in exercise (18,19), but it does not conserve glycogen stores (20).

There are two ways to maintain blood glucose levels: by preexercise snacks or by carbohydrate feedings during exercise. Coyle et al. (21) found that exercisers receiving a carbohydrate feeding every 20 min maintained blood glucose levels better and exercised longer compared with exercisers receiving no carbohydrate. Muscle glycogen was depleted in both groups at the same rate, but the exogenous carbohydrate source allowed exercise to proceed for a longer time period. Therefore, the recommendation for all exercisers is that 30–75 g of carbohydrate/h be consumed throughout exercise so that 1 g of carbohydrate/min will be delivered to the tissues when fatigue would set in (18).

For the exerciser with diabetes whose blood glucose levels may drop

Table 9.4. Nutritive Analysis of Fluid Replacement Beverages

	PORTION	CALORIES	CARBO-HYDRATE (g)	SODIUM (mg)	POTASSIUM (mg)	CARBO-HYDRATE CONCEN-TRATION (%)
All Sport Body Quencher	8 fl oz	70	20	55	55	8
Exceed Energy Drink Powder	2 Tbsp + 8 fl oz water	70	17	50	45	7
Gatorade Thirst Quencher	8 fl oz	50	14	110	30	6
PowerAde Thirst Quencher	8 fl oz	70	19	55	30	8
Soft drinks	8 fl oz	110–130	27–32	9–30	Trace	10–13
Fruit juice	8 fl oz	120–180	30–45	0–15	61–510	12–18

sooner, faster, and to lower levels, carbohydrate feedings during exercise take on added importance. In general, during events of a long duration, a minimum of 30–60 g of carbohydrate should be consumed every hour, distributed at 15- to 30-min intervals. Along with carbohydrate feedings, appropriate adjustments in insulin doses are needed. This allows hepatic glycogenolysis to proceed, thus decreasing the risk of hypoglycemia and lessening the need for supplemental food to manage exercise.

Solid or liquid forms of carbohydrate may be consumed. Mason et al. (22) found that athletes consuming 25 g of either a solid or liquid carbohydrate every 30 min performed equally well. Each form has its advantages: liquids provide fluid for hydration, whereas solids may prevent hunger. However, for exercise lasting longer than 60–90 min, a liquid carbohydrate form is most often chosen and recommended because it is practical and contributes to adequate hydration (23). Rapid gastric emptying allows fluids into the plasma and glucose into cells as quickly as possible. Gastric emptying is affected by temperature, volume, osmolarity, and sugar content of the solution. As volume increases, so does the rate of gastric emptying. The higher the sugar content, the slower the rate of emptying. Cold fluids pass through the stomach more quickly than warm ones (24).

Solutions containing 8% carbohydrate empty from the stomach as quickly as plain water. Drinks with a concentration of carbohydrate or sugars >10% can cause osmotic problems and lead to gastrointestinal upset, such as cramps, nausea, diarrhea, or bloating (25). Fruit juice and most regular soft drinks contain about 12% carbohydrate and need to be diluted with an equal amount of water. For the exerciser with diabetes, diluted fruit juice or fluid replacement beverages can provide both needed fluids and a source of carbohydrate (Table 9.4).

Carbohydrate Intake After Exercise

Combining carbohydrate before and during events increases performance ability, but of equal importance is carbohydrate intake after exercise. Consuming carbohydrate immediately after exercise compared with waiting 2 h has been shown to replete carbohydrate stores more efficiently. To optimize repletion of muscle glycogen following exhaustive exercise, 1.5 g of carbohydrate/kg body wt within 30 min after exercise should be consumed, and a second 1.5 g of carbohydrate/kg body wt should be consumed 1–2 h later (26). This is a time when high-carbohydrate feedings may be most useful (Table 9.5). When muscle glycogen is depleted, a carbohydrate-rich diet will restore glycogen to its preexercise levels within 24 h (27).

Replacing carbohydrate following exercise is absolutely essential for the exerciser with diabetes who is at great risk for late-onset hypoglycemia (28). It is often more important to replace carbohydrate after exercising than before. Blood glucose levels should be monitored at 1- or 2-h intervals to assess the response to exercise and to make the necessary adjustments in insulin and food intake.

FLUIDS

During exercise, water should be consumed on a set schedule. Because the thirst mechanism is blunted with exercise, it is essential for athletes and trainers to monitor and meet fluid needs. Cool, plain water is the recommended beverage for fluid replacement before, during, and after short-term moderate exercise. Athletes should note weight changes from fluid losses during exercise and drink 2 cups of water for every pound lost.

While sedentary people lose a quart of water daily from sweating, athletes engaged in strenuous activity may lose 2 or more quarts (4 pounds)/h. To prevent dehydration, the following guidelines are provided for athletes (2).

Drink 3 cups of cold water 2 h before an event. In hot weather, adequate hydration helps to prevent the rise in core temperature and to reduce heat-induced stress in the cardiovascular system.

Drink 1–2 cups more of water 10–15 min before the event. Continue drinking small amounts (1/2 to 1 cup) of fluid at 10- to 20-min intervals throughout the competition. This is necessary to replace sweat losses and maintain blood volume. Although larger volumes empty rapidly from the stomach, many athletes are uncomfortable when exercising with a nearly full stomach.

Table 9.5. Nutritive Analysis of High-Carbohydrate Beverages

	SERVING SIZE	CALORIES	CARBO-HYDRATE (g)	SODIUM (mg)	CARBO-HYDRATE (%)
■ Exceed High Carbohydrate Drink Powder	6 Tbsp + 8 fl oz water	230	59	115	24
■ GatorLode	12 fl oz	283	71	95	20
■ Carbo Energizer	8 fl oz	237	59	130	25
■ Carbo Powder	16 fl oz	339	85	100	18

For exercise sessions of up to about 60–90 min (for exercisers with diabetes, 60 min), plain water is usually the best replacement beverage. For exercise lasting longer than 60–90 min, water and extra carbohydrate may be needed. Fruit juices (diluted with water) and fluid replacement beverages are good sources of fluids and carbohydrate.

After competition or training, athletes should continue to drink water periodically until weight has been regained. Lost fluids need to be fully replaced at the time the fluid deficit occurs. Delayed rehydration fails to restore the body's altered fluid compartments well into the next day.

NUTRITIONAL GUIDELINES

Although guidelines can help exercisers get started, it is important to emphasize that each athlete is an individual. Everyone varies in his or her response to training and physical stress. Adjustments that work for one person may not work for another. Both awareness of the signals the body provides and blood glucose monitoring allow the person with diabetes to become expert at interpreting this information and to exercise safely.

REFERENCES

1. Franz MJ: Nutrition: can it give athletes with diabetes a boost? *The Diabetes Educator* 17:163–72, 1991
2. Position of The American Dietetic Association and The Canadian Dietetic Association: Nutrition for physical fitness and athletic performance for adults. *J Am Diet Assoc* 93:691–96, 1993
3. National Research Council: *Recommended Dietary Allowances.* 10th ed. Washington DC, National Academy Press, 1989, p. 29
4. Sherman WM, Doyle JA, Lamb DR, Strauss RH: Dietary carbohydrate, muscle glycogen, and exercise performance during 7 d of training. *Am J Clin Nutr* 57:27–31, 1993
5. Wasserman DH, Lacy DB, Goldstein RS, William PE, Cherrington AD: Exercise-induced fall in insulin and hepatic carbohydrate during exercise. *Am J Physiol* 256: E500–508, 1989
6. Wasserman DH, Spalding JS, Lacy DBB, Colburn CA, Goldstein RE, Cherrington AD: Glucagon is a primary controller of the increments in hepatic glycogenolysis and gluconeogenesis during exercise. *Am J Physiol* 257:E108–17, 1989
7. Neuffer PD, Costill DL, Flyn MG, Kirwan JP, Mitchell JB, Houmard J: Improvements in exercise performance: effects of carbohydrate feeding and diet. *J Appl Physiol* 62:983–88, 1987
8. Wright DA, Sherman WM, Dernbach AR: Carbohydrate feedings before, during, or in combination improve cycling endurance performance. *J Appl Physiol* 71:1082–88, 1991
9. Sherman WM, Costill DL, Fink WJ, Miller JM: The effect of exercise and diet manipulation on muscle glycogen and its subsequent use during performance. *Int J Sports Med* 2:114–18, 1981
10. Coleman E: Update on carbohydrate: solid versus liquid. *Int J Sports Nutr* 4:80–88, 1994
11. Costill DL: Carbohydrate nutrition before, during, and after exercise. *Fed Proc* 44:364–68, 1985
12. Nathan DN, Madnek S, Delahanty L: Programming pre-exercise snacks to prevent post-exercise hypoglycemia in intensively treated insulin-dependent diabetics. *Ann Intern Med* 4:483–86, 1985
13. Zinman B, Zunuga-Guajardo S, Kelly D: Comparison of the acute and long-term effects of exercise on glucose control in type I diabetics. *Diabetes Care* 7:515–19, 1984
14. Wallberg-Henriksson H, Gunnarsson R, Henriksson J, DeFronzo R, Felig P, Ostman J, Wahren J: Increased peripheral insulin sensitivity and muscle mitochondrial enzymes but unchanged blood glucose control in type I diabetes after physical training. *Diabetes* 11:311–17, 1982
15. Wasserman DH, Zinman B: Exercise in individuals with IDDM

(Technical Review). *Diabetes Care* 17:924–37, 1994

16. Schiffrin A, Parikh S: Accomodating planned exercise in type I diabetic patients on intensive treatment. *Diabetes Care* 8:337–43, 1985

17. Wahren J, Felig P, Hagenfeldt L: Physical exercise and fuel homeostasis in diabetes metabolism. *Diabetologia* 14:213–22, 1978

18. Coggan AR, Coyle EF: Carbohydrate ingestion during prolonged exercise: effects on metabolism and performance. *Exercise Sport Sci Rev* 19:1–40, 1991

19. Coggan AR, Swanson SC: Nutritional manipulation before and during endurance exercise: effects on performance. *Med Sci Sports Exercise* 24:S331–35, 1992

20. Coyle EF, Coggan AR, Hemmert MK, Ivy JL: Muscle glycogen utilization during prolonged strenuous exercise when fed carbohydrate. *J Appl Physiol* 61:165–72, 1986

21. Coyle EF, Hagberg JM, Hurley BF, Martin WH, Ehsani AA, Holloszy JO: Carbohydrate feeding during prolonged strenuous exercise can delay fatigue. *J Appl Physiol* 55: 230–35, 1983

22. Mason WL, McConell G, Hargreaves M: Carbohydrate ingestion during exercise: liquid vs. solid feedings. *Med Sci Sports Exercise* 25:966–69, 1993

23. Coyle EF, Montain SJ: Benefits of fluid replacement with carbohydrate during exercise. *Med Sci Sports Exercise* 24:S324–30, 1992

24. Lamb DR, Brodowicz GR: Optimal use of fluids of varying formulations to minimize exercise-induced disturbances in homeostasis. *Sports Med* 3:247–74, 1986

25. Wagenmakers AJM, Brouns F, Saris WHM, Halliday D: Oxidation rates of orally ingested carbohydrates during prolonged exercise in men. *J Appl Physiol* 75:2774–80, 1993

26. Ivy JL, Katz SL, Cutler CL, Sherman WM, Coyle EF: Muscle glycogen synthesis after exercise: effect of time of carbohydrate ingestion. *J Appl Physiol* 64:1480–85, 1988

27. Zachwieja J, Costill DL, Pascoe DD, Roberts RA, Fink WJ: Influence of muscle glycogen depletion on the rate of resynthesis. *Med Sci Sports Exercise* 23:44–48, 1991

28. MacDonald MJ: Postexercise late-onset hypoglycemia in insulin-dependent diabetic patients. *Diabetes Care* 10:584–88, 1987

10. Exercise and Weight Control

Highlights
Exercise and Weight Control

- Weight loss is presumably important in the treatment and prevention of type II diabetes.
- The combination of diet, exercise, and behavior modification is the most effective approach to weight control.
- Exercise may also help prevent weight gain in individuals with type I diabetes on intensive therapy.
- Current dietary interventions focus on reducing calories and dietary fat.

- Low-intensity, long-duration exercise is recommended for weight loss.
- A combination of lifestyle exercise and programmed exercise is recommended.
- Behavioral approaches, which teach patients to rearrange their environment to support healthy eating and exercise behaviors, are important for long-term maintenance of behavior change.

Exercise and Weight Control

RENA R. WING, PhD

INTRODUCTION

The majority of patients with type II diabetes are overweight. For these individuals, weight loss is an important component of treatment. Lowering body weight can improve glycemic control, reduce insulin resistance, and improve coronary heart disease (CHD) risk factors in patients with type II diabetes. Modest weight losses of 15–30 lb (7–14 kg) are often sufficient to improve glycemic control and cardiovascular risk factors.

EXERCISE AS AN ADJUNCT TO DIET IN TYPE II DIABETES

The most successful approach to long-term weight control involves the combination of diet, exercise, and behavior modification. University-based research programs using such combinations of diet, exercise, and behavior modification typically produce weight losses of 20–30 lb at the end of a 20-week program. Forty to sixty percent of this weight loss (10–15 lb) is maintained over a year of follow-up (1).

Exercise is an important aspect of weight control intervention because the energy expenditure associated with regular activity has the potential to create a state of negative energy balance. However, when exercise is used as a sole treatment approach, the results are very limited. This is because most overweight individuals increase their exercise only modestly, leading to small energy deficits. Moreover, the increase in physical activity may be compensated for by increases in caloric intake and changes in activity patterns after exercise. Ballor and Keesey (2) found that 10–16 weeks of exercise alone produced weight losses of only 0.6 kg in women and 1.3 kg in men.

Exercise is far more effective when used as a component of weight-loss intervention, in combination with caloric restriction, rather than as a sole treatment modality. The combination of diet plus exercise has been shown to improve weight loss compared with diet alone. The benefits of diet plus exercise, relative to diet alone, are most apparent in studies using moderate caloric restriction rather than very-low-calorie diets (VLCDs) and in the maintenance of weight loss rather than initial weight loss. For example, Dahlkoetter et al. (3) compared the effects of diet alone, exercise alone, and the combination of diet plus exercise. At the end of the 8-week program, weight losses were –3.2, –2.8, and –6.0 kg for diet, exercise, and the combination, respectively. At 6-month follow-up, weight losses were 2.1, 2.8, and 7.3 kg, respectively. Likewise, in a study with overweight patients with type II diabetes, Wing et al. (4) found that subjects in a diet only group lost 5.6 kg at the end of treatment and maintained a weight loss of 3.8 kg at 1 year. Far better results were obtained for the diet plus exercise condition, where weight losses averaged 9.3 kg at the end of treatment and 7.9 kg at 1 year. A recent review of this literature concluded that the average long-term weight loss was 4.9 kg in five studies of exercise only, 4.0 kg in four diet studies, and 7.2 kg in three diet plus exercise studies (5).

The combination of diet plus exercise has also been shown to minimize the loss of lean body mass and the decrease in resting metabolic rate that accompanies weight loss (6). Again, these positive effects of diet plus exercise versus diet alone are greatest when exercise is combined with moderate calorie restriction. Smaller benefits of exercise are observed in studies using VLCDs, where the severity of the caloric restriction seems to overshadow the potential benefits of exercise.

Finally, the combination of diet plus exercise produces greater improvement in CHD risk factors than diet alone. Wood et al. (7) conducted a year-long study of diet only versus diet plus exercise in a sample of 132 men and 132 women. Men in the diet plus exercise group lost 8.7 vs. 5.1 kg in the diet only group; in women, the weight losses were 5.1 and 4.1 kg, respectively, a nonsignificant difference. Men in the diet plus exercise group showed greater reduction in the waist-to-hip ratio and in triglycerides and greater increases in high-density lipoprotein (HDL) cholesterol than those in the diet only group; these differences resulted in far greater reductions in the estimated 12-year CHD risk for men in the diet plus exercise versus diet only group (–21.8 vs. –12.9 estimated events/1,000 people). For women, the diet plus exercise program also produced significantly greater improvements in HDL cholesterol and in the estimated 12-year CHD risk than diet only.

The combination of diet plus exercise may also be important in the prevention of diabetes. Both weight loss and exercise have been shown to be independently related to the risk of developing type II diabetes. Changes in weight and exercise behaviors can reduce insulin resistance and visceral abdominal fat.

EXERCISE AS A WAY TO PREVENT WEIGHT GAIN IN PATIENTS ON INTENSIVE INSULIN THERAPY

Several recent studies have suggested that weight gain is a potential negative effect of intensified insulin therapy in subjects with type I diabetes (8). Moreover, the effect of intensive insulin treatment on body weight is related to the degree of improvement in glycemic control. Thus, patients who are initially in poorest control, and apparently wasting a large number of calories in glycosuria, experience the greatest weight gain with intensive therapy. Efforts to prevent weight gain in these individuals have not been systematically investigated, but it would appear that the combination of increased exercise and moderate caloric restriction would again be most successful in these individuals, as in other overweight individuals.

DEVELOPING AN EFFECTIVE WEIGHT-LOSS PROGRAM

Given that the combination of diet, exercise, and behavior modification is most effective for long-term weight loss, each of these components will be briefly discussed below.

Modifying Dietary Intake to Promote Weight Loss

The dietary component of behavioral weight-loss programs focuses on both decreasing overall caloric intake and lowering the amount of dietary fat. Traditionally, most behavioral weight-loss programs have used a diet of 1,200–1,500 kcal/day. Subjects are taught to self-monitor the foods they consume and to calculate the calories in those foods. A great deal of flexibility is provided to subjects in selecting the foods to consume as long as they stay within their calorie goal. Exchange system diets have also been used in many treatment programs to produce weight loss and ensure a balanced dietary intake.

Recently, behavioral treatment programs have placed more emphasis on lowering dietary fat intake. Subjects are given dietary fat goals in the range of 20–30% of calories from fat. Restriction of fat intake has been shown to produce weight loss in and of itself (9). Moreover, a recent study found that a weight-loss treatment program that focused on both lowering dietary fat and overall calorie intake was more effective for weight loss than a program focusing on caloric restriction alone (10).

VLCDs, defined as diets of <800 kcal/day, have also been used in the treatment of overweight patients in general and overweight individuals with type II diabetes in particular (11). VLCDs appear safe when used with carefully selected patients and appropriate medical management. Moreover, they are extremely effective in producing initial weight losses and improving glycemic control. Unfortunately, however, techniques are not yet available to help patients maintain these weight losses; consequently, when studied at 1-year follow-up, subjects treated with behavior modification and a VLCD maintain weight losses comparable to those treated with behavior modification and a more moderate 1,000–1,500 kcal/day regimen. As noted above, the effects of exercise are more apparent in programs combining exercise with moderate caloric restriction than in programs with VLCDs.

Modifying Physical Activity Patterns to Promote Weight Loss and Maintenance

The physical activity component of weight-loss programs is designed to increase overall calorie expenditure. Consequently, the types of activities emphasized are those of low intensity (50% of maximum) and long duration (1 h/session), such as walking, bicycling, or swimming. Subjects are encouraged to exercise frequently (initially 5 times/week), since frequent exercise has been shown to be most effective for weight loss. No additional benefits in terms of weight loss are seen with high-intensity exercise (6). Moreover, high-intensity exercise may increase the risk of injuries and attrition.Walking is recommended for the typical overweight patient with type II diabetes (60 years of age and 200 lb). Participants are encouraged to start exercise very slowly, walking about 1/2 mile for 5 days/week. The distance is gradually increased until participants reach a goal of 2 miles/day for 5 days/week.

The major issue in developing an exercise program for overweight patients with type II diabetes is the problem of long-term adherence. As noted in other sections of this book, few people are willing to maintain exercise habits long term, and clearly, long-term exercise habits are required to produce long-term weight control. To increase long-term adherence to exercise, the following suggestions are offered:

■ **Encourage lifestyle exercise in addition to programmed exercise.** A distinction can be made between increasing daily physical activity (e.g., using stairs instead of elevators and parking further from one's destination) versus programmed exercise (setting aside a time each day for the purpose of exercise). Most behavioral weight-loss programs encourage both types of exer-

cise to produce the greatest overall change in caloric expenditure.
■ **Supervised exercise may help patients begin exercise.** Providing supervised exercise at the start of a weight-loss program has been shown to improve weight loss and maintenance (12). This supervised exercise may entail simply leading a group of overweight patients on a walk. The group format and the support of the leader may be helpful in maximizing the initial reinforcement value of exercise.
■ **Help patients identify barriers to exercise and teach strategies to reduce these barriers.** Patients often identify fatigue, lack of time, bad weather, and competing responsibilities as reasons for lack of exercise. It is helpful to work with each patient individually to determine the reasons for poor adherence and to help patients identify solutions to these problems.

Behavior Modification

The third component of an effective weight-loss program is behavior modification. Behavior modification techniques are designed to help patients change their behavior by changing the cues and reinforcers in their environment. Behavioral strategies are usually taught to patients during a series of 16–24 weekly group sessions. Key behavioral strategies include the following:
■ **Self-monitoring.** Participants are instructed to record both the foods they consume and the physical activity they perform. By determining the caloric value of each, patients learn to identify problem foods and patterns in their eating and exercise habits. These records provide helpful feedback to patients on their behavior changes. For example, they can see gradual increases in the number of calories expended through exercise each week. These records can also be used by the therapist to identify behaviors that require further attention.

- **Stimulus control.** Participants are taught to increase cues for appropriate behaviors and decrease cues for inappropriate behaviors. Specifically in the area of exercise, patients may be encouraged to leave out their exercise shoes to remind them to take a walk and/or to move the television (a cue for inappropriate behavior) to a more distant location.
- **Goal setting and reinforcement.** Participants are encouraged to set short-term, realistic goals (e.g., walking 2 miles/day on 5 days this week) and to reinforce themselves when they achieve these goals. Reinforcers can be simple things such as buying a special magazine, or patients can put aside $1.00 for each mile walked until sufficient money is accrued for a larger reward.
- **Continued contact.** One of the key components of a behavioral treatment program is the contact between the patient, the therapist, and the other individuals in the treatment group. Recent studies have shown that continued contact over extended periods of time (biweekly for 18 months) can help overweight patients maintain their weight loss over time (13). Even phone contacts have been shown to be helpful in maintaining exercise behaviors long term (14).

REFERENCES

1. Wadden TA: The treatment of obesity: an overview. *Obesity: Theory and Therapy*. Stunkard AJ, Wadden TA, Eds. New York, Raven, 1993, p. 197–218
2. Ballor DL, Keesey RE: A meta-analysis of the factors affecting exercise-induced changes in body mass, fat mass and fat-free mass in males and females. *Int J Obes* 15:717–26, 1991
3. Dahlkoetter J, Callahan EJ, Linton J: Obesity and the unbalanced energy equation: exercise versus eating habit change. *J Consult Clin Psychol* 47:898–905, 1979
4. Wing RR, Epstein LH, Paternostro-Bayles M, Kriska A, Nowalk MP, Gooding W: Exercise in a behaviour-al weight control programme for obese patients with type 2 (non-insulin-dependent) diabetes. *Diabetologia* 31:902–909, 1988
5. King AC, Tribble DL: The role of exercise in weight regulation in nonathletes. *Sports Med* 11:331–49, 1991
6. Bouchard C, Depres J-P, Tremblay A: Exercise and obesity. *Obes Res* 1:133–47, 1993
7. Wood PD, Stefanick ML, Williams PT, Haskell WL: The effects on plasma lipoproteins of a prudent weight-reducing diet, with or without exercise, in overweight men and women. *N Engl J Med* 325:461–66, 1991
8. Carlson MG, Campbell PJ: Intensive insulin therapy and weight gain in IDDM. *Diabetes* 42:1700–707, 1993
9. Henderson MM, Kushi LH, Thompson DJ, Gorbach SL, Clifford CK, Insull W Jr, Moskowitz M, Thompson RS: Feasibility of a randomized trial of a low-fat diet for the prevention of breast cancer: dietary compliance in the Women's Health Trial Vanguard Study. *Prev Med* 19:115–33, 1990
10. Wing RR, Pascale R, Butler B: Low-fat diet improves weight loss in obese NIDDMs without adverse effects on lipids or glycemic control (Abstract). *Diabetes* 42 (Suppl.1): 140A, 1993
11. National Task Force on the Prevention and Treatment of Obesity: Very-low-calorie diets. *JAMA* 270: 967–74, 1993
12. Craighead LW, Blum MD: Supervised exercise in behavioral treatment for moderate obesity. *Behav Ther* 20:49–59, 1989
13. Perri MG, McAdoo WG, Spevak PA, Newlin DB: Effect of a multicomponent maintenance program on long-term weight loss. *J Consult Clin Psychol* 52:480–81, 1984
14. King AC, Frey-Hewitt B, Dreon DM, Wood PD: The effects of minimal intervention strategies on long-term outcomes in men. *Arch Intern Med* 149:2741–46, 1989

11. Adjustment of Insulin Therapy

Highlights
Adjustment of Insulin Therapy

- Hypoglycemia in patients with insulin-treated diabetes may occur both during and after exercise.
- Rational strategies for its prevention are based on adjustments of insulin therapy.
- Specific insulin adjustments need to be individualized for a given patient based on his or her experience and the intensity and duration of the exercise.
- To make adjustments in insulin dosage, the patient must have a sound knowledge of basic principles and must monitor his or her blood glucose frequently.
- Exercise-induced hypoglycemia usually cannot be avoided by changing the insulin injection site.
- Patients on intensive insulin therapy should, in general, be able to participate in sports without an excessively high risk of exercise-induced hypoglycemia.

Adjustment of Insulin Therapy

MICHAEL BERGER, MD

INTRODUCTION

The dramatic changes in insulin sensitivity that occur during and after exercise require that diabetic patients adjust their insulin therapy in order to prevent hypoglycemia. Also contributing to this need to adjust insulin is the fact that the stimulation of hepatic glucose production, which is essential for maintaining normal blood glucose levels during exercise, is blocked or partially inhibited by the hyperinsulinemia resulting from exogenous insulin substitution (1). In addition, the physiological decrease of circulating insulin levels (due to decreased ß-cell secretion) at the beginning of physical exercise, which is instrumental in allowing for the increased hepatic glucose production, cannot take place in patients on insulin treatment. All of these events contribute to the risk of exercise-induced hypoglycemia in insulin-treated diabetic patients.

Hypoglycemia induced by exercise has been recognized as a threat to people with diabetes ever since insulin treatment became available. Unfortunately, it has prevented some young diabetic patients from participating in sports and games for decades. Usually, this is because of their own or their teachers' and parents' fear of exercise-induced hypoglycemia and their inability to prevent it. Even today, a high percentage of reported episodes of severe hypoglycemia in children and adolescents occur as a result of exercise (2,3). It is the author's belief that this highlights the lack of understanding of all concerned of the means to prevent exercise-induced hypoglycemia, especially by appropriate adjustments of insulin therapy.

Exercise-induced hypoglycemia was described with admirable clarity by R.D. Lawrence in 1926 (4) as a phenomenon whereby physical activity acts as a potentiator of the hypoglycemic action of insulin. Based on a single experiment with one diabetic patient, combined with his clinical experience with two others, Lawrence developed his decisive recommendations to prevent exercise-induced hypoglycemia almost 70 years ago. He stated that before vigorous or prolonged exercise, the insulin dose may have to be reduced substantially, often by as much as 50%.

Lawrence also pointed out that the insulin dosage after exercise needs to be reduced to avoid postexercise episodes of hypoglycemia. According to his experience, these basic recommendations could easily be included in an appropriate educational program: "Patients should and do easily learn to reduce their insulin before unaccustomed exercise or activity. Even after exercise . . . it is usually advisable to reduce the next dose of insulin." It remains unexplained why such sophisticated guidance based on solid clinical research and experience has failed to make its way into routine clinical practice for so long.

ADJUSTMENT OF INSULIN THERAPY BEFORE AND AFTER EXERCISE

Any rational strategy to prevent exercise-induced hypoglycemia in insulin-treated patients must be based on an adjustment of insulin therapy. Such adjustments are intended to mimic the fall of serum insulin levels early during exercise, and to allow for the increased insulin sensitivity during and after physical activity, by reducing the iatrogenic hyperinsulinemia at these times (5). If it appears impossible or unnecessary to make such adjustments of insulin therapy (e.g., in case physical exercise was not anticipated or was of a duration of <30 min), supplemental carbohydrates before and during exercise may be used to counterbalance the iatrogenic hyperinsulinemia (see Chapter 9).

If physical exercise exceeds 30 min, planned adjustments in insulin therapy will be required to ensure optimal performance and to minimize the risk of hypoglycemia. In practice, physicians need to calculate the percentage by which patients need to reduce their dosages of regular and prolonged insulin preparations or insulin infusion rates at times before, during, and after their physical activity. Numerous investigators have directed their attention to this question, and an impressive number of publications have attempted to work out precise and practical recommendations and guidelines. Some of them are described in the following sections.

ALTERING THE INSULIN INJECTION SITE

Following reports in the 1970s of a paradoxical increase of serum insulin levels in patients exercising shortly after insulin injection, attempts were made to avoid exercise-induced hypoglycemia by changing the site of the insulin injection to parts of the body that were not involved or were substantially less involved in the planned exercise (6). Thus, it was widely suggested that patients inject their insulin dose into the abdomen or the arm instead of the leg if they were about to jog or ride their bicycles. However, with the possible exception of vigorous exercise initiated within the first 30 min after an injection of regular insulin, this recommendation turned out to be quite useless and, in fact, potentially dangerous. Exercise-induced hypoglycemia cannot be avoided by simply changing the insulin injection site (7).

If the plasma insulin level is high for any reason, hypoglycemia is likely to occur. With regard to the insulin injection site, it needs to be added that the intramuscular application of insulin should be meticulously avoided, since contractions will accelerate the absorption of insulin into the circulation from the musculature (8). Also, the ambient temperature of the injection site needs to be taken into account, because a hot environment may quite profoundly accelerate insulin absorption kinetics during exercise (9).

DECREASING INSULIN DOSAGES

In principle, diabetologists and their patients have returned to the basic recommendations of Lawrence (4) in an effort to develop strategies to prevent exercise-induced hypoglycemia. In practice, variables such as type of exercise, mode of insulin therapy, clinical characteristics, and condition of the patient have made the formulation of precise, effective, and safe rules difficult (10). Nevertheless, a number of basic principles for the prevention of exercise-induced hypoglycemia have been worked out.

In anticipation of a long period of exercise (e.g., hiking, bicycle touring, long distance running, or cross-country skiing) that begins during the morning hours, the prebreakfast insulin dosage will have to be reduced by more than 50%. On a day of marathon running, insulin dosages may have to be reduced by more than 80%. A postexercise reduction of insulin dosages is often necessary after prolonged endurance exercise, even on the following day. The amount by which the insulin dose is decreased in these circumstances will also depend on the type of insulin treatment used by the patient. Thus, in patients predominantly treated with long-acting insulin preparations, it may even be necessary to withhold insulin on the morning of a day when prolonged and intense exercise is planned. In type I diabetic patients on more modern types of insulin treatment, i.e. intensified insulin therapy (at least 50% of daily insulin requirements administered as regular insulin), a withdrawal of insulin for the entire day of extraordinary physical activity will not be possible without risk of potentially harmful degrees of hyperglycemia.

The longer the physical activity and the better the patient is physically trained and adapted to exercise, the more drastic the insulin dosage reduction needs to be. Shorter-term, exhaustive, and stressful forms of exercise (such as certain highly competitive sports) may lead to transient phases of hyperglycemia, especially so in the less well-trained individuals. If not adequately informed, these patients may be surprised and disturbed by postexercise hyperglycemia and may wrongly decide to inject extra insulin in this situation. The biological effect of such an extra injection of insulin will often coincide with the postexercise increase in insulin sensitivity, and an episode of potentially severe hypoglycemia can result.

Several authors have tried to link the risk of exercise-induced hypoglycemia to the time of day when the exercise is performed. Obviously, the risk of hypoglycemia is particularly low if patients with insulin-dependent diabetes mellitus (IDDM) exercise before their morning insulin injection. In this situation, strenuous exercise might very well precipitate substantial hyperglycemia because of potential hypoinsulinemia at this time of the day.

It is not unexpected that the risk of nocturnal hypoglycemia is particularly high when exercise is performed in the evening hours. To prevent this, a reduction of the evening insulin dosages by 50% or more may be required. Some physicians are hesitant to have their patients exercise in the evening hours because of the risk of nocturnal hypoglycemia. However, a great number of our patients can only exercise in the evening, at least on workdays; hence, appropriate adjustments for evening exercise need to be worked out for and with them.

Obviously, the time span between the onset of exercise and the previous insulin injection, the type of insulin preparation used, and the strategy for insulin substitution are all of importance for the fine adjustment of insulin dosage to maintain glycemic homeostasis during and after exercise. Patients also will have to take into account their preferences with regard to the consumption of extra carbohydrates when deciding on the insulin dosage adjustments they have to make. For examples of adjustments of insulin dosage to avoid insulin-induced hypoglycemia, see Table 11.1.

For IDDM patients treated predominantly with long-acting insulin preparations (conventional insulin therapy), insulin adjustments for exercise can prove difficult. In particular, insulin preparations with longer half-lives, by causing sustained hyperinsulinemia, interfere with glycemic control during and after intense, prolonged exercise. Accordingly, diabetic athletes in the U.S. opted for intensified insulin therapy to ensure optimal and safe performance long before this form of treatment became generally accepted. Because intensified insulin therapy is gradually becoming the standard treat-

Table 11.1. Examples of Insulin Adjustments for two Patients on Intensive Insulin Therapy

DAY	INSULIN U (REGULAR/NPH)				SMBG (mg/dl)				REMARKS
	Morning R/NPH	Pre-lunch R	Pre-dinner R	Bedtime NPH	Morning	Pre-lunch	Pre-dinner	Bedtime	
M	6/10	6	6	8	110	90	130	140	
T	6/10	6	3	6	130	100	120	100	Tennis
W	6/10	6	8	8	110	120	100	120	Dinner party
F	8/14	4	6	8	120	110	100	140	
S	4/6	0	3	4	130	100	90	130	Hiking
Su	6/10	4	6	8	90	130	120	130	

Tennis for 2 h at 7:30 P.M. Hiking all day on the flat.

ment for IDDM patients, comments on potential adjustments of other insulin substitution strategies can be restricted.

For patients with IDDM or non-insulin-dependent diabetes mellitus (NIDDM) on conventional (twice daily) insulin therapy, the duration and intensity of physical exercise may need to be limited if performance and safety are to be kept at optimal levels. This is because the possibilities to adjust insulin dosages to reflect the changing insulin requirements during and after exercise are restricted because of the kinetics of intermediate- and long-acting insulin preparations. Table 11.2 gives some examples of insulin dose adjustments in connection with exercise for patients on conventional insulin regimens.

Even more complex and unpredictable is the situation for patients with NIDDM on combination therapies: e.g., NPH or ultralente insulin in the evening and a sulfonylurea drug in the morning. If such a patient plans to exercise in the morning, the use of two different hypoglycemic principles with independent mechanisms of action and varying half-lives makes it next to impossible to recommend a rational and effective adjustment of insulin/sulfonylurea dosages to mimic a near-physiological insulinemia. Because these therapeutic regimens seem to be restricted to elderly patients for whom only mild-intensity exercise is appropriate, a reduction (or omission) of the morning sulfonylurea dose, along with some extra carbohydrates, may suffice to counter the increased peripheral glucose requirements resulting from physical activities.

For patients who want to enjoy physical exercise of prolonged duration and a high degree of intensity, or who want to exercise irregularly according to changing daily schedules and preferences, or who are competitive athletes and need intensive physical training, it must be concluded that the necessary adjustments of insulin dosages can only be made in the framework of intensified insulin therapy.

EXERCISE IN IDDM PATIENTS ON CONTINUOUS SUBCUTANEOUS INSULIN INFUSION (CSII)

Particular efforts have been undertaken to determine how to prevent exercise-induced hypoglycemia in IDDM patients who treat themselves with CSII (11). In a study from our laboratory, several adaptations proved to be necessary to maintain glucose homeostasis during and after exercise (12). The premeal insulin bolus had to be reduced by 50% when 1 h of bicycle exercise was to be performed beginning 2 h after the meal. In addition, it proved necessary both to stop the insulin infusion completely during exercise and to reduce the insulin infusion by 25% for several hours after exercise. Only when these complex adaptations were carried out could exercise-induced hypoglycemia be effectively prevented.

Note that during the very cumbersome experimental protocol of this study, all other potentially confounding factors were kept constant—a situation not present in day-to-day life with its

Table 11.2. Example of Insulin Adjustments for a Patient on Conventional Insulin Therapy

DAY	INSULIN U (30% REGULAR/70% NPH)		SMBG (mg/dl)			REMARKS
	Morning	Predinner	Morning	Prelunch	Predinner	
T	32	16	140		130	
W	28	14	130	100	90	Gardening
Th	32	16	120	120	140	

Exercise is mild-intensity gardening between 9 A.M. and noon.

necessary and welcome spontaneity. However, it became clear that even during CSII, a relatively standardizable form of insulin substitution therapy, it is difficult to calculate precisely to what degree the insulin dosage needs to be decreased to prevent exercise-induced hypoglycemia.

CONCLUSIONS

Patients need to adjust their insulin therapy on the basis of their personal experiences in order to avoid exercise-induced hypoglycemia. This adjustment requires a sound knowledge of basic principles and frequent self-monitoring of blood glucose (SMBG). SMBG remains the patients' primary yardstick for managing how to effectively and safely participate in sports and games.

In the author's experience, a structured treatment and teaching program that includes instruction on how to deal with exercise-induced hypoglycemia has proven very useful. Intensified insulin therapy in an unselected group of ~700 consecutive IDDM patients resulted after 3 years in a fall of HbA_{1c} levels to a mean of 7.6% and a significant decrease in the incidence of severe hypoglycemia to 0.13 cases/patient/year (13). In patients with severe hypoglycemia, exercise played only a minor role as a precipitating factor.

This study suggests that patients on intensified insulin therapy should, in general, be able to participate in sports without an excessively high risk of exercise-induced hypoglycemia, pro-vided they have participated in an adequate treatment and teaching program. The educational program may need to include a discussion of hypoglycemia risks, due to such factors as hypoglycemia unawareness, nephropathy, early pregnancy, or other factors specific to the individual patient. Suggested general guidelines for patients are given in Table 11.3.

In addition to building up a personal body of experience and growing self-confidence, diabetic patients who are active and ambitious in sports have learned much from each other. The International Diabetic Athletes Association (IDAA) is a unique and effective example of a self-help group of diabetic patients experienced and successful in sports and athleticism (see RESOURCES) (14). Among its members are numerous diabetic individuals of international reputation, including several Olympic Gold Medal winners. Within this group, a wealth of personal experiences, ideas, and hints that could never have been provided by the medical profession or by diabetes educators are exchanged.

It is not surprising that almost all of the members of IDAA are on intensified insulin therapies. Wherever possible, a member of the IDAA (which has chapters in many countries) should be asked to participate in the specific education and counseling of patients who want to begin exercise or competitive sports, or who want to continue their careers as amateur or professional athletes despite having developed diabetes.

Table 11.3. General Guidelines to Avoid Exercise-Induced Hypoglycemia

- Measure blood glucose before, (during), and after exercise.
- Unplanned exercise should be preceded by extra carbohydrates, e.g. 20–30 g/30 min of exercise; insulin may have to be decreased after exercise.
- If exercise is planned, insulin dosages must be decreased before and after exercise, according to the exercise intensity and duration as well as the personal experience of the patient; insulin dosage reductions may amount to 50–90% of daily insulin requirements.
- During exercise, easily absorbable carbohydrates may have to be consumed.
- After exercise, an extra carbohydrate-rich snack may be necessary.
- Diabetic patients interested in sports need a specific education program for self-treatment; they should contact the IDAA.

REFERENCES

1. Zinman B, Murray FT, Vranic M, McClean PA, Albisser AM, Leibel BS, Marliss EB: Glucoregulation during moderate exercise in insulin-treated diabetics. *J Clin Endocrinol Metab* 45:641–52, 1977

2. McDonald MJ: Post-exercise late-onset hypoglycemia in insulin-dependent diabetic patients. *Diabetes Care* 10:584–88, 1987

3. Bergada I, Suissa S, Dufrense J, Schiffrin A: Severe hypoglycemia in children. *Diabetes Care* 12: 239–44, 1989

4. Lawrence RD: The effect of exercise on insulin action in diabetes. *Br Med J* i:648–50, 1926

5. Zinman B, Vranic M, Albisser AM, Leibel BS, Marliss EB: The role of insulin in the metabolic response to exercise in diabetic man. *Diabetes* 28 (Suppl. 1): 76–81, 1979

6. Koivisto VA, Felig P: Effects of leg exercise on insulin absorption in diabetic patients. *N Engl J Med* 298:77–83, 1978

7. Kemmer FW, Berchtold P, Berger M, Starke A, Cüppers HJ, Gries FA, Zimmermann H: Exercise-induced fall of blood glucose in insulin-treated diabetics unrelated to alteration of insulin mobilization. *Diabetes* 28:1131–37, 1979

8. Frid A, Östman J, Linde B: Hypoglycemia risk during exercise after intramuscular injection of insulin in the thigh in IDDM. *Diabetes Care* 13:473–77, 1990

9. Rönnemaa T, Koivisto VA: Combined effect of exercise and ambient temperature on insulin absorption and postprandial glycemia in type I diabetic patients. *Diabetes Care* 11:769–73, 1988

10. Kemmer FW: Prevention of hypoglycemia during exercise in type I diabetes. *Diabetes Care* 15 (Suppl. 4):1732–35, 1992

11. Schiffrin A, Parikh S: Accommodating planned exercise in type I diabetic patients on intensive treatment. *Diabetes Care* 8:337–42, 1985

12. Sonnenberg GE, Kemmer FW, Berger M: Exercise in type I (insulin-dependent) diabetic patients treated with continuous subcutaneous insulin infusion: prevention of exercise-induced hypoglycaemia. *Diabetologia* 33:696–703, 1990

13. Jörgens V, Grüsser M, Bott U, Mühlhauser I, Berger DM: Effective and safe translation of intensified insulin therapy to general internal medicine departments. *Diabetologia* 36:99–105, 1993

14. Thurm U, Harper P: I'm running on insulin. *Diabetes Care* 15 (Suppl. 4):1811–13, 1992

12. Long-Term Exercise Programs

Highlights
Long-Term Exercise Programs

- Patients with type II diabetes often have poor aerobic exercise capacity.
- Regular exercise in those with type II diabetes is associated with improved glucose control that can be maintained for years.
- Exercise improves glucose control primarily by its effects on insulin sensitivity.
- Regular exercise has not been shown to be effective in improving long-term glucose control in people with type I diabetes.
- Much of the effect of regular exercise on glucose and lipids is the result of the summed effects of individual exercise bouts and, in some cases, significant changes in body composition rather than the trained state.
- Regular exercise is associated with a reduction in triglyceride-rich lipoprotein particles and smaller more atherogenic low-density lipoprotein (LDL) particles. Effects on high-density lipoprotein cholesterol and LDL cholesterol are less consistent.
- Regular exercise may improve blood pressure, particularly in patients with insulin resistance and hyperinsulinemia.
- Regular exercise may improve fibrinolytic activity in some patients with diabetes.
- It is possible to develop exercise programs that patients will adhere to for months to years with a reasonable degree of safety.

Long-Term Exercise Programs

STEPHEN H. SCHNEIDER, MD

INTRODUCTION

Regular physical activity is currently recommended by the American Diabetes Association as part of the treatment plan for type II diabetes mellitus (1). However, formal exercise programs are relatively expensive and labor intensive. It is important, therefore, to consider carefully the long-term risks and benefits of such programs as well as to what extent they represent a practical approach to treatment. This task is made difficult by the fact that most of our current understanding is based on studies in which small numbers of selected patients were followed for limited periods of time. Concurrent interventions and the effects of exercise on other health-related behaviors in most studies make it difficult to attribute benefits to exercise per se. Observations related to the long-term outcomes of exercise-based treatment programs are presented in this chapter. Since the vast majority of patients studied have had type II diabetes, observations will be limited to that group, except where specifically indicated.

There are potentially many benefits of adding exercise to other therapies in patients with type II diabetes. As discussed elsewhere in this book, exercise may improve glucose control. In addition, exercise is advocated as a means of improving insulin sensitivity in the hope that this will diminish hyperinsulinemia and related cardiovascular risk factors, including dyslipidemia, hypertension, and coagulation abnormalities. Exercise may also improve an individual's self-image and quality of life. It could be useful in the prevention of diabetes, and it may result in weight loss and favorable changes in body composition. Many of these issues have not been well addressed in the available long-term studies, which have focused primarily on metabolic effects.

FITNESS

To assess the long-term value of exercise, it is necessary to study the changes in fitness during physical training and to distinguish the initial training response from the metabolic state obtained with a maintenance exercise program. Most studies suggest that patients with type II diabetes have a lower (10–15%) aerobic exercise capacity (VO_{2max}) than do sedentary nondiabetic control subjects (2). This low level of aerobic fitness points to the special value exercise might have in the treatment of this population. Physical training causes similar percentage increases of maximal oxygen uptake in patients with type II diabetes and control subjects. However, because of the lower initial value, the absolute improvement is more modest in the patient with type II diabetes. Indeed, the VO_{2max} commonly obtained during exercise maintenance is similar to that of untrained control subjects. In contrast, uncomplicated patients with type I diabetes are at least as fit as their nondiabetic peers, and the effects of physical training in the two groups are indistinguishable. These differences in fitness and achievable training intensities may help to explain some of the differences in the long-term results of exercise programs in patients with the two types of diabetes.

Most of the longer term studies of physical training in diabetes utilize regimens of aerobic exercise at an intensity of 50–85% VO_{2max} 3–4 times/week for 30–60 min/session. With these regimens, typical increases in VO_{2max} range from 10 to 20%, with the larger increases being observed with exercise of greater intensity and duration. Longitudinal studies suggest that most of the improvement in VO_{2max} occurs within the first 6–12 weeks of training. Thereafter, levels of fitness tend to plateau in patients with type II diabetes and, to a lesser extent, in those with type I diabetes, as well as nondiabetic subjects. The level of fitness of both control and diabetic patients tends to decline with increasing age, but the relative improvement in fitness is at least partially maintained for many years if subjects continue to exercise. A conservative view would be to consider studies of more than 3 months duration to examine changes that can be expected to persist in the maintenance phase of long-term exercise-based interventions. It should be kept in mind that fitness and physical activity are related but distinct measures. It is not clear that changes in aerobic fitness, as measured by VO_{2max}, accurately reflect all of the benefits that can be conferred by regular physical activity.

GLUCOSE CONTROL

Long-term studies demonstrate a sustained improvement in glucose control for as long as regular exercise is maintained in most patients with type II diabetes (Table 12.1). Saltin et al. (3) studied 25 men with mild type II diabetes during 3 months of training and found improved glucose tolerance and de-

Table 12.1. Effects of Long-Term Physical Training on Patients With Type II Diabetes

REFER-ENCE	NUMBER OF PATIENTS	AGE	DURATION	TYPE OF EXERCISE	GLUCOSE	LIPID	BP
2	111	55 ± 1	1 year	Aerobic (60–75%) 40–60 min 4 times/week	↓ HbA$_{1c}$ ↓FBS	↓TG	↓sBP
6	78	54 ± 6	1 year	Aerobic, home–based (~70%) 30–60 min 4 times/week	↓ HbA$_{1c}$ ↓ FBS	↓ TG higher HDL	?
4	46	50 ± 2	3 months	Aerobic (80–90%) 50 min 3 times/week	POGTT and glucose disposal improved	No change	↓sBP during work only
7	41	48 ± 1	6 years	Aerobic, home-based ? intensity 3 times/week	POGTT improved	↓TG and choles-terol	↓sPB and dBP
3	25	48 ± 2	3 months	Aerobic (60–90%) 45 min 2 times/week	↓FBS and insulin improved POGTT	?	?
5	30	42 ± 10	1 year	Aerobic ?intensity 2–3 times/week	↓FBS	?	?
21	8	59 ± 1	2 years	Aerobic (75%) 45 min 3 times/week	No change	No change	No change

Age is mean ± SE. BP, blood pressure; FBS, fasting blood sugar; TG, triglyceride; sBP, systolic blood pressure; POGTT, post oral glucose tolerance test; dBP, diastolic blood pressure.

creased insulin levels. Krotkiewski et al. (4) studied 46 men and women and found improved glucose tolerance after 3 months and unchanged fasting insulin levels. In the Zuni diabetes project, free aerobic exercise sessions were offered daily under the supervision of Zuni volunteers (5). Thirty self-selected participants had a significantly greater decrease in fasting plasma glucose levels than did matched control subjects for an average follow-up of 50 weeks; 29% were able to discontinue oral hypoglycemic agents compared with only 7% among nonparticipants (see Chapter 26). Vanninen et al. (6) studied 78 patients in a largely unsupervised exercise-based program for 1 year. This is one of the few studies in which an attempt was made to prospectively randomize patients. Improved glucose and insulin levels persisted for a full year and were associated with a decreased level of HbA_{1c} of ~12%. Changes were greatest in the patients reporting higher intensity exercise. Schneider et al. (2) exercised 111 patients with type II diabetes for 3–4 months. Levels of HbA_{1c} continued to improve over a 3-month training period, and a decrease of 10–15% was maintained in a smaller number of subjects who continued to exercise regularly for 1 year. In the Malmo Study, 41 patients with type II diabetes and 207 with impaired glucose tolerance were evaluated during a 5-year, largely unsupervised exercise program (7). Improvements in glucose tolerance were found and were well maintained throughout the 5 years of this study. To what extent these improvements were due to changes in body composition during these studies is difficult to estimate, because direct measures of adiposity are not available. However, weight loss (2–4 kg) and decreases in body mass index (1–3 kg/m^2) were modest and of borderline significance compared with control subjects.

GLUCOSE CONTROL IN TYPE I DIABETES

The beneficial effects of exercise in those with type I diabetes are less clear.

While long-term studies are few, it appears that physical training is not consistently associated with improved glucose control (8–10). On the other hand, a study of 10 patients over an 8-month period by Peterson et al. (11) suggests that it is possible to obtain a sustained decrease in HbA_{1c} with exercise in selected patients. It is likely that the relatively high incidence of hypoglycemia related to exercise in patients with type I diabetes results in increased carbohydrate intake and decreased insulin dosage and that this largely compensates for the effect of exercise to enhance glucose disposal. Schneider et al. (2) noted a mild initial improvement in glucose control in 25 type I diabetic patients trained for more than 3 months that was lost by the 3rd month of observation, despite continued adherence to the exercise regimen, in contrast to patients with type II diabetes in the same program. Whether the 10–20% reduction in insulin requirements commonly seen in such patients is of long-term value remains to be proven.

INSULIN SENSITIVITY

An increase in insulin sensitivity is probably the major mechanism by which regular physical activity improves glucose control. In most exercise programs for patients with type II diabetes, a significant decrease in fasting plasma glucose is often observed in the face of decreased or unchanged levels of insulin. After a meal, insulin levels are often decreased to an even greater degree. There are many mechanisms by which regular physical activity could improve insulin sensitivity, including changes in body composition, muscle mass, and capillary density, which are discussed elsewhere in this book. Whether the improvement in insulin sensitivity is related to the trained state per se is not clear. Following a single glycogen-depleting bout of exercise, insulin sensitivity may be enhanced for as long as 48 h, and, in fact, much of the decrease in HbA_{1c} in patients who exercise regularly may be explained by the summed effects of the individual bouts of exercise rather than the trained state

(12). Studies of detraining on insulin sensitivity are consistent with this in that the improvement in insulin sensitivity in physically active individuals dissipates within 3–4 days of inactivity following many months of physical training long before other measures of aerobic fitness have decreased (3). Additional effects of the trained state, when present, are probably related to increases in the number or activity of GLUT4 glucose transporters in muscle and changes in body composition.

HYPERLIPIDEMIA

In addition to improved glucose control, one of the potential benefits of exercise in the treatment of diabetes is a reduction in the risk of premature coronary artery disease. Kohn et al. (13), in a prospective study of 8,715 men, showed a decreased age-adjusted death rate, particularly for cardiovascular disease, in patients with impaired glucose tolerance and mild type II diabetes who were more aerobically fit. In type II diabetes in particular, glucose intolerance is associated with a cluster of risk factors for atherosclerotic vascular disease, including dyslipidemia, hypertension, and coagulation defects. The hyperlipidemia most commonly associated with diabetes includes elevated levels of triglyceride-rich lipoproteins and, in type II (but not type I) diabetes, decreased levels of high-density lipoprotein (HDL) cholesterol. The most consistent effect of regular exercise is a decrease in plasma triglyceride levels. Decreases in plasma triglyceride levels of as much as 20–30% are often, but not always, noted. Changes in total low-density lipoprotein (LDL) cholesterol have not been consistently demonstrated, but exercise does appear to diminish the concentration of a small dense subclass of LDL that may be more closely associated with atherosclerotic vascular disease (14). Effects are greatest in the more insulin-resistant hypertriglyceridemic patients.

Some of the effects of exercise on triglyceride levels are quite transient and mirror effects of carbohydrate metabolism. Improved triglyceride clearance correlates with an acute increase in lipoprotein lipase activity in some, but not all, studies. Thus, after a short delay following a single bout of activity, triglyceride levels fall and remain suppressed for at least 48 h (15). This effect of exercise is maintained and results in a stable decrease in plasma triglyceride levels when activity is performed on a regular basis. Triglyceride levels measured within a few days of the last bout of exercise were found to be decreased by ~25% after 3–4 months in the study by Schneider et al. (2) and for up to 6 years in the Malmo Study (7). Most studies have failed to demonstrate significant increases in HDL cholesterol, even when triglyceride levels are significantly decreased. The major exception is the 1-year study of Vanninen et al. (6), in which HDL cholesterol levels rose and stayed higher for the entire year of study. In nondiabetic populations, increased HDL cholesterol is found only with intense exercise over a prolonged period of time. The poor exercise capacity of many patients with type II diabetes and the resulting modest levels of physical activity achieved may explain, in part, the apparent lack of an effect. No effect of exercise on lipoprotein(a) concentrations has been demonstrated. Detraining studies in patients with diabetes have not been done. To the extent that maintenance exercise results in a loss of intra-abdominal fat and lowers insulin levels in the portal circulation, it is likely to be associated with decreased hepatic lipid synthesis.

HYPERTENSION

Essential hypertension is commonly associated with type II diabetes. In long-term exercise-based programs in the general population, physical training is associated with a modest (5–10 mmHg) decrease in systolic and diastolic blood pressure and a modest decrease in the percentage of patients who go on to require antihypertensive medication (16). In the study by Schneider et al. (2), a modest but significant decrease in systolic blood pressure of 5 mm was noted in a group with type II diabetes. Benefits are at least as good and possibly better in older subjects (17) and women (18). Improvements are most likely to be noted in insulin-resistant hyperinsulinemic patients (19,20). Both resting pressure and the blood pressure response to exercise at a constant absolute workload are reduced in trained subjects. It is likely that the blood pressure responses to stress and integrated blood pressure levels across the day are improved to a greater degree than resting levels, but this has not been demonstrated in a population with diabetes. In some studies, the expected decrease in resting pulse rates seen with physical training is absent in patients with diabetes. This may be related to subclinical autonomic neuropathy and decreased parasympathetic tone.

COAGULATION

Coagulation abnormalities, including enhanced platelet function and impaired fibrinolytic activity, are frequently found in diabetes and are associated with premature large vessel disease. However, long-term studies on the effects of physical training on the coagulation system in diabetic patients are few. Some cross-sectional studies suggest that the enhanced platelet activation often found in patients with diabetes is related to poor fitness. Other studies suggest that PAI-1 (plasminogen-activating inhibitor), a major inhibitor of fibrinolytic activity, which is often elevated in type II diabetes, may be reduced in more fit individuals. Clearly, prospective studies need to be done to better assess this effect. Most long-term studies have failed to demonstrate consistent changes in the elevated levels of fibrinogen- and factor VIII–related activities reported in patients with type II diabetes.

CANDIDATES FOR EXERCISE-BASED PROGRAMS

Exercise-based treatment programs for type II diabetes appear to be practical for most patients. A major exception

was noted in a study by Skarfors et al. (21), in which only 8 of 48 potential candidates did not have other diseases or treatments that made long-term physical training impractical. This has not been the experience in other studies in which participants were drawn from the clinic population with type II diabetes. Note that subjects in most of these studies had milder forms of type II diabetes and, for the most part, did not require insulin therapy. The duration of diabetes is not always clear, but the known duration for most subjects was <10 years. In screening potential participants in an exercise program, Schneider et al. (2) found that 6% had previously undiagnosed ischemic heart disease, 14% had peripheral vascular disease, 42% had hypertension, 8% had proteinuria, and 16% had background retinopathy. Few of these problems were severe enough to exclude patients from monitored exercise, although these findings do emphasize the need for a thorough evaluation before starting patients on an exercise program.

COMPLIANCE WITH EXERCISE-BASED PROGRAMS

Adherence to programs of physical training over the long term have been remarkably variable. Results range from the 12% retention rate at 6 months in the study by Skarfors et al. (11) to the 90% adherence rate over 5 years in the Malmo Study. In most clinical studies, participation in formal exercise sessions begins to fall off after 6 weeks, with a significant dropout rate by 3 months. On the other hand, if the success of these programs is assessed by self-reported changes in physical activity outside the formal setting, the results are much more encouraging. In the program reported by Schneider et al. (2) for example, in which attendance at monitored sessions was encouraged, only ~60% of patients were attending regularly beyond 4 months. On the other hand, after 1 year, 73 of 100 patients reported engaging in meaningful exercise at least twice a week at home. Higher aerobic fitness compared with controls suggests that these self-reports had some validity. The two Finnish studies (7,9) that had the highest retention rates largely used informal and unmonitored exercise protocols. It should be noted, however, that inexpensive exercise facilities are much more readily available in Scandinavia than in the U.S. In general, it appears that formal exercise sessions may be of value in the initial assessment of patients for possible complications and for training patients in exercise techniques. On the other hand, maintenance of exercise beyond 3 months is best performed outside the formal setting with regular, but less frequent, assessments and self-monitoring of exercise activity.

It would be of interest to be able to identify patients likely to do well on exercise-based programs in advance. In one study, self-referral to the program was the best predictor of long-term adherence, and spousal participation was also helpful. Women and older patients were also more likely to continue in at least the formal exercise session (2). Factors such as the level of metabolic control, weight, education, and type of diabetes were not useful predictors. Patients with newly diagnosed diabetes or those undergoing major life stress at the time of entry did poorly. Willingness to maintain an exercise log appears to be a good predictor early on of long-term success in a number of studies (Table 12.2).

Many epidemiological studies suggest that low to moderate levels of lifestyle-related physical activity may be associated with a decreased risk of premature cardiovascular disease. Whether this lower level lifestyle-type activity would be effective in the treatment of type II diabetes and whether adherence to such a program would be greater than that of more traditional programs in patients with diabetes is not clear. Recent studies by King et al. (22) suggest that programs of moderate physical activity ($\sim$50% VO_{2max}) result in improvements similar to those of programs involving more intense activity. On the other hand, overall rates of adherence to moderate- and high-intensity programs were similar. In addition, studies by Maehlum et al. (23) suggest that subsequent improvements in glucose disposal are not seen at exercise intensities below 30–40% of VO_{2max}. This is consistent with the general observation that glycogen-depleting exercise is required for at least the acute effects of exercise on insulin sensitivity. Thus, the role of very-low-intensity lifestyle-type activities in the treatment of type II diabetes remains unclear.

PRECAUTIONS

Major complications requiring hospitalization (other than hypoglycemia) have rarely been reported during long-term physical training in properly selected patients. Schneider et al. (2) noted a 12% incidence of musculoskeletal injuries, possibly related in some degree to neuropathy. Minor foot lesions were common. There was one nonfatal ischemic event during the study but no episodes of sudden death. Of 30 subjects with proliferative retinopathy, 3 suffered retinal hemorrhage associated with inappropriate activities, and no patient with background retinopathy developed retinal hemorrhage. Whether or not the relatively high incidence of postexercise proteinuria (29%) is of concern is not clear. In patients with

---

Table 12.2. Factors That May Influence Success in a Long-Term Exercise Program

Positive
    Self-referral
    Spousal participation
    Female sex
    Older patients
    Maintenance of an exercise log
Negative
    Recent diagnosis
    Severe anxiety
Neutral
    Degree of glucose control
    Weight
    Educational background
    Type of diabetes

type I diabetes, hypoglycemia was common; it occurred in virtually all patients at some point. However, only two episodes of hypoglycemia were severe enough to require assistance in the emergency room.

SUMMARY

The available data on long-term exercise-based interventions supports their use in patients with type II diabetes. Improvements in glucose disposal, insulin sensitivity, lipid profiles, and blood pressure are achievable and can be maintained for months to years. Whether these improvements will be associated with a decreased mortality remains to be determined. Risks are acceptable and can be minimized with a complete preexercise evaluation and proper physical training techniques. The effects of long-term exercise on type I diabetes require more study. In addition, little is known about long-term exercise as a treatment for diabetes in special groups, such as minorities and children. Finally, a great deal needs to be learned about the effects of different types of exercise. Small studies suggest that resistance exercise alone or in combination with aerobic activities could contribute to improved glucose tolerance and risk factor reduction and may offer special benefits for weight reduction. On the other hand, epidemiological studies suggest that exercise at intensities lower than that used traditionally in the treatment of diabetes is associated with decreased cardiovascular mortality in the general population. The long-term effects of low-intensity exercise, as well as whether such regimens really do result in improved adherence, need to be examined in populations with diabetes. Until such studies are available, the ADA guidelines (1) form a reasonable basis for the use of exercise-based programs in the treatment of diabetes mellitus.

REFERENCES

1. American Diabetes Association: Diabetes mellitus and exercise (Position Statement). *Diabetes Care* 13:804–805, 1990
2. Schneider SH, Khachadurian AK, Amorosa LF, Clemow L, Ruderman NB: Ten-year experience with an exercise-based outpatient lifestyle modification program in the treatment of diabetes mellitus. *Diabetes Care* 15 (Suppl. 4):1800–10, 1992
3. Saltin B, Lindgarde F, Lithell H, Eriksson KF, Gad P: Metabolic effects of long-term physical training in maturity-onset diabetes. *Excerpta Med Amsterdam* 9:345–50, 1980
4. Krotkiewski M, Lonnroth P, Mondroukas K, Wroblewski Z, Rebuffe-Scrive M, Holm G, Smith U, Bjorntorp P: Effects of physical training on insulin secretion and effectiveness and on glucose metabolism in obesity and type II (non-insulin-dependent) diabetes mellitus. *Diabetologia* 28:881–90, 1985
5. Heath GW, Wilson RH, Smith J, Leonard BE: Community-based exercise and weight control: diabetes risk reduction and glycemic control in Zuni Indians. *Am J Clin Nutr* 53:S1642–46, 1991
6. Vanninen E, Uusitupa M, Siitonen O, Laitinen J, Lansimies E: Habitual physical activity, aerobic capacity, and metabolic control in patients with newly diagnosed type II diabetes mellitus: effect of a 1-year diet and exercise intervention. *Diabetologia* 35:340–46, 1992
7. Eriksson KF, Lindgarde F: Prevention of type II (non-insulin-dependent) diabetes mellitus by diet and physical exercise: the 6-year Malmo Feasibility Study. *Diabetologia* 34:891–98, 1991
8. Landt KW, Campaigne BN, James FW, Sperling M: Effects of exercise training on insulin sensitivity in adolescents with type I diabetes. *Diabetes Care* 8:461–65, 1985
9. Wallberg–Henriksson H, Gunnarsson R, Jenriksson J, DeFronzo R, Feliz P, Ostman J, Wahren J: Increased peripheral insulin sensitivity and muscle mitochondrial

enzymes but unchanged blood glucose control in type I diabetics after physical training. *Diabetes* 31:1044–50, 1982

10. Stratton R, Wilson D, Endres RK, Goldstein DE: Improved glycemic control after supervised 8-wk exercise program in insulin-dependent diabetic adolescents. *Diabetes Care* 10:589–93, 1987

11. Peterson CM, Jones RL, Dupuis A, Levine BS, Bernstein R, O'Shea M: Feasibility of improved blood glucose control in patients with insulin-dependent diabetes mellitus. *Diabetes Care* 2:329–35, 1979

12. Schneider SH, Amorosa LF, Khachadurian AK, Ruderman NB: Studies on the mechanism of improved glucose control during regular exercise in type II diabetes. *Diabetologia* 26:355–60, 1984

13. Kohn HW, Gordon NF, Villegas JA, Blair SN: Cardiorespiratory fitness, glycemic status, and mortality risk in men. *Diabetes Care* 15:184–92, 1992

14. Houmard JA, Bruno NJ, Bruner RK, McCammon MR, Israel RG, Barakal HA: Effects of exercise training on the chemical composition of plasma LDL. *Atheroscler Thromb* 14:325–30, 1994

15. Holloszy JO, Skinner JS, Toro G, Cureton TK: Effects of a 6-month program of endurance exercise on serum lipid levels of middle-aged men. *Am J Cardiol* 14:753–60, 1964

16. Tipton CM: Exercise training and hypertension. In *Exercise and Sports Science Reviews.* Vol 19. Holloszy JO, Ed. Philadelphia, Williams & Wilkins, 1991, p. 462–63

17. Hagberg JM, Montain ST, Martin WH, Ehsani AA: Effect of exercise training in 60- to 69-year-old persons with essential hypertension. *Am J Cardiol* 64:348–53, 1989

18. Kiwoshita A, Urata H, Tanabe Y: What type of hypertensives respond better to mild exercise therapy. *J Hypertension* 6 (Suppl. 4):5631–33, 1988

19. Krotkiewski M, Mandroukas K, Sjostrom L: Effects of long-term physical training on body fat, metabolism, and blood pressure in obesity. *Metabolism* 28:650–58, 1979

20. Rocchini AP, Katch U, Schork A, Kelch RP: Insulin and blood pressure during weight loss in obese adolescents. *Hypertension* 10:267–73, 1987

21. Skarfors ET, Wegener TA, Lithell H, Selinas I: Physical training as a treatment for type II (non-insulin-dependent) diabetes in elderly men. *Diabetologia* 30:930–33, 1987

22. King AC, Haskell WL, Taylor CB, Kraemer HC, DeBusk RF: Home-based exercise training in healthy older men and women. *JAMA* 266:1535–42, 1991

23. Maehlum S, Pruett EDR: Muscular exercise and metabolism in male juvenile diabetics. *Scand J Clin Lab Invest* 32:149–53, 197

III. Exercise in Patients With Diabetic Complications

13. The Diabetic Foot

Highlights
The Diabetic Foot

- Exercise programs play an important role in the management of diabetes.
- Most exercise programs involving the lower extremity are weight-bearing.
- Many people with diabetes have peripheral arterial disease (PAD) and peripheral neuropathy (PN), which can limit such activities.
- The diabetic patient with PN and loss of protective sensation should not engage in repetitive weight-bearing exercises, such as prolonged walking, treadmill, or jogging. Such activity in these patients may result in blistering, ulceration, and fractures. Patients with previous plantar foot ulceration may have a recurrence.
- Patients with insensate feet can engage in non–weight-bearing exercises, such as swimming, bicycling, chair exercises, and arm exercises.
- Exercise programs for patients with PAD and PN should be prescribed by a physician and closely supervised.

The Diabetic Foot

MARVIN E. LEVIN, MD

INTRODUCTION

An exercise program usually requires the use of the lower extremities. Diabetic patients frequently have peripheral arterial disease (PAD) and peripheral neuropathy (PN). These complications may limit the exercise program. Therefore, evaluation of PAD and PN should be carried out before prescribing an exercise program involving the lower extremities.

PERIPHERAL ARTERIAL DISEASE

Evaluation of PAD is based on signs and symptoms (Table 13.1) and on noninvasive vascular laboratory findings. Intermittent claudication is one of the most common symptoms of PAD. Patients with this complication are frequently limited in the amount of exercise they can do. It should be kept in mind that people with diabetes may have significant PAD but no symptoms of intermittent claudication because PN has prevented the sensation of ischemic pain. The basic treatment for intermittent claudication is nonsmoking and a supervised exercise program. This should be carried out under the direction of a physician, and a clearly defined program should be established. If patients are instructed simply to do a walking exercise, it may be incomplete and unsuccessful.

A walking program for intermittent claudication may improve not only collateral circulation but also muscle metabolism. Hiatt et al. (1) have shown that exercise increases the formation of acylcarnitine from carnitine and acyl-CoA. This substance can produce pain. In Hiatt's series, those who were in a walking exercise program had less formation of acylcarnitine and less pain (1). In this group of patients, the decrease in pain was not associated with an increase in blood flow.

Rest pain and night pain are indicative of severe PAD, and their presence is an absolute contraindication for any walking exercise program.

The presence of a dorsalis pedis and posterior tibial pulse does not rule out ischemic changes in the forefoot. Because exercise puts added strain on the forefoot and toes, careful evaluation of the blood flow to these areas should be made. If there is any question about this on physical examination, toe pressures as well as Doppler pressures at the ankle should be carried out.

The vascular laboratory findings can be very helpful in the evaluation of PAD. In most instances, a simple hand-held Doppler can provide significant information regarding peripheral vascular status. An ankle-brachial index of 0.9 or less confirms the presence of PAD. Intermittent claudication usually begins when the ankle-brachial index is 0.75 or less. However, there is a wide range of values before a patient actually detects ischemic claudication. In the diabetic patient, the Doppler may give an erroneously high value because of calcification in the vessels, which decreases the

Table 13.1. Signs and Symptoms of Peripheral Arterial Disease

- Intermittent claudication
- Cold feet
- Nocturnal pain
- Rest pain
- Nocturnal and rest pain relieved with dependency
- Absent pulses
- Blanching on elevation
- Delayed venous filling after elevation
- Dependent rubor
- Atrophy of subcutaneous fatty tissue
- Shiny appearance of skin
- Loss of hair on foot and toes
- Thickened nails, often with fungal infection
- Gangrene
- Miscellaneous
    Blue toe syndrome
    Acute vascular occlusion

compressibility. In the final analysis, a good history relating to ischemic symptoms as well as the experienced hand and eye can give an accurate evaluation of PAD.

PERIPHERAL NEUROPATHY

Significant PN is an indication to limit weight-bearing exercise. PN with motor nerve involvement and muscle atrophy can result in foot deformities, particularly cocked-up or claw toes. This can lead to ulceration at the top and/or tip of the toes unless special in-depth foot wear with a protective insole is used. This muscle imbalance can also cause a thinning or shifting of the protective fat pad under the first metatarsal head. Continued walking or exercising on these unprotected, vulnerable areas can lead to ulceration.

Sensory loss is a common problem, leading to painless trauma. Repetitive exercise on insensitive feet can ultimately lead to ulceration and fractures. Evaluation of PN can be made by checking the deep tendon reflexes, vibratory sense, and position sense. Touch sensation can best be evaluated by using inexpensive Semmes-Weinstein monofilaments. The inability to detect sensation using the 5.07 monofilament is indicative of the loss of protective sensation. Patients with this degree of insensitivity should have their weight-bearing exercises markedly limited. Sensory involvement leading to the Charcot foot, either in the acute stage or with deformity, is an absolute contraindication for weight-bearing exercise.

DIABETIC FOOT ULCERS

Diabetic plantar foot ulcers result from repetitive stress on insensitive feet that have increased plantar pressure. The presence of a diabetic foot ulcer is an absolute contraindication to any weight-bearing exercise. Diabetic patients with PN have increased pressure; those with ulceration tend to have the highest pressures. Plantar pressures are increased for three reasons: foot deformity, callus build-up, and limited joint mobility with a decrease in flexibility of the foot due to glycosylation of tendons and ligaments.

RELIEVING FOOT PRESSURES

For the patient performing weight-bearing exercise, decreasing foot pressure provides protection against callus buildup and ulceration. A variety of approaches are used to relieve foot pressures. Simply removing the callus will reduce pressure in that area by close to 30%. The use of running or walking shoes decreases the rate of callus buildup (2), because the cushioning that is usually found in this type of shoe decreases pressure. Cavanagh and Ulbrecht (3) found that a cushioned shoe could reduce barefoot pressure by 45%. The Thor-Lo Company had developed an experimental hosiery that reduced foot pressures by 30%. However, this stocking required special fitting and special shoes to accommodate the stocking and is no longer marketed. Thor-Lo tennis hosiery reduces peak pressures by 27% compared with going barefoot. This hosiery is very similar to the company's experimental hosiery and is available in many stores that sell sporting goods (4).

Table 13.2. Contraindicated Exercises for Diabetic Patients With Loss of Protective Sensation

- Treadmill
- Prolonged walking
- Jogging
- Step exercises

CONTRAINDICATED EXERCISE IN PEOPLE WITH DIABETES AND PERIPHERAL NEUROPATHY

Some of the exercises that are contraindicated in diabetic patients with loss of protective sensation are listed in Table 13.2. For people with diabetes and PN and insensate feet, prolonged walking, running, jogging, and use of the treadmill are contraindicated. Figure 13.1 shows the areas of maximum pressures with walking. The maximum pressure is on the forefoot, particularly the metatarsal head, at 20 lb/in^2. Comparing this with the pressure of riding a stationary bicycle at 20 miles/h, with minimal resistance, we find that the pressure is only 11 lb/in^2 (Fig. 13.2). Step exercises may be contraindicated in people with an insensate foot. The repetitive stress and pressure from this type of exercise can result in blisters and ulceration.

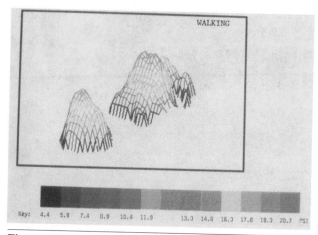

Figure 13.1. Foot pressure, when walking in ordinary shoes, is 20 lb/in^2 on the forefoot and toes.

EXERCISES FOR PEOPLE WITH DIABETES AND PERIPHERAL NEUROPATHY

Exercises recommended for patients with PN and loss of sensation are listed in Table 13.3. These include swimming, bicycling, rowing, chair exercises, and arm exercises. Swimming is an excellent exercise, but certain precautions must be taken. Diabetic patients who go swimming where there is a hot sandy beach or hot cement around a swimming pool must be cautioned to wear protective footwear to prevent severe burns to insensate feet. Swimming pools frequently have rough cement bottoms. Abrasion of the skin of the feet can occur. Unless the bottom of the pool is tiled, the patient should wear protective footwear in the pool. Long exposure to the water can lead to maceration of the skin, making it more susceptible to trauma. Chair exercises, shown in Fig. 13.3, can also involve lifting the legs. Arm exercises, shown in Fig. 13.4, may be helpful.

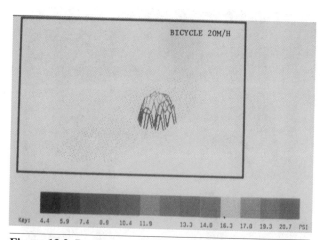

Figure 13.2. Pressure on the forefoot, while riding a stationary bicycle with minimal resistance, is 11 lb/in^2.

EXERCISE AND AMPUTATION LEVEL

Unfortunately, amputation is a common occurrence in individuals with diabetes. Exercise for the amputee represents a major problem. Velocity in walking is significantly impaired. Pinzur (5) has shown that a normal walking speed is 50 m/min or ~2 miles/h, but in a below-the-knee amputee, it is reduced to 40 m/min or ~1.6 miles/h.

Table 13.3. Exercises for Diabetic Patients With Loss of Protective Sensation

- Non–weight-bearing
- Swimming
- Bicycling
- Rowing
- Chair exercises
- Arm exercises

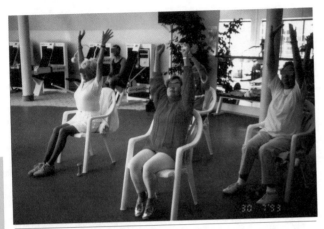

Figure 13.3. Chair exercises.

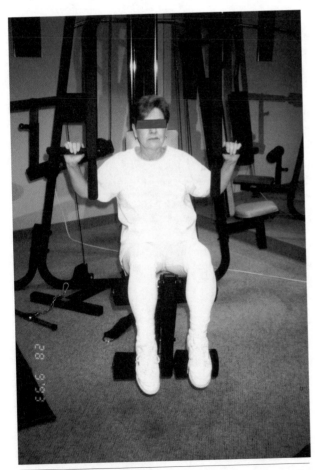

Figure 13.4. Arm exercises.

A nonamputee's maximum walking speed is 80 m/min. A below-the-knee amputee's maximum walking speed is reduced to 55 m/min (5). The energy cost of ambulation is also markedly increased (Table 13.4) (6,7). Therefore, walking exercises in the diabetic amputee are extremely limited. In addition, prolonged walking may subject the patient to trauma and ulceration of the stump.

FOOT CARE

The instructions for foot care (Table 13.5) are especially important for diabetic patients with PAD and PN and should be observed under all circumstances. Those diabetic patients who are doing weight-bearing exercises should pay particular attention to the instructions.

SUMMARY

Exercise is an important modality in the management of diabetes. However, because of complications of PAD and PN, with the development of the insensate foot, foot deformities, and increased foot pressure, weight-bearing exercises may need to be curtailed in these patients. The presence of an active foot ulcer is an absolute contraindication for weight-bearing exercise. Patients who have a previously healed ulcer must take special precautions when exercising. Scar tissue is very vulnerable to the sheer forces of walking. Patients with PAD, PN, and insensate feet can perform a variety of exercises, such as swimming, bicycling, rowing, chair exercises, and upper body exercises.

Diabetic patients with previous ulcerations, particularly those with PAD and PN, should have specific detailed instructions in foot care and in techniques for decreasing foot pressure before an exercise program is undertaken. Physical therapists and the personnel in exercise centers should discuss with the referring physician the type of exercise program the diabetic patient can undertake.

Table 13.4. Energy Cost of Ambulation

SUBJECTS	OPTIMAL SPEED (m/min)	ENERGY COST	
		$(ml\ O_2 \cdot min^{-1} \cdot kg^{-1})$	$(ml\ O_2 \cdot m^{-1} \cdot kg^{-1})$
Normal (6)	82	13.0	0.16
Syme (7)	54	11.5	0.21
Below-the-knee (7)	45	11.7	0.26
Above-the-knee (7)	36	12.6	0.35
Crutches (normal subjects) (6)	40	13.7	0.25

Adapted from Steinberg FU: Rehabilitation of the diabetic amputee and neuropathic disabilities. In *The Diabetic Foot*. 4th ed. Levin ME, O'Neal LW, Eds. St. Louis, Mosby, 1988, p. 310–32.

Table 13.5. Patient Instructions for the Care of the Diabetic Foot

- Do not smoke.
- Inspect feet daily for blisters, cuts, and scratches. The use of a mirror can aid in seeing the bottom of the feet. Always check between the toes.
- Wash feet daily. Dry carefully, especially between the toes.
- Avoid extremes of temperatures. Test water with hand or elbow before bathing.
- If feet feel cold at night, wear socks. Do not apply hot water bottles or heating pads. Do not soak feet in hot water.
- Do not walk on hot surfaces, such as sandy beaches or the cement around swimming pools.
- Do not walk barefoot.
- Do not use chemical agents for the removal of corns and calluses. Do not use corn plasters. Do not use strong antiseptic solutions on your feet.
- Do not use adhesive tape on your feet.
- Inspect the insides of shoes daily for foreign objects, nail points, torn lining, and rough areas.
- If vision is impaired, have a family member inspect your feet daily, trim nails, and buff down calluses.
- Do not soak feet.
- For dry feet, use a very thin coat of a lubricating oil, such as baby oil. Apply this after bathing and drying the feet. Do not put the oil or cream between the toes. Consult your physician for detailed instructions.

- Wear properly fitting stockings. Do not wear mended stockings. Avoid stockings with seams. Change stockings daily.
- Do not wear garters.
- Shoes should be comfortable at the time of purchase. Do not depend on them to stretch out. Shoes should be made of leather. Running shoes may be worn after checking with your physician.
- Do not wear shoes without stockings.
- Do not wear sandals with thongs between the toes.
- Take special precautions in wintertime. Wear wool socks and protective footgear, such as fleece-lined boots.
- Cut toenails straight across.
- Do not cut corns and calluses. Follow instructions from your physician or podiatrist.
- See your physician regularly and be sure that your feet are examined at each visit.
- Notify your physician or podiatrist at once should you develop a blister or sore on your foot.
- Be sure to inform your podiatrist that you have diabetes.

Adapted from Levin ME: Pathogenesis and management of diabetic foot lesions. In *The Diabetic Foot*. 5th ed. Levin ME, O'Neal LW, Bowker JH, Eds. St. Louis, Mosby, 1993, p. 19–60.

REFERENCES

1. Hiatt WR, Regensteiner JG, Hargarten ME, Wolfel EE, Brass EP: Benefit of exercise conditioning for patients with peripheral arterial disease. *Circulation* 81:602–609, 1990
2. Soulier SM: The use of running shoes in the prevention of plantar diabetic ulcers. *J Am Podiatr Med Assoc* 76:395–400, 1986
3. Cavanagh PR, Ulbrecht JS: Biomechanics of the foot in diabetes mellitus. In *The Diabetic Foot*. 5th ed. Levin ME, O'Neal LW, Bowker JH, Eds. St. Louis, Mosby, 1993, p. 199–232
4. Murray HJ, Veves A, Young MJ, Richie DH, Boulton AJM, American Group for the Study of Experimental Hosiery in the Diabetic Foot: Role of experimental socks in the care of the high-risk diabetic foot: a multicenter patient evaluation study. *Diabetes Care* 16:1190–92, 1993
5. Pinzur MS: Amputation level selection in the diabetic foot. *Clin Orthop Relat Res* 296:68–70, 1993
6. Fisher SV, Gullickson G: Energy cost of ambulation in health and disability: a literature review. *Arch Phys Med Rehabil* 59:124–33, 1978
7. Waters RL, Perry J, Antonelli D, Hislop H: Energy cost of walking of amputees: the influence of level of amputation (Abstract). *J Bone Jt Surg* 58A:42–46, 1978

14. Retinopathy

Highlights
Retinopathy

- Regularly performed exercise is useful in controlling the diabetic condition.
- In general, exercise and physical exertion have no negative impact on the risk of vision loss in cases of diabetic macular edema and nonproliferative diabetic retinopathy.
- In cases of very severe nonproliferative diabetic retinopathy and proliferative diabetic retinopathy, especially when vitreous hemorrhage and/or fibrous retinal traction is present, some types of exercise and physical exertion may be contraindicated because of a risk of traction retinal detachment or vitreous hemorrhage.
- It is advisable to determine accurately the level of retinopathy before suggesting an exercise program for patients with diabetes mellitus.

Retinopathy

LLOYD M. AIELLO, MD, JERRY CAVALLERANO, OD, PhD, LLOYD P. AIELLO, MD, PhD, AND SVEN-ERIK BURSELL, PhD

INTRODUCTION

Nearly 100 years ago, Dr. Elliott P. Joslin identified diet, exercise, and proper medical management as the cornerstones of appropriate diabetes care. Despite the subsequent discovery of insulin and innumerable advances in the understanding and treatment of diabetes mellitus, these cornerstones remain fundamental to this day. Nevertheless, the appropriate role of exercise in diabetes management is not fully appreciated.

One area of ongoing concern involves possible adverse effects of exercise and physical exertion on the microvascular complications of diabetes in general and diabetic retinopathy in particular. Physical exercise could have potentially detrimental effects on diabetic retinopathy and vision, either by raising systolic blood pressure through exertion, with possible subsequent vitreous hemorrhage, or by decreasing already compromised circulating oxygen levels. Conversely, exercise can have positive effects through its action on hormonal levels, high-density lipoprotein (HDL) concentrations, and retinal microcirculatory changes, or by optimization of blood glucose levels.

Despite such conflicting theoretical effects, clinicians and researchers generally agree that appropriate, individually tailored exercise regimens are beneficial in the management of diabetes and in reducing complications of the disease.

OCULAR PHYSIOLOGY

Diabetic retinopathy is the most sight-threatening ocular complication of diabetes. The retina is a highly vascularized, light-sensitive tissue that transforms light focused through the refractive media of the eye into neural messages that the brain interprets as vision. The human eye (and its retina) is an extension of the brain, each originating embryologically from the same neural tissue.

The retina is composed of rod cells, cone cells, and a variety of neural cells that receive, process, and transmit neural signals to the occipital lobe of the brain in response to the light image focused on the retina. Within the retina are numerous arteries and veins that provide the blood supply for the retinal tissue.

RETINAL ABNORMALITIES IN DIABETES MELLITUS

Diabetes can damage the retinal vessels, causing leakage of blood and blood products into the retina and impairing the blood's circulation through the retina. The retinal vessels undergo ultrastructural damage, such as pericyte or mural cell degeneration and retinal blood flow autoregulatory impairment. These changes result from complex hormonal and biochemical alterations mediated by metabolic abnormalities associated with elevated blood glucose levels. These processes can alter vessel contractility and permeability and, ultimately, normal physiological function. Changes in vessel permeability may lead to diabetic macular edema. In diabetic macular edema, fluid collects in the macula, which is the area of the retina responsible for our most acute vision. Changes in retinal blood flow or nutrient delivery to the retina may result in relative retinal hypoxia that, in the most severe stages, may ultimately lead to new vessel growth and diabetic retinopathy.

Diabetic retinopathy can be broadly classified as nonproliferative diabetic retinopathy (NPDR) and proliferative diabetic retinopathy (PDR). Diabetic macular edema can be present with either NPDR or PDR and must always be considered in addition to the level of retinopathy (Table 14.1). NPDR can be further classified as mild, moderate, severe, or very severe, based on the degree of retinal changes (Table 14.2). Each level poses a risk of progression to PDR. Accurate diagnosis of a patient's retinopathy level is critical, because the risk of progression to PDR and high-risk PDR varies depending on the specific NPDR level. It is the level of retinopathy that dictates appropriate examination schedules and therapeutic regimens (Table 14.3).

Table 14.1. Clinically Significant Diabetic Macular Edema

■ Thickening of the retina located ≤500 μm from the center of the macula or
■ Hard exudates with thickening of the adjacent retina located ≤500 μm from the center of the macula or
■ A zone of retinal thickening, 1 disk area or larger in size located ≤1 disk diameter from the center of the macula

Clinically significant diabetic macular edema may be present with any level of retinopathy. Specific evaluation for diabetic macular edema requires careful evaluation by a qualified examiner using fundus biomicroscopy through dilated pupils on at least an annual basis.

Table 14.2. Levels of Retinopathy

NPDR
A. Mild NPDR
■ At least 1 hemorrhage/microaneurysm (H/MA)
■ Definition not met for B, C, D, E, F

B. Moderate NPDR
■ H/MA of a moderate degree
■ Soft exudates, venous beading (VB), and intraretinal microvascular abnormalities (IRMA) definitely present
■ Definition not met for C, D, E, F

C. Severe NPDR
■ H/MA of a moderate degree in 4 retinal quadrants or
■ VB in 2 or more retinal quadrants or
■ IRMA of moderate degree in at least 1 quadrant

D. Very severe NPDR
■ Any 2 or more of C above
■ Definition not met for E, F

PDR
E. Early PDR
■ New vessels present
■ Definition not met for E

F. High-risk PDR
■ NVD ≥1/3–1/2 disk area or
■ NVD and vitreous or pre-retinal hemorrhage or
■ NVE ≥1/2 disk area and pre-retinal or vitreous hemorrhage

PDR is composed of NVD or NVE in the retina, pre-retinal or vitreous hemorrhage, and fibrous tissue proliferation. Specific grading of level of retinopathy requires careful retinal evaluation by a qualified examiner through dilated pupils on at least an annual basis.

Retinopathy marked by new vessel growth on the optic nerve (neovascularization at the disk; NVD), elsewhere in the retina (neovascularization elsewhere; NVE), or by proliferation of fibrous tissue on the retina is classified as PDR. In the proliferative stage of diabetic retinopathy, new blood vessels form on the surface of the retina, presumably in an attempt to deliver more oxygenated blood to areas of the retina that experience relative hypoxia. These fragile new vessels do not relieve the relative hypoxia and can leak or burst, causing vitreous hemorrhage. Physical exertion, especially Valsalva-type maneuvers, and elevated systolic blood pressure may put added stress on these weakened vessel walls, possibly increasing the risk of vitreous hemorrhage. Furthermore, these vessels are usually accompanied by glial tissue, which may contract and cause traction on the retina and subsequent retinal detachment. Physical straining can potentiate this traction, leading to retinal detachment.

The 5-year risk of severe vision loss (best vision of 5/200 or worse) for eyes with high-risk PDR may be as high as 60%. This risk can be reduced to <5% over 5 years by proper and timely laser photocoagulation. The 3-year risk of moderate vision loss (e.g., a loss of vision from 20/20 to 20/40 or from 20/50 to 20/100) is 25–30%. This risk can be reduced 50% by timely and appropriate laser photocoagulation. Regular eye evaluations are crucial to determining the level of retinopathy, the need for laser photocoagulation, and the impact, if any, of retinopathy on a choice of exercise program (Tables 14.3 and 14.4).

RETINAL AND OCULAR CONSIDERATIONS DURING EXERCISE

Insulin-Dependent Diabetes Mellitus (IDDM)

Several studies have investigated the relationship of exercise to the development of PDR (1–4). In people diagnosed with diabetes before 30 years of age, of whom most are expected to have IDDM, there is a suggestion that higher levels of physical activity may result in a reduced risk of PDR in women (1). Women evaluated in the study who either participated in team sports in high school or college or considered their level of activity to be strenuous were less likely to have PDR when compared with women who did not participate in team sports or consider themselves to be physically active (1). No such relationship, however, was found in male participants in the study. Other studies did not identify any positive effects of exercise in preventing PDR in men or women (2–4). It has been postulated that the positive effect of exercise in preventing PDR in women may be the result of hormonal influences. Significantly, none of the studies noted a deleterious effect of exercise on the development of PDR.

Although the beneficial effects of exercise for people with diabetes are generally accepted, one area of controversy surrounds the effects of exercise on growth hormone (GH). Potentially adverse effects of GH on diabetic retinopathy have been suggested by studies involving diabetic individuals with pituitary ablation and dwarfism (5,6). In subsequent studies, measures of the plasma level of GH rose in individuals who had severe diabetic retinopathy, but did not rise significantly for those who exhibited no diabetic retinopathy, suggesting that GH might contribute to the development of diabetic retinopathy

(7,8). Because it is postulated that GH secretion increases in people with diabetes (7,9) and microangiopathy under conditions such as muscular exercise, the theoretical potential adverse effects of exercise on diabetic retinopathy have been raised. However, most clinicians and researchers agree that the beneficial effect of an appropriate exercise regimen for people with diabetes outweighs any theoretical detriment.

Non-Insulin-Dependent Diabetes Mellitus (NIDDM)

The National Institutes of Health, in its consensus paper on diet and exercise in NIDDM, consider the cornerstone of therapy for NIDDM to be a "style of life centered around diet and supplemented, if needed, by insulin or oral agents" (10). Exercise is recognized as an auxiliary means to facilitate caloric loss, assist in glucose regulation, and reverse insulin resistance at insulin target tissues, such as the liver, skeletal muscle, and adipose tissue. The consensus panel recognized potential complications of exercise in patients with NIDDM, including cardiac disease, bone and soft tissue injuries, and eye disease, particularly PDR. The ocular risks include retinal detachment and vitreous hemorrhage, especially during exercise "that requires straining and breath holding (such as weight lifting)" (10).

Table 14.3. Eye Examination Schedule

	RECOMMENDATION TIME OF FIRST EXAM	ROUTINE MINIMUM FOLLOW-UP
IDDM	5 years after onset or at puberty or pregnancy	Yearly
NIDDM	At time of diagnosis	Yearly
Gestational	Before pregnancy	Early in the 1st trimester, and each trimester or more frequently as indicated, and 3–6 months postpartum

Abnormal findings will dictate more frequent follow-up examinations.

General Considerations

In general, exercise and physical activity have not been shown to accelerate retinopathy. There is some indication that physical exercise has a positive effect on reducing the risk of diabetic complications by either direct or indirect mechanisms. In both IDDM and NIDDM patients, aerobic exercises improve or maintain cardiovascular function, increase levels of HDLs, aid in weight control, increase insulin sensitivity, and reduce risk factors for vascular disease (11–16). Studies of people with diabetic retinopathy have shown that cardiovascular training with moderate levels of exercise results in significant improvements in cardiovascular health (11).

For patients who have PDR that is active, strenuous activity may precipitate vitreous hemorrhage or traction retinal detachment (17,18). Although one retrospective study (19) involving 72 diabetic patients presenting with 95 episodes of vitreous hemorrhage showed that 80 of the hemorrhages were associated with exercise no more strenuous than walking, it is our philos-

Table 14.4. Considerations for Activity Limitation in Diabetic Retinopathy

LEVEL OF DR	ACCEPTABLE ACTIVITIES	DISCOURAGED ACTIVITIES	OCULAR AND ACTIVITY REEVALUATION
No DR	Dictated by medical status	Dictated by medical status	12 months
Mild NPDR	Dictated by medical status	Dictated by medical status	6–12 months
Moderate NPDR	Dictated by medical status	Activities that dramatically elevate blood pressure: ■ Power lifting ■ Heavy Valsalva maneuvers	4–6 months
Severe NPDR and very severe NPDR	Dictated by medical status	Limit systolic blood pressure, Valsalva maneuvers, and active jarring: ■ Boxing ■ Heavy competitive sports	2–4 months (may require laser surgery)
PDR	Low-impact, cardiovascular conditioning: ■ Swimming (not diving) ■ Walking ■ Low-impact aerobics ■ Stationary cycling ■ Endurance exercises	Strenuous activity, Valsalva maneuvers, pounding, or jarring: ■ Weight lifting ■ Jogging ■ High-impact aerobics ■ Racquet sports ■ Strenuous trumpet playing	1–2 months (may require laser surgery)

ophy that people with PDR should avoid anaerobic exercise and exercise that involves straining, jarring, such as high-impact aerobics and jogging, or Valsalva-type maneuvers. A rise in systolic blood pressure that accompanies strenuous exercise can increase pressure on damaged retinal capillaries and neovascular tufts, resulting in intraretinal, pre-retinal, and vitreous hemorrhage. In the long term, however, before the onset of PDR, physical activity and exercise may reduce the risk of PDR and diabetic macular edema indirectly by its effect on blood pressure and HDL, which are both associated with retinopathy (20,21).

SPECIAL PRECAUTIONS

Table 14.4 summarizes exercise activities that may be appropriate based on level of retinopathy. These guidelines reflect the approach to exercise taken at the Beetham Eye Institute and, as such, are suggestions rather than explicit medical directives. In all cases, decisions are based on the patient's individual needs, condition, and physician recommendation.

We suggest that people with PDR avoid exercise regimens that result in systolic blood pressure >170 mmHg (22). Note, however, that this recommendation is arbitrary, and based on other studies (11), limiting the blood pressure increase to only 170 mmHg may have little, if any, exercise benefit. This latter study (11) suggested that blood pressure increase be limited to <50 mmHg above resting levels or to a maximum systolic blood pressure of 200 mmHg for those patients having residual vision and to 240 mmHg for those patients having no residual light perception. The suggestions recommended in this study, however, were also arbitrary, because it was determined that no adverse ophthalmologic events could be directly related to the exercise program over the 2-year duration of the study. Thus, it appears that the blood pressure restrictions given above should be taken as conservative estimates. We do suggest, however, that concurrent monitoring of blood pressure and level

of retinopathy is necessary once a person has advanced beyond mild to moderate levels of NPDR.

It has also been demonstrated that people with severe diabetic retinopathy and IDDM have impaired cardiovascular response to exercise, which is reflected in decreased heart rate, decreased left ventricular ejection factor, and decreased muscle blood flow (23). In addition, a recently published article (24) demonstrated abnormalities in the autonomic regulation of the ophthalmic circulation during exercise. These considerations, taken together with suggestions regarding blood pressure elevations, should have an impact on the level of exercise chosen and the potential therapeutic benefit derived for patients with severe diabetic retinopathy.

Other general restrictions for patients with PDR include avoiding activities that lower the head below waist level, Valsalva-type maneuvers that result in increased blood pressure, and near maximal isometric contractions (12,17,18). Similarly, weight lifting with high resistance and low repetitions and exercises that force a person to hold his or her breath should be avoided. Vigorous bouncing, including jogging, high-impact aerobics, and contact sports is contraindicated because of the risk of retinal tears, retinal detachment, or vitreous hemorrhage in eyes with retinal neovascularization, fibrous tissue proliferation, or retinal traction (12). Strenuous upper extremity exercises, such as rowing and army cycle ergometry, likewise are contraindicated (12).

Beneficial low-risk exercises include endurance exercise, stationary cycling, low-intensity machine rowing, swimming, and walking. Even patients who have lost vision should attempt to maintain some level of regular physical exercise. With appropriate hemodynamic and glucose monitoring, patients with diabetic retinopathy and autonomic neuropathy may exercise safely (25–27).

CONCLUSIONS

In most cases, exercise is an important component of diabetes care. A person's exercise regimen should be carefully crafted and monitored by his or her health-care team, including the exercise physiologist, nutritionist, internist, and eye doctor experienced in the management of diabetic eye disease. Currently, diabetic retinopathy cannot be prevented, but careful evaluation, follow-up, and timely and appropriate laser photocoagulation can reduce the 5-year risk of severe visual loss from PDR to <5% and cut the risk of moderate vision loss from diabetic macular edema by 50% or more. Because even serious retinopathy frequently causes no visual symptoms, especially in the most treatable stages, regular eye examinations are indicated to establish the level of retinopathy. These regular examinations must be obtained at least yearly and will provide the clinical information that determines an appropriate exercise program for people with diabetes.

REFERENCES

1. Cruickshanks KJ, Klein R, Moss SE, Klein BEK: Physical activity and proliferative diabetic retinopathy in people diagnosed with diabetes before age 30 yr. *Diabetes Care* 15:1267–72, 1992
2. LaPorte RE, Dorman JS, Tajima N, Cruickshanks KJ, Orchard TJ, Cavender DE, Becker DJ, Drash AL: Pittsburgh Insulin-Dependent Diabetes Mellitus and Mortality Study: physical activity and diabetic complications. *Pediatrics* 78: 1027–33, 1986
3. Kriska AM, LaPorte RE, Patrick SL, Kuller LH, Orchard TJ: The association of physical activity and diabetic complications in individuals with insulin-dependent diabetes mellitus: The Epidemiology of Diabetes Complications Study VII. *J Clin Epidemiol* 44:1207–14, 1991
4. Orchard TJ, Dorman JS, Maser RE, Becker DJ, Ellis D, LaPorte RE, Kuller LH, Wolfson SK Jr, Drash AL: Factors associated with avoidance of severe complications after 25 yr of IDDM: Pittsburgh Epidemiology of Diabetes Com- plications Study I. *Diabetes Care* 13:741–47, 1990
5. Kohner EM, Joplin GF, Blach RK, Cheng H, Fraser TR: Pituitary ablation in the treatment of diabetic retinopathy (a randomized trial). *Trans Ophthalmol Soc* 92:79–90, 1972
6. Merimee TJ: A follow-up study of vascular disease in growth-hormone-deficient dwarfs with diabetes. *N Engl J Med* 298:1217–22, 1978
7. Passa P, Gauville C, Canivet J: Influence of muscular exercise on plasma level of growth hormone in diabetics with and without retinopathy. *Lancet* 342:72–74, 1994
8. Alzaid AA, Dinneen SF, Melton LJ, Rizza RA: The role of growth hormone in the development of diabetic retinopathy. *Diabetes Care* 17:531–34, 1994
9. Hansen AP: Abnormal serum growth hormone response to exercise in maturity-onset diabetics. *Diabetes* 22:619–28, 1973
10. National Institutes of Health: Consensus development conference on diet and exercise in non-insulin-dependent diabetes mellitus. *Diabetes Care* 10:639–44, 1987
11. Bernbaum M, Albert S, Cohen JD, Drimmer A: Cardiovascular conditioning in individuals with diabetic retinopathy. *Diabetes Care* 12:740–42, 1989
12. Graham C, Lasko-McCarthey P: Exercise options for people with diabetic complications. *Diabetes Educator* 16:212–20, 1990
13. Vranic M, Berger M: Exercise and diabetes. *Diabetes* 28:147–63, 1979
14. Delio D: Aerobic exercise programs and the management of diabetes. *Pract Diabetol* 4:12–20, 1985
15. Franz MJ: Exercise and diabetes: fuel metabolism, benefits, risks and guidelines. *Clin Diabetes* 6: 58–70, 1988
16. Horton ES: Role and management of exercise in diabetes mellitus. *Diabetes Care* 11:201–11, 1988

17. Sharuk GS, Stockman ME, Krolewski AS, Aiello LM, Rand LI: Patient activity and the risk of vitreous hemorrhage in eyes with proliferative diabetic retinopathy (Abstract). *Invest Ophthalmol* 27 (Suppl.):5, 1986

18. Sharuk GS, Stockman ME, Krolewski AS, Aiello LM, Rand LI: Patient activity and the risk of vitreous hemorrhage in eyes with proliferative diabetic retinopathy (Abstract). *Invest Ophthalmol* 28 (Suppl.):246, 1987

19. Anderson B Jr: Activity and diabetic vitreous hemorrhages. *Ophthalmology* 87:173–75, 1980

20. Klein R, Klein BEK, Moss SE, Davis MD, DeMets DL: Is blood pressure a predictor of the incidence or progression of diabetic retinopathy? *Arch Intern Med* 149: 2427–32, 1989

21. Klein BEK, Moss SE, Klein R, Surawicz TS: The Wisconsin Epidemiologic Study of Diabetic Retinopathy. XIII. Relationship of serum cholesterol to retinopathy and hard exudate. *Ophthalmology* 98:1261–65, 1991

22. Greenlee G: Exercise options for patients with retinopathy and peripheral vascular disease. *Pract Diabetol* 6:9–11, 1987

23. Margonato A, Gerundini P, Vicedomini G, Gilardi M, Pozza G, Fazio F: Abnormal cardiovascular response to exercise in young asymptomatic diabetic patients with retinopathy. *Am Heart J* 112: 554–60, 1986

24. Albert SG, Gomez CR, Russell S, Chaitman BR, Bernbaum M, Kong BA: Cerebral and ophthalmic artery hemodynamic responses in diabetes mellitus. *Diabetes Care* 16: 476–82, 1993

25. Bernbaum M, Albert SG, Cohen JD: Exercise training in individuals with diabetic retinopathy and blindness. *Arch Phys Med Rehabil* 70:605–11, 1989

26. Bernbaum M, Albert SG, Brusca SR, Drimmer A, Duckro P: Promoting diabetes self-management and independence in the visually impaired: a model clinical program. *Diabetes Educator* 14: 51–54, 1988

27. Bernbaum M, Albert SG, Brusca SR, Drimmer A, Duckro P, Cohen JD, Trindade MC, Silverberg AB: A model clinical program for patients with diabetes and vision impairment. *Diabetes Educator* 15: 325–30, 1989

15. Cardiovascular Complications

Highlights
Cardiovascular Complications

- Atherosclerotic heart disease and hypertension are common in patients with diabetes and are a major cause of morbidity and mortality.
- Silent myocardial ischemia is more common in the patient with diabetes and may be associated with autonomic dysfunction.
- Autonomic neuropathy is associated with an increased mortality from myocardial infarction and sudden death and may be a marker for clinically unrecognized cardiac disease.
- Exercise may decrease cardiovascular risk in patients with diabetes.
- Before starting an individualized exercise program, the patient with diabetes should undergo a thorough history and physical examination to detect any signs of cardiovascular disease. A graded exercise test is necessary if the patient is at high risk for underlying cardiovascular disease.
- Exercise of moderate intensity is usually recommended for individuals with stable coronary artery disease and/or hypertension.
- Patients with a recent cardiac event should be stratified according to risk for exercise and should follow a cardiac rehabilitation program.

Cardiovascular Complications

SERGIO WAXMAN, MD, AND RICHARD W. NESTO, MD

CARDIOVASCULAR DISEASE AND DIABETES

Diabetes constitutes a major risk factor for the development of cardiovascular disease; indeed, its effect greatly exceeds that of many standard risk factors for atherosclerosis, particularly in women and young adults (1–4). Data from the Framingham Heart Study have demonstrated that cardiovascular mortality is more than doubled in men and more than quadrupled in women who have diabetes compared with their nondiabetic counterparts (5). The relative risk of myocardial infarction is 50% greater in diabetic men and 150% greater in diabetic women. Myocardial infarction accounts for as many as 30% of all deaths in IDDM patients (6). Coronary atherosclerosis is more extensive, as well as more prevalent, in diabetic than in nondiabetic individuals (7). Silent myocardial ischemia is also more common in patients with diabetes (8,9). It may be associated with autonomic dysfunction (10), and appears to be more prevalent in individuals on insulin therapy who have retinopathy (11). During exercise, the anginal perceptual threshold is prolonged compared with that of nondiabetic individuals, possibly due to the presence of autonomic neuropathy (12,13).

In addition to atherosclerosis, hypertension is more common and, alone or in combination with coronary artery disease, is a major cause of morbidity and mortality in people with diabetes (1). The most common type of hypertension in patients with type II diabetes is essential hypertension, which may be related to obesity, central adiposity, and insulin resistance (the latter possibly due to increased sympathetic activity [14,15] and sodium retention in the kidney [16]). In type I diabetes, diabetic nephropathy and renal artery stenosis due to an increased prevalence of generalized atherosclerosis (17) are also common causes of hypertension.

Cardiac disease may also be present in patients with diabetes in the absence of coronary artery disease. Diabetic cardiomyopathy is associated with abnormalities of systolic and diastolic left ventricular function (18). Pathological findings in diabetic cardiomyopathy include myocardial enlargement, hypertrophy, and fibrosis, as well as an increase in basement membrane thickening (19,20). Even in the absence of clinical signs of cardiac impairment, left ventricular function may be impaired in diabetic patients during exercise by mechanisms that are not completely understood but that may involve the presence of microangiopathy or autonomic dysfunction (21–23) or inadequate systemic venous return with limitation in left ventricular filling (24).

Autonomic neuropathy is frequently present in patients with diabetes (25, see also Chapter 18). It is associated with increased mortality from myocardial infarction and sudden death, and it may be a marker for clinically unrecognized cardiac disease. Alterations in autonomic regulation may lead to ischemia by a number of mechanisms that include: 1) increasing myocardial oxygen demand because of higher resting heart rates, 2) reducing myocardial blood flow by increasing coronary vascular tone at sites of coronary stenosis, 3) reducing coronary perfusion pressure during orthostatic hypotension, and 4) eliminating early warning signs of ischemia (26).

CARDIOVASCULAR PHYSIOLOGY—BENEFITS OF EXERCISE FOR DECREASING CARDIOVASCULAR RISK

Exercise decreases cardiovascular risk in the general population (27–30), and its effects are likely to be equally beneficial in the diabetic patient (see Chapters 4 and 24). The potential mechanisms for the decrease in cardiovascular risk associated with exercise are shown in Table 15.1. Exercise is associated with changes in insulin sensitivity and lipid metabolism, events that are likely to have long-term effects on the development of cardiovascular complications. In people at high risk

Table 15.1. Changes Associated With Exercise That May Decrease Cardiovascular Risk

- Decreased blood pressure
- Increased HDL cholesterol level
- Decreased triglyceride level
- Reduced weight
- Increased fibrinolysis in response to thrombotic stimuli
- Increased insulin sensitivity
- Reduced susceptibility to serious ventricular arrhythmias
- Associated behavioral changes (smoking cessation, diet, stress reduction)
- Psychological effects (decreased depression and anxiety)

for developing type II diabetes, exercise may prevent the onset of diabetes (31) and may affect the course of atherosclerosis-related disease.

Aerobic exercise benefits patients with coronary artery disease by modulating physiological changes that enable the patient to achieve a higher functional state. In previously sedentary individuals, maximal oxygen uptake may increase by 15–25% over baseline after a few months of regular aerobic exercise performed at 60–80% of maximum aerobic capacity for 20–60 min 3–5 days/week (32). This level of exercise benefits the cardiovascular system by decreasing heart rate at rest and during submaximal exercise, increasing stroke volume at rest and with submaximal and maximal exercise, and increasing maximal cardiac output (33–35). These changes result in reduced myocardial oxygen demand during submaximal exercise and allow the patient with coronary artery disease to perform a higher workload despite impaired coronary flow reserve. This, in turn, increases the amount of work that can be done at the anginal or ischemic threshold (36).

In contrast to aerobic physical activity, isometric exercise produces an acute pressor response that is related to the size of muscle mass and the degree of muscular tension exerted. This imposes a greater pressure than volume overload on the left ventricle in relation to the body's ability to supply oxygen. The marked rise in blood pressure is related to an increase in cardiac output with little or no decrease in total peripheral resistance. Because the response to activation of a small muscle group is similar to the response to a large muscle group, the cardiovascular response to this form of exercise is difficult to grade. Although physicians have been hesitant to prescribe isometric exercise for their patients, some studies suggest that regimens incorporating moderate levels of resistance and high repetitions may be safe for patients with coronary artery disease (37), may favorably alter cardiovascular risk factors such as high-density lipoprotein (HDL) cholesterol, and may improve insulin sensitivity (38–40). Its use in elderly individuals is described in Chapter 22.

Exercise following myocardial infarction has been associated with decreased mortality (41), a benefit that may be related to a significant reduction in sudden death. Performance of exercise at regular intervals has also been noted to decrease the risk of myocardial infarction (42). Sedentary individuals experience a higher relative risk of myocardial infarction following an episode of heavy exertion compared with individuals who exercise 5 or more times/week (42).

Despite these benefits, exercise may have risks and be contraindicated in certain patients with diabetes. Some risks, however, can be minimized if patients and physicians have a comprehensive knowledge of medical condition, physical limitations, and safe and appropriate exercises.

SPECIAL PROBLEMS IN PATIENTS WITH DIABETES

Coronary Artery Disease

The exercise prescription for the patient with diabetes and coronary artery disease differs little from that for the nondiabetic patient and is influenced to a great extent by the presence of other complications of diabetes. The ischemic response to exercise, ischemic threshold, and the propensity to arrhythmias during exercise should be evaluated. In many cases, left ventricular systolic function at rest and its response to exercise should also be assessed. This information can be used to modify an exercise prescription dependent on the overall risk for subsequent cardiac events, which is based on the presence of ischemia, left ventricular function, and/or arrhythmias.

Exercise of moderate intensity is usually recommended for patients with known coronary artery disease in the absence of ischemia or significant arrhythmias (43). This level of exercise can be targeted to 60–80% of the maximum heart rate corresponding to 50–74% of the maximum oxygen consumption (44). In patients with angina, exercise training increases functional capacity at the anginal threshold. For these patients, the target heart rate during aerobic exercise should be set at no less than 10 beats below the ischemic threshold (45). Sublingual nitroglycerin before exercise may allow patients with low anginal thresholds to achieve higher levels of exercise. In patients without angina, targeting a specific level of activity may be more complicated; in these patients, the ischemic threshold should be determined by exercise electrocardiographic monitoring. Particular attention should be paid to these patients, because a lack of angina in the setting of ischemia can be due to autonomic neuropathy, which may also be an indicator of more severe coronary disease, left ventricular dysfunction, and a poor overall cardiovascular prognosis.

Isometric exercise, as discussed earlier, may be beneficial for patients with coronary artery disease; in particular, those with normal or near-normal left ventricular function. Programs that include 8–12 repetitions of loads corresponding to 40–50% of maximum strength appear safe for these patients (46).

Hypertension

Exercise reduces blood pressure by 5–10 mmHg in some patients with essential hypertension (47,48), and its effects are usually noted within 10 weeks of training (49). Although the mechanism for the antihypertensive effects of exercise is unknown, possible explanations may include the attenuation of sympathetic nervous system activity with subsequent reduction in peripheral vascular resistance (40) and improved insulin sensitivity with a reduction in circulating insulin (50). The latter may decrease sodium reabsorption by the renal tubules (51).

Before starting an exercise program, the hypertensive patient requires adequate blood pressure control because exercise causes acute increases in systolic pressure, and this increase may be exaggerated in the diabetic patient (52). The blood pressure response to exercise should be monitored initially, and adjustments in therapy should be made accordingly. Exercise should be performed with a frequency of at least 4 times/week, with each session lasting between 30 and 60 min. Exercise of moderate intensity is generally recommended for the individual with hypertension (43). This level of exercise can be targeted to 60–80% of the maximum heart rate, which corresponds to 50–74% of the maximum oxygen consumption (44). High-intensity and isometric exercises should be minimized because they can cause a significant pressor response.

Autonomic Neuropathy

The presence of autonomic neuropathy may be a marker for severe but clinically unrecognized cardiac disease. Therefore, exercise for these patients should be prescribed with extreme caution (see Chapter 18).

Parasympathetic function is usually impaired before sympathetic function. This is characteristically manifested as a higher basal heart rate; although, during exercise, the heart rate and blood pressure responses tend to be blunted (53,54). Such abnormalities in the regulation of heart rate and peripheral vascular resistance result in decreased cardiac output with exertion and may account for a reduced exercise capacity. In addition, left ventricular systolic and diastolic function at rest and during exercise may be abnormal even in the absence of coronary artery disease as a result of diabetic cardiomyopathy. The effects of exercise on the cardiovascular system in diabetic patients with autonomic neuropathy are unknown, although low levels of exercise may be beneficial and safe for some of these patients. Periodic evaluations should be made in the diabetic patient with autonomic neuropathy to detect signs of cardiovascular disease.

Orthostatic hypotension may be present in some patients with autonomic dysfunction, and patients should be screened for it before an exercise regimen is prescribed. The evaluation should be done at rest, and if orthostatic hypotension is present in the absence of symptoms, long warm-up and cooldown periods of low-intensity exercise are recommended before and after each training session. The patient should be educated to recognize early signs of neurocirculatory collapse and report any symptoms to his/her regular physician.

EVALUATION OF THE DIABETIC PATIENT DURING EXERCISE

Before starting an individualized exercise program, the person with diabetes should undergo a thorough interview and physical examination to detect any signs of cardiovascular disease. A graded exercise test is necessary if the patient is at high risk for underlying cardiovascular disease, based on the following criteria:

- Non-insulin-dependent diabetes mellitus of >10 years duration or in those >35 years of age
- Any additional risk factor for coronary artery disease
- Presence of microvascular disease (retinopathy, nephropathy, including proteinuria)
- Peripheral vascular disease
- Autonomic neuropathy

The exercise stress test should be performed in such patients for evaluation of ischemia, arrhythmias, abnormal hypertensive response to exercise, or an abnormal orthostatic response during or after exercise. The stress test also provides information regarding initial levels of working capacity, specific precautions that may need to be taken, and heart rates used to prescribe activities. In women and in selected patients who are likely to have nonspecific electrocardiographic changes in response to exercise (such as individuals with hypertension and left ventricular hypertrophy), or nonspecific ST and T wave changes on the resting electrocardiogram, or in those taking diuretics, alternative tests, such as radionuclide or echocardiographic stress testing, should be performed.

The exercise stress test should be done near the time of day the patient would normally exercise to determine safety and to assess the need to modify the exercise prescription. It should also be performed while the patient is taking any antianginal or antihypertensive medications. ß-blockers and calcium-channel blockers may attenuate the heart rate and blood pressure responses to exercise, lessening diagnostic accuracy, and may need to be held the morning of the test. Vasodilator medications, such as calcium-channel blockers and angiotensin-converting enzyme inhibitors, may be associated with postexercise hypotension. In these patients, prolonged cooldown periods may be required. Patients on chronic diuretic therapy may have low serum potassium levels and an increased potential for arrhythmias during exercise. Serum potassium levels should be monitored periodically in these patients.

CARDIAC REHABILITATION

Patients with exercise-induced ischemia, heart failure, or a recent cardiac event, such as myocardial infarction, coronary angioplasty, or bypass surgery, should participate in a cardiac rehabilitation program. The risk of cardiac rehabilitation is very low, with one major cardiovascular complication (cardiac arrest or myocardial infarction) per 81,101 patient-hours and one fatality per 783,972 patient-hours (55). The prevalence of these complications is related to the degree of left ventricular dysfunction and the severity of heart disease. Initial physical activity should be monitored by a professional to record symptoms, heart rate, blood pressure, and rating of perceived exertion. When tolerance and safety are documented, the individual can perform that activity without supervision.

The exercise test is an important part of the rehabilitative process. It provides reassurance to the patient, risk stratification, and information about exercise capacity that is important in determining a safe level of exercise. A symptom-limited exercise test is usually performed 4–8 weeks after hospital discharge, and if no further studies are indicated, a regular conditioning program can be initiated. Low-risk patients (Table 15.2) can participate in a home exercise program. Duration and intensity should be low initially and gradually increased in the absence of symptoms. Because ischemia is frequently asymptomatic in the patient with diabetes, an objective assessment of ischemia should be done periodically as the level of exercise increases. An exercise test is used for this purpose. Patients at moderate to high risk for cardiac complications during exercise (Table 15.2) should participate in a medically supervised program. For a more detailed review on cardiac rehabilitation, see the American Heart Association's Exercise Standards (43).

THE CARDIOLOGIST'S ROLE IN PRESCRIBING EXERCISE FOR PATIENTS WITH DIABETES

Formulating an exercise prescription for the patient with diabetes should be a multidisciplinary effort involving all members of the health-care team and the patient. The cardiologist, as part of the team, should *1)* act as a consultant, providing information on the benefits, potential risks, and appropriateness of exercise for each particular patient; *2)* educate the health-care team and patient to be aware of and recognize signs, symptoms, and clinical conditions that are associated with coronary artery disease. *3)* work in conjunction

with the team to screen the patient and formulate an individualized exercise program; and *4)* monitor the patient's progress.

Table 15.2. Classification of Risk Related to Vigorous Exercise in Patients With Coronary Artery Disease

Low risk (but slightly greater than for apparently healthy individuals)

Known CAD and the following clinical characteristics:
■ New York Heart Association class 1 or 2
■ Exercise capacity >6 METs
■ No evidence of heart failure
■ Free of ischemia or angina at rest or on the exercise test at ≤6 METs
■ Appropriate rise in systolic blood pressure during exercise
■ No sequential ectopic ventricular contractions
■ Ability to satisfactorily self-monitor intensity of activity

Moderate to high risk

Known CAD and any of the following clinical characteristics:
■ History of two or more myocardial infarctions
■ New York Heart Association class 3 or 4
■ Exercise capacity <6 METs
■ Ischemic horizontal or downsloping ST depression of ≥4 mm or angina during exercise
■ Fall in systolic blood pressure with exercise
■ Presence of a life-threatening medical problem
■ History of a primary cardiac arrest
   Ventricular tachycardia at a workload of ≥6 METs

CAD, coronary artery disease. Known CAD is defined as history of myocardial infarction, coronary bypass surgery, angioplasty, angina pectoris, abnormal exercise test, or an abnormal coronary angiogram. Adapted from the American Heart Association (43).

REFERENCES

1. Garcia MJ, McNamara PM, Gordon T, Kannel WB: Morbidity and mortality in diabetics in the Framingham population. *Diabetes* 23: 105–11, 1974
2. Barrett-Connor E, Orchard TJ: Diabetes and heart disease. In *Diabetes in America*. Harris MJ, Hamman RF, Eds. Bethesda, MD, National Institutes of Health, National

Diabetes Data Group, 1985 (NIH publ. no. 85–1468)

3. Barrett-Connor E, Wingard DL: Sex differential in ischemic heart disease mortality in diabetics: a prospective population-based study. *Am J Epidemiol* 118:489–96, 1983

4. Jarrett RJ, McCartney P, Keen H: The Bedford survey: ten-year mortality rates in newly diagnosed diabetics, borderline diabetics and normoglycaemic controls and risk indices for coronary heart disease in borderline diabetics. *Diabetologia* 22:79–84, 1982

5. Kannel W, McGee D: Diabetes and cardiovascular disease: the Framingham Study. *JAMA* 241:2035–38, 1979

6. Barrett-Connor E, Orchard T: Insulin-dependent diabetes mellitus and ischemic heart disease. *Diabetes Care* 8:65–70, 1985

7. Robertson W, Strong J: Atherosclerosis in persons with hypertension and diabetes mellitus. *Lab Invest* 18:538–51, 1968

8. Zarich S, Waxman S, Freeman R, Mittleman M, Hegarty P, Nesto RW: Effect of autonomic nervous system dysfunction on the circadian pattern of myocardial ischemia in diabetes mellitus. *J Am Coll Cardiol* 24:956–62, 1994

9. Nesto RW, Phillips RT, Kett KG, Hill T, Perper E, Young E, Leland OS Jr: Angina and exertional myocardial ischemia in diabetic and nondiabetic patients: assessment by exercise thallium scintigraphy. *Ann Intern Med* 108:170–75, 1988

10. Langer A, Freeman RM, Josse RG, Steiner G, Armstrong PW: Detection of silent myocardial ischemia in diabetes mellitus. *Am J Cardiol* 67:1073–78, 1991

11. Naka M, Hiramatsu K, Aizawa T, Momose A, Yoshizawa K, Shigematsu S, Ishihara F, Niwa A, Yamada T: Silent myocardial ischemia in patients with non-insulin-dependent diabetes mellitus as judged by treadmill exercise testing and coronary angiography. *Am Heart J* 123:46–53, 1992

12. Umachandran V, Ranjadayalan K, Ambepityia G, Marchant B, Kopelman PG, Timmis AD: The perception of angina in diabetes: relation to somatic pain threshold and autonomic function. *Am Heart J* 121:1649–54, 1991

13. Ambepityia G, Kopelman PG, Ingram D, Swash M, Mills PG, Timmis AD: Exertional myocardial ischemia in diabetes: a quantitative analysis of anginal perceptual threshold and the influence of autonomic function. *J Am Coll Cardiol* 15:72–77, 1990

14. Rowe JW, Young JB, Minaker KL, Stevens AL, Pallota J, Landsberg L: Effect of insulin and glucose infusions on sympathetic nervous system activity in normal men. *Diabetes* 30:219–25, 1981

15. Goldstein DS: Plasma catecholamines and essential hypertension: an analytic review. *Hypertension* 5:86–99, 1983

16. DeFronzo RA: The effect of insulin on renal sodium metabolism. *Diabetologia* 21:165–71, 1981

17. The Working Group on Hypertension in Diabetes: Statement on hypertension in diabetes mellitus. Final report. *Arch Intern Med* 147:830–42, 1987

18. Zarich S, Nesto R: Diabetic cardiomyopathy. *Am Heart J* 118:1000–12, 1989

19. Rubler S, Dlugash J, Yuceoglu YZ, Kumral T, Branwood AW, Grisham A: New type of cardiomyopathy associated with diabetic glomerulosclerosis. *Am J Cardiol* 30:595–602, 1972

20. Fein F: Diabetic cardiomyopathy. *Diabetes Care* 13:1169–79, 1990

21. Vered Z, Battler A, Segal P, Liberman D, Yerushalmi Y, Berezin M, Neufeld HN: Exercise induced left ventricular dysfunction in young men with asymptomatic diabetes mellitus (diabetic cardiomyopathy). *Am J Cardiol* 54:633–37, 1984

22. Mustonen JN, Uusitupa MI, Tahvanainen K, Talwar S, Laasko M, Lansimies E, Kuikka JT, Pyorala K: Impaired left ventricular systolic function during exercise in middle-aged insulin-dependent and non-

insulin-dependent diabetic subjects without clinically evident cardiovascular disease. *Am J Cardiol* 62: 1273–79, 1988

23. Takahashi N, Iwasaka T, Sugiura T, Hasegawa T, Tarumi N, Matsutani M, Onoyama H, Inada M: Left ventricular dysfunction during dynamic exercise in non-insulin-dependent diabetic patients with retinopathy. *Cardiology* 78:23–30, 1991

24. Borow KM, Jaspan JB, Williams KA, Neumann A, Wolinski-Walley P, Lang R: Myocardial mechanics in young adult patients with diabetes mellitus: effects of altered load, inotropic state and dynamic exercise. *J Am Coll Cardiol* 15:1508–17, 1990

25. Nesto RW: Diabetes and heart disease. In *World Book of Diabetes in Practice*. Vol. 3. Krall LP, Ed. Elsevier, 1988

26. Jacoby RM, Nesto RW: Acute myocardial infarction in the diabetic patient: pathophysiology, clinical course and prognosis. *J Am Coll Cardiol* 20:736–44, 1992

27. Paffenbarger RS, Hyde RT, Wing AL, Hsieh C: Physical activity, all-cause mortality, and longevity of college alumni. *N Engl J Med* 314:605–13, 1986

28. Leon AS, Connett J, Jacobs DR, Rauramaa R: Leisure-time physical activity levels and risk of coronary artery disease and death: the Multiple Risk Factor Intervention Trial. *JAMA* 258:2388–95, 1987

29. Powell KE, Thompson PD, Caspersen CJ, Kendrick JS: Physical activity and the incidence of coronary heart disease. *Annu Rev Public Health* 8:253–87, 1987

30. Blair SN, Kohl HW III, Paffenbarger RS Jr, Clark DG, Cooper KH, Gibbons IW: Physical fitness and all-cause mortality—a prospective study of healthy men and women. *JAMA* 262:2395–401, 1989

31. Helmrich SP, Ragland DR, Leung RW, Paffenbarger RS Jr: Physical activity and reduced occurrence of non-insulin-dependent diabetes mellitus. *N Engl J Med* 325:147–52, 1991

32. American College of Sports Medicine: The recommended quantity and quality of exercise for developing and maintaining cardiorespiratory and muscular fitness in healthy adults. *Med Sci Sports Exercise* 22:265–74, 1990

33. Blomquist CG: Cardiovascular adaptations to physical training. *Annu Rev Physiol* 45:169–89, 1983

34. Clausen JP: Circulatory adjustments to dynamic exercise and effect of physical training in normal subjects and in patients with coronary artery disease. *Prog Cardiovasc Dis* 18: 459–95, 1976

35. Paterson DH, Shephard RJ, Cunningham D, Jones NL, Andrew G: Effects of physical training on cardiovascular function following myocardial infarction. *J Appl Physiol* 47:482–89, 1979

36. Redwood DR, Roring DR, Epstein SE: Circulatory and symptomatic effects of physical training in patients with coronary artery disease and angina pectoris. *N Engl J Med* 286:959–65, 1972

37. Ghilarducci LE, Holly RG, Amsterdam EA: Effects of high resistance training in coronary artery disease. *Am J Cardiol* 64:866–70, 1989

38. Hurley BF, Hagberg JM, Goldberg AP, Seals DR, Ehsani AA, Brennan RE, Holloszy JO: Resistive training can reduce coronary risk factors without altering VO_{2max} or percent body fat. *Med Sci Sports Exercise* 20:150–54, 1988

39. Hurley BF, Kokkinos PF: Effects of weight training on risk factors for coronary artery disease. *Sports Med* 4:231–38, 1987

40. Jennings G, Nelson L, Nestel P, Esler M, Korner P, Burton D, Bazelmans J: The effects of changes in physical activity on major cardiovascular risk factors, hemodynamics, sympathetic function, and glucose utilization in man: a controlled study of four levels of activity. *Circulation* 73:30–40, 1986

41. O'Connor GT, Buring JE, Yusuf S, Goldhaber SZ, Olmstead EM, Paffenbarger RS Jr, Hennekens CH: An overview of randomized trials of

rehabilitation with exercise after myocardial infarction. *Circulation* 80:234–44, 1989

42. Mittleman MA, Maclure M, Tofler GH, Sherwood JB, Goldberg RJ, Muller JE: Triggering of acute myocardial infarction by heavy physical exertion. *N Engl J Med* 329:1677–83, 1993

43. American Heart Association Writing Group: Exercise standards: a statement for health professionals from the American Heart Association (Special Report). *Circulation* 91: 580–615, 1995

44. Pollock ML, Wilmore JH (Eds.): *Exercise in Health and Disease: Evaluation and Prescription of Exercise for Prevention and Rehabilitation.* 2nd ed. Philadelphia, PA, Saunders, 1990, p. 105

45. American College of Sports Medicine: *Guidelines for Exercise Testing and Prescription.* 4th ed. Philadelphia, PA, Lea & Febiger, 1991

46. Butler RM, Beierwaltes WH, Rogers FJ: The cardiovascular response to circuit weight-training in patients with cardiac disease. *J Cardiopulm Rehab* 7:402–409, 1987

47. Blackburn H: Physical activity and hypertension. *J Clin Hypertens* 2: 154–62, 1986

48. Seals DR, Hagberg JM: The effect of exercise on human hypertension: a review. *Med Sci Sports Exercise* 16:207–15, 1984

49. Martin JE, Dubert PM, Lushman WC: Controlled trial of aerobic exercise in hypertension. *Circulation* 81:1560–67, 1990

50. Krotkiewski M, Lonnroth P, Mandroukas K, Wroblewski Z, Rebuffe-Scrive M, Holm G, Smith U, Bjorntorp P: The effects of physical training on insulin secretion and effectiveness and on glucose metabolism in obesity and type 2 (non-insulin-dependent) diabetes mellitus. *Diabetologia* 28:881–90, 1985

51. Leon AS: Effects of exercise conditioning on physiologic precursors of coronary heart disease. *J Cardiopulm Rehab* 11:46–57, 1991

52. Schneider SH, Khachadurian AK, Amorosa LF, Clemow L, Ruderman NB: Ten-year experience with an exercise-based outpatient lifestyle modification program in the treatment of diabetes mellitus. *Diabetes Care* 15:1800–10, 1992

53. Kahn J, Zola B, Juni J, Vinik A: Decreased exercise heart rate and blood pressure response in diabetic subjects with cardiac autonomic neuropathy. *Diabetes Care* 9:389–94, 1986

54. Hilsted J, Galbo H, Christensen N: Impaired cardiovascular responses to graded exercise in diabetic autonomic neuropathy. *Diabetes Care* 28:313–19, 1979

55. Van Camp SP: The safety of cardiac rehabilitation. *J Cardiopulm Rehab* 11:64–70, 1991

16. Nephropathy: Early

Highlights
Nephropathy: Early

- Many diabetic patients have a normal albumin excretion rate (<20 µg/min). In some patients, moderate exercise provokes albuminuria, but whether exercise-induced albuminuria in these individuals predicts progression is not yet known.
- The major factors for progression from normo- to microalbuminuria are poor metabolic control and high normal albumin excretion rate (10–20 µg/min).
- Good metabolic control reduces exercise-induced albuminuria.
- In patients with microalbuminuria (20–200 µg/min), albuminuria increases considerably with light to moderate exercise.
- Increases in baseline albuminuria without exercise are related to blood pressure elevation. With physical exercise, acute increases in albuminuria are also related to acute increases in blood pressure.

- Antihypertensive treatment decreases not only baseline blood pressure but also exercise-induced blood pressure elevation and abnormal albuminuria.
- In overt diabetic renal disease (albumin excretion >200 µg/min), there are marked changes in blood pressure at baseline. These changes are further aggravated by physical exercise, during which blood pressure may reach high levels.
- In the clinical setting, pragmatic guidelines are proposed. Patients with diabetes, especially with microalbuminuria and overt renal disease, should probably perform only moderate exercise; severe and erratic exercise may have a deleterious effect not only on metabolic control but also on vascular and renal disease, although such adverse effects have not been documented in clinical trials.

Nephropathy: Early

CARL ERIK MOGENSEN, MD

INTRODUCTION

Exercise proteinuria has been known for many years. There are early descriptions of the phenomenon, but the first published report was that of Collier in 1907, describing "functional albuminuria" in athletes (1). Since then, many papers on this topic related to normal renal physiology have been published (2–19). The first to describe comprehensively the hemodynamic effects of exercise on such parameters as heart rate and blood pressure in patients with diabetes was published in 1966 by the Swedish investigator T. Karlefors (20). A new era began around 1970 after the introduction of radioimmunoassay or other immuno-based techniques (21,22) as exact measurements of urinary albumin excretion rate.

Regular physical exercise is usually recommended as part of the clinical care of diabetic patients. Apart from its benefits, exercise may also have important implications for vascular function and disease. It is well known that diabetic nephropathy eventually may develop in about 1/3 of patients with insulin-dependent diabetes mellitus (IDDM) (23,24) and in a considerable number of patients with non-insulin-dependent diabetes mellitus (NIDDM). Patients with incipient and overt diabetic nephropathy are known to manifest generalized vascular complications, which could be exaggerated or complicated by the impact of exercise. Antihypertensive treatment and good metabolic control seem to be the most effective intervention measures in postponing progression of early and late renal disease (15,23). In this context, it is also important that exercise-induced blood pressure elevation be reduced during antihypertensive treatment (15,25–29).

RENAL AND BLOOD PRESSURE RESPONSE TO EXERCISE IN HEALTHY INDIVIDUALS

Numerous studies have explored the acute and prolonged effects of exercise on renal hemodynamics, albuminuria, and blood pressure. It is well known that exercise (e.g., on a bicycle ergometer) considerably increases blood pressure in direct relation to the exercise load (11,30,31). At the same time, exercise can cause pronounced changes in renal function (32). An outline of an exercise test is shown in Table 16.1. With severe acute exercise, some decline in the glomerular filtration rate (GFR) and an even more pronounced reduction in renal plasma flow (RPF) occur. Thus, the filtration fraction is considerably increased (32), and filtration pressure over the glomerular membrane is very likely increased. The

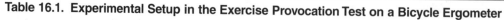

Table 16.1. Experimental Setup in the Exercise Provocation Test on a Bicycle Ergometer

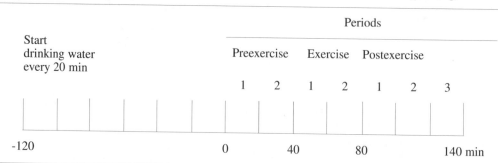

		Periods				
	Preexercise		Exercise		Postexercise	
Start drinking water every 20 min	1	2	1	2	1	2	3

-120   0   40   80   140 min

Heart rate was measured by counting the pulse rate; blood pressure by auscultatory technique; urinary albumin excretion and urinary ß₂-microglobulin excretion by radioimmunoassay; and GFR/RPF was optional.

Reproduced from Mogensen CE, Christensen CK, Vittinghus E: The stages of diabetic renal disease with emphasis on the stage of incipient diabetic nephropathy. *Diabetes* 32 (Suppl. 2):64–78, 1983.

latter may lead to an increase in urinary albumin excretion rate, especially with severe or prolonged exercise, even in normal individuals (31). Such exercise-induced changes in renal function are transient, and usually after 1 h at rest the hemodynamic pattern is again reversed (31,32). There are no reports indicating that exercise-induced changes in renal function in otherwise healthy individuals are deleterious in the long run. In other words, healthy individuals exposed to long-term exercise through their jobs or their sport activities do not appear to be more likely to develop renal disease.

RENAL AND BLOOD PRESSURE RESPONSE TO EXERCISE IN IDDM PATIENTS

Karlefors, many years ago, examined the hemodynamic response to exercise

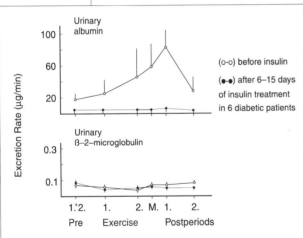

Exercise loads: 450 and 600 kpm/min.

M = mean of 2. exercise and 1. postperiod.

Figure 16.1 Urinary albumin and ß₂-microglobulin excretion at the onset of IDDM in young patients, before and after insulin treatment, as described in Table 16.1. Urinary albumin excretion indicates glomerular proteinuria; ß₂-microglobulin excretion indicates tubular proteinuria. The latter is not found.

Reproduced from Mogensen CE, Christensen CK, Vittinghus E: The stages of diabetic renal disease with emphasis on the stage of incipient diabetic nephropathy. *Diabetes* 32 (Suppl. 2):64–78, 1983.

in diabetic individuals with complications (20). Since then, numerous studies have been performed to explore the renal and blood pressure response to exercise in diabetic individuals (10–14,16,27,28,30–49a), especially after it became possible to measure urinary proteins in small concentrations (21,22). This review will focus on IDDM, because little information is available on the effect of exercise on renal function in patients with NIDDM (12,50,51).

Usually the baseline urinary albumin excretion rate is increased in newly diagnosed IDDM patients, at least in those with very poor glycemic control (31) (Fig. 16.1). This increase in albumin excretion rate is amplified by light and moderate physical exercise (31). ß₂-microglobulin excretion, a marker of tubular proteinuria, is normal, suggesting that the changes are of glomerular origin (10). It is also clear that glomerular hyperfiltration is often found at the time hyperglycemia is first diagnosed. With proper insulin treatment for a few weeks, these renal abnormalities are normalized, although some glomerular hyperfiltration usually persists. Most IDDM patients exhibit a normal baseline albumin excretion rate for the first 5 years after diagnosis (24), although new studies suggest that this is not universally the case (23).

NORMOALBUMINURIC DIABETIC INDIVIDUALS

In normoalbuminuric IDDM individuals, changes in GFR and RPF in response to exercise are similar to those in healthy people without diabetes. As in people without diabetes, exercise causes a slight reduction in GFR during exercise and a more pronounced reduction in plasma flow, resulting in an increased filtration fraction. Usually, filtration fraction is already increased at baseline in IDDM patients, and this abnormality is amplified by exercise (32). It is therefore not surprising that exercise may lead to an increased albumin excretion rate in a considerable proportion of patients with IDDM (Fig.

16.2). Exercise-induced microalbuminuria in diabetes was first described in 1975 (11). It soon became clear that the greatest increase occurred immediately after exercise (10) (Fig. 16.1). It was also apparent that this increase in albumin excretion is of glomerular origin, because ß$_2$-microglobulin excretion is not increased by exercise in these patients (Fig. 16.2). Thus, the exercise test reveals early glomerular changes or abnormalities (10).

In some studies, exercise-induced albuminuria was not different in normoalbuminuric patients with IDDM and healthy control subjects (36). This may reflect differences in diabetes duration and also the nature of the exercise test. Some investigators used a fixed exercise load, while others used a submaximal exercise load related to a calculated maximal exercise level (36).

It has been suggested that exercise-induced albuminuria (in normoalbuminuric individuals) could be a predictor of the later development of microalbuminuria in IDDM patients. However, no proper prospective long-term study has been conducted to clarify this issue. Furthermore, the considerable variability in exercise-induced albuminuria in patients with normal baseline values suggests this test may not be a valid predictor. Resting baseline values (e.g., overnight collections or early morning urine) show a gradual increase in albumin excretion with time in patients who progress to microalbuminuria or overt renal disease. For these reasons, longitudinal measurements of baseline values may provide more useful information than the exercise test, both in the clinical setting and in research projects. It should be remembered that baseline values for albumin excretion at rest may also show considerable variability; however, it is easy to do many repeated measurements. A potential use of the exercise test might be to study the response to antihypertensive treatment. It may be considered beneficial if administration of a drug not only protects against an exercise-induced blood pres-

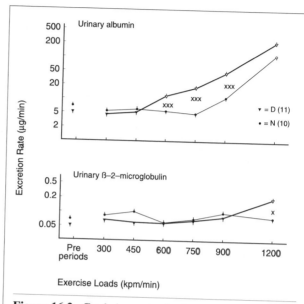

Figure 16.2. Graded exercise in diabetic and normal men; measurements of urinary proteins are in periods with increasing exercise.

Reproduced from Mogensen CE, Christensen CK, Vittinghus E: The stages of diabetic renal disease with emphasis on the stage of incipient diabetic nephropathy. *Diabetes* 32 (Suppl. 2):64–78, 1983.

sure elevation, but also ameliorates exercise-induced albuminuria (26–29).

Because exercise may induce microalbuminuria in normoalbuminuric individuals, care should be taken that urine samples collected after exercise are not used in the clinical follow-up of patients; early morning urine should be used instead (23).

MICROALBUMINURIC DIABETIC INDIVIDUALS

IDDM patients with microalbuminuria (urinary albumin excretion rates >20 µg/min) or incipient diabetic nephropathy usually show some increase in blood pressure in the basline resting situation. This increase is further aggravated by physical exercise, and usually there is a correlation between the albuminuria (Fig. 16.3) and the blood pressure increase (Fig. 16.4) induced by exercise (30). As in patients with normoalbuminuria, exer-

Whether the increased albuminuria caused by this mechanism promotes further renal damage is unknown, although it has been proposed that albuminuria in its own right may contribute to renal structural damage (23). To date, there is no evidence that short-term periods of exercise, by provoking proteinuria, cause renal damage. However, this possibility cannot be excluded.

INDIVIDUALS WITH DIABETES AND OVERT PROTEINURIA

Overt proteinuria is characterized by large increases in urinary albumin excretion to rates >200 μg/min. With the development of proteinuria, the decline in GFR usually starts. It has been shown that exercise increases blood pressure abnormally in proteinuric diabetic individuals (20). The clearance of large molecular dextran is also enhanced by exercise in these individuals (33). This has been attributed to depletion of negative charges on the glomerular capillary wall; however, whether this phenomenon influences exercise-induced proteinuria is unknown. The influence of exercise on the clinical status of patients with overt nephropathy has been poorly investigated and warrants further study.

THE DAILY LIFE EXERCISE SITUATION AND RENAL PROGNOSIS

As indicated, there may be a potential risk of more rapid progression of nephropathy in individuals who exercise intensively on a regular basis and thus have more exercise-induced albuminuria and blood pressure increases during their daily life situation. There are no definitive studies that address this important clinical issue. A study from Japan in a small series of patients suggests no difference in clinical outcome between individuals with diabetes who exercised to a limited extent and those who exercised heavily in their daily life situation (52). Less

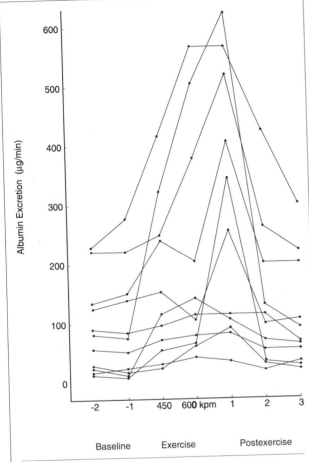

Figure 16.3. Urinary albumin excretion during exercise in young diabetic men with incipient diabetic nephropathy (baseline urinary albumin excretion at screening: 20–200 μg/min).

Reproduced from Mogensen CE, Christensen CK, Vittinghus E: The stages of diabetic renal disease with emphasis on the stage of incipient diabetic nephropathy. *Diabetes* 32 (Suppl. 2):64–78, 1983.

cise-induced albuminuria in patients with microalbuminuria at rest is of glomerular origin (10,30,31). It is likely that the increased systemic blood pressure response in microalbuminuric individuals is to some extent transmitted to the glomerulus, inducing a stretching effect on the glomerular structure and thus producing an increased glomerular passage of plasma protein molecules, in particular, albumin.

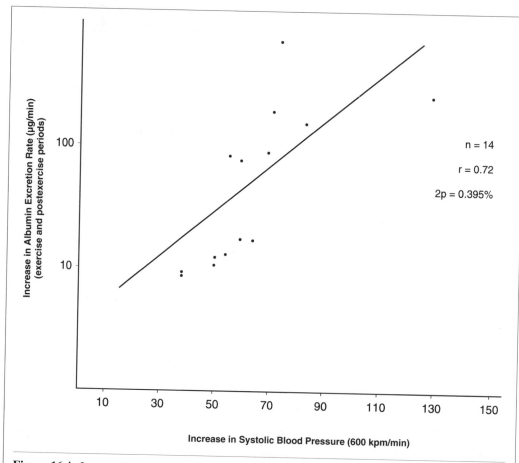

Figure 16.4. Increase in albumin excretion rate during exercise plotted against increase in systolic blood pressure during exercise (600 kpm/min) (patients as shown in Fig. 16.3).

Reproduced from Mogensen CE, Christensen CK, Vittinghus E: The stages of diabetic renal disease with emphasis on the stage of incipient diabetic nephropathy. *Diabetes* 32 (Suppl. 2):64–78, 1983.

questionable is the potential risk of severe exercise in patients with nephropathy who also have proliferative retinopathy. These patients may experience retinal hemorrhages as a result of substantial elevations in blood pressure (see Chapter 14).

EFFECT OF INTERVENTION PROGRAMS ON EXERCISE-INDUCED ALBUMINURIA

It has been documented that exercise-induced albuminuria can be reduced by good metabolic control in patients with IDDM (31,43,48). Exercise-induced albuminuria in IDDM patients can also be reduced in the short term as well as in the long term by antihypertensive treatment (26–28). An example is shown in Fig. 16.5. A similar effect of antihypertensive agents has also been observed in patients with essential hypertension (15,25,29). Exercise-induced albuminuria may be reduced by aspirin and dipyridamole, but further studies are needed to confirm this finding (40). A similar effect using picotamide in NIDDM patients was obtained by

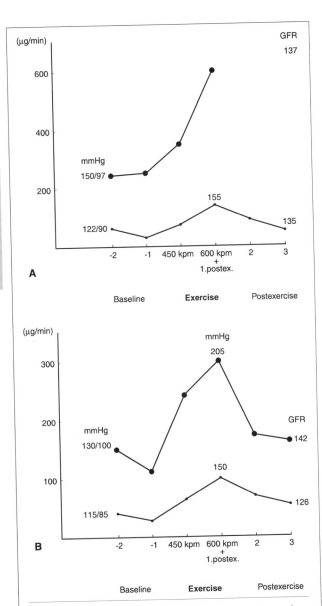

A

Baseline   **Exercise**   Postexercise

B

Baseline   **Exercise**   Postexercise

Figure 16.5. Albumin excretion before and after antihypertensive treatment. Data from exercise provocation tests.

Reproduced from Mogensen CE, Christensen CK, Vittinghus E: The stages of diabetic renal disease with emphasis on the stage of incipient diabetic nephropathy. *Diabetes* 32 (Suppl. 2):64–78, 1983.

Giustina et al. (53). Indomethacin seems also to reduce exercise-induced albuminuria (54).

PRAGMATIC EXERCISE RECOMMENDATIONS IN PATIENTS WITH IDDM AND NEPHROPATHY

It is questionable whether specific exercise recommendations are needed for most patients with incipient or overt nephropathy. In patients with overt nephropathy, there is usually self-limitation, because their exercise capacity is generally diminished. Clearly, however, it would not be prudent to recommend severe exercise or excessive sport activities in these individuals. On the other hand, there is no reason light to moderate exercise should be excluded from the patient's usual daily activities. Such exercise may be useful for other reasons, and it is unlikely to have any harmful effect on renal function.

NOTES REGARDING NIDDM

There are only a few studies about exercise-induced albuminuria in patients with NIDDM (12,50,51). Light to moderate exercise may induce microalbuminuria in these patients, and good control may ameliorate the abnormality (12). However, moderate-intensity exercise can be of importance in the clinical management of NIDDM patients, and there is no evidence that it has an adverse effect on renal prognosis. Rather, it should be encouraged. In the long run, such an exercise program may reduce the associated hypertension, although there are no clinical trials in this area. Note that patients with NIDDM are often quite sedentary, and in the clinical management of their disease, it is usually more advisable to propose, rather than discourage, exercise.

REFERENCES

1. Collier W: Functional albuminuria in athletes. *Br Med J* 1:4–6, 1907
2. Campanacci L, Faccini L, Englaro E, Rustia R, Guarnieri GF, Barat R, Carraro M, De Zotti R, Micheli W: Exercise-induced proteinuria. *Contrib Nephrol* 26:31–41, 1981
3. Castenfors J: Renal function during exercise with special reference to

exercise proteinuria and the release of renin (Abstract). *Acta Physiol Scand* 70 (Suppl.):293, 1967

4. Clerico A, Giammattei C, Cecchini L, Lucchetti A, Cruschelli L, Penno G, Gregori G, Giampietro O: Exercise-induced proteinuria in well-trained athletes. *Clin Chem* 36: 562–64, 1990

5. Houser MT, Jahn MF, Kobayashi A, Walburn J: Assessment of urinary protein excretion in the adolescent: effect of body position and exercise. *J Pediatr* 109:556–61, 1986

6. Houser MT: Characterization of recumbent, ambulatory, and postexercise proteinuria in the adolescent. *Pediatr Res* 21:442–46, 1987

7. Huttunen N-P, Käär M-L, Pietiläinen M, Vierikko P, Reinilä M: Exercise-induced proteinuria in children and adolescents. *Scand J Clin Lab Invest* 41:58–87, 1981

8. Kachadorian WA, Johnson RE: Renal responses to various rates of exercise. *J Appl Physiol* 28:748–52, 1970

9. Krämer BK, Kernz M, Ress KM, Pfohl M, Müller GA, Schmülling R-M, Risler T: Influence of strenuous exercise on albumin excretion. *Clin Chem* 34:2516–18, 1988

10. Mogensen CE, Vittinghus E, Sølling E: Abnormal albumin excretion after two provocative renal tests in diabetes: physical exercise and lysine injection. *Kidney Int* 16: 385–93, 1979

11. Mogensen CE, Vittinghus E: Urinary albumin excretion during exercise in juvenile diabetes: a provocative test for early abnormalities. *Scand J Clin Lab Invest* 35:295–300, 1975

11a.Dahlquist G, Aperia A, Carlsson L, Linne T, Persson B, Thoren C, Wilton P: Effect of metabolic control and duration on exercise-induced albuminuria in diabetic teenagers. *Acta Paediatr Scand* 72:895–902, 1983

12. Mohamed A, Wilkin T, Leatherdale BA, Rowe D: Response of urinary albumin to submaximal exercise in newly diagnosed non-insulin-dependent diabetes. *Br Med J* 288: 1342–43, 1984

13. Nordgren H, Freyschuss U, Persson B: Blood pressure response to physical exercise in healthy adolescents and adolescents with insulin-dependent diabetes mellitus. *Clin Sci* 86:425–32, 1994

14. Osei K: Ambulatory and exercise-induced blood pressure responses in type I diabetic patients and normal subjects. *Diabetes Res Clin Pract* 3:125–34, 1987

15. Pedersen EB, Mogensen CE, Larsen JS: Effects of exercise on urinary excretion of albumin and β_2-microglobulin in young patients with mild essential hypertension without treatment and during long-term propranolol treatment. *Scand J Clin Lab Invest* 41:493–98, 1981

16. Poortmans J, Dorchy H, Toussaint D: Urinary excretion of total proteins, albumin, and β_2-microglobulin during rest and exercise in diabetic adolescents with and without retinopathy. *Diabetes Care* 5:617–23, 1982

17. Poortmans JR: Postexercise proteinuria in humans: facts and mechanisms. *JAMA* 253:236–40, 1985

18. Robertshaw M, Cheung CK, Fairly I, Swaminathan R: Protein excretion after prolonged exercise. *Ann Clin Biochem* 30:34–37, 1993

19. Taylor A: Some characteristics of exercise proteinuria. *Clin Sci* 19: 209–17, 1960

20. Karlefors T: Circulatory studies during exercise with particular reference to diabetics. *Acta Med Scand* 180 (Suppl.):449, 1966

21. Keen H, Chlouverakis C: Urinary albumin excretion and diabetes mellitus. *Lancet* ii:1155–56, 1964

22. Miles DW, Mogensen CE, Gundersen HJG: Radioimmunoassay for urinary albumin using a single antibody. *Scand J Clin Lab Invest* 26:5–11, 1970

23. Mogensen CE: Definition of diabetic renal disease in insulin-dependent diabetes mellitus based on renal function tests. In *The Kidney and Hypertension in Diabetes*

Mellitus. 2nd ed. Mogensen CE, Ed. Boston, Dor-drecht, London, Kluwer Academic Publishers, p. 1–14, 1994

24. Mogensen CE: Microalbuminuria, early blood pressure elevation, and diabetic renal disease. *Curr Opin Endocrinol Diabetes* 1:239–47, 1994

25. Christensen CK, Krusell LR: Acute and long-term effect of antihypertensive treatment on exercise-induced microalbuminuria in essential hypertension. *J Clin Hypertens* 3:704–12, 1987

26. Christensen CK, Mogensen CE: Acute and long-term effect of antihypertensive treatment on exercise-induced albuminuria in incipient diabetic nephropathy. *Scand J Clin Lab Invest* 46:553–59, 1986

27. Romanelli G, Giustina A, Bossoni S, Caldonaxxo A, Cimino A, Cravarezza P, Giustina G: Short-term administration of captopril and nife-dipine and exercise-induced albuminuria in normotensive diabetic patients with early-stage nephropathy. *Diabetes* 39:1333–38, 1990

28. Romanelli G, Giustina A, Cimino A: Short-term effect of captopril on microalbuminuria induced by exercise in normotensive diabetics. *Br Med J* 298:284–88, 1989

29. Samuelsson O, Rångemark C, Lind H, Lindholm L, Pennert K, Hedner T: Lisinopril lowers postexercise albuminuria more effectively than atenolol in uncomplicated, primary hypertension. *J Hypertens* 12 (Suppl. 3):S43, 1994

30. Christensen CK: Abnormal albuminuria and blood pressure rise in incipient diabetic nephropathy induced by exercise. *Kidney Int* 25: 819–23, 1984

31. Vittinghus E, Mogensen CE: Graded exercise and protein excretion in diabetic man and the effect of insulin treatment. *Kidney Int* 21: 725–29, 1982

32. Vittinghus E, Mogensen CE: Albumin excretion and renal haemodynamic response to physical exercise in normal and diabetic man.

Scand J Clin Lab Invest 41: 627–32, 1981

33. Ala-Houhala I: Effects of exercise on glomerular passage of macromolecules in patients with diabetic nephropathy and in healthy subjects. *Scand J Clin Lab Invest* 50:27–33, 1990

34. Brouhard BH, Allen K, Sapire D, Travis LB: Effect of exercise on urinary N-acetyl-ß-D-glucosaminidase activity and albumin excretion in children with type I diabetes mellitus. *Diabetes Care* 8:466–72, 1985

35. Chase HP, Garg SK, Harris S, Marshall G, Hoops S: Elevation of resting and exercise blood pressures in subjects with type I diabetes and relation to albuminuria. *J Diabetic Complications* 6:138–42, 1992

36. Feldt-Rasmussen B, Baker L, Deckert T: Exercise as a provocative test in early renal disease in type 1 (insulin-dependent) diabetes: albuminuric, systemic and renal haemodynamic responses. *Diabetologia* 28:389–96, 1985

37. Garg SK, Chase HP, Harris S, Marshall G, Hoops S, Osberg I: Glycemic control and longitudinal testing for exercise microalbuminuria in subjects with type I diabetes. *J Diabetic Complications* 4:154–58, 1990

38. Groop L, Stenman S, Groop PH, Mäkipernaa A, Teppo AM: The effect of exercise on urinary excretion of different size proteins in patients with insulin-dependent diabetes mellitus. *Scand J Clin Lab Invest* 50:525–32, 1990

39. Hermansson G, Ludvigsson J: Renal function and blood-pressure reaction during exercise in diabetic and non-diabetic children and adolescents. *Acta Paediatr Scand* 283 (Suppl.):86–94, 1980

40. Hopper AH, Tindall H, Urquhart S, Davies JA: Reduction of exercise-induced albuminuria by aspirin-dipyridamole in patients with diabetes mellitus. *Horm Metab Res* 19:210-13, 1987

41. Huttunen N-P, Käär M-L, Puukka R, Åkerblom HK: Exercise-induced

proteinuria in children and adolescents with type 1 (insulindependent) diabetes. *Diabetologia* 21:495–97, 1981

42. Jefferson JG, Greene SA, Smith MA, Smith RF, Griffin NKG, Baum JD: Urine albumin to creatinine ratio response to exercise in diabetes. *Arch Dis Child* 60:305, 1985

43. Koivisto VA, Huttunen N-P, Vierikko P: Continuous subcutaneous insulin infusion corrects exercise-induced albuminuria in juvenile diabetes. *Br Med J* 282:778–79, 1981

44. Rubler S, Arvan SB: Exercise testing in young asymptomatic diabetic patients. *Angiology* 27:539–48, 1976

45. Torffvit O, Castenfors J, Bengtsson U, Agardh CD: Exercise stimulation in insulin-dependent diabetics, normal increase in albuminuria with abnormal blood pressure response. *Scand J Clin Lab Invest* 47:253–59, 1987

46. Townsend JC: Increased albumin excretion in diabetes. *J Clin Pathol* 43:3–8, 1990

47. Viberti GC, Jarrett RJ, McCartney M, Keen M: Increased glomerular permeability to albumin induced by exercise in diabetic subjects. *Diabetologia* 14:293–300, 1978

48. Viberti GC, Pickup JC, Bilous RW, Keen H, Mackintosh D: Correction of exercise-induced microalbuminuria in insulin-dependent diabetics after 3 weeks of subcutaneous insulin infusion. *Diabetes* 30:818–23, 1981

49. Watts GF, Williams I, Morris RW, Mandalia S, Shaw KM, Polak A: An acceptable exercise test to study microalbuminuria in type 1 diabetes. *Diabetic Med* 6:787–92, 1989

49a. Bognetti E, Meschi F, Pattarini A, Zoja A, Chiumello G: Postexercise albuminuria does not predict microalbuminuria in type 1 diabetic patients. *Diabetic Med* 11:850–56, 1994

50. Fujita Y, Matoba K, Takeuchi H, Ishii K, Yajima Y: Anaerobic threshold can provoke microalbuminuria in non-insulin-dependent diabetics. *Diabetes Res Clin Pract* 22:155–62, 1994

51. Inomata S, Oosawa Y, Itoh M, Inoue M, Masamune O: Analysis of urinary proteins in diabetes mellitus with reference to the relationship between microalbuminuria and diabetic renal lesions. *J Jpn Diabetic Soc* 30:429–35, 1987

52. Matsuoka K, Nakao T, Atsumi Y, Takekoshi H: Exercise regimen for patients with diabetic nephropathy. *J Diabetic Complications* 5:98–100, 1991

53. Giustina A, Bossoni S, Cimino A, Comini MT, Gazzoli N, Leproux GB, Wehrenberg WB, Romanelli G, Giustina G: Picotamide, a dual TXB synthetase inhibitor and TXB receptor antagonist, reduces exercise-induced albuminuria in microalbuminuric patients with NIDDM. *Diabetes* 42:178–82, 1993

54. Rudberg S, Sätterström G, Dahlquist R, Dahlquist G: Indomethacin but not metoprolol reduces exercise-induced albumin excretion rate in type 1 diabetic patients with microalbuminuria. *Diabetic Med* 10:460–64, 1993

ADDENDUM: RECENT REVIEWS ON OTHER ASPECTS OF RENAL DISEASE IN DIABETES

1. Mogensen CE: Systemic blood pressure and glomerular leakage with particular reference to diabetes and hypertension. *J Intern Med* 235:297–316, 1994

2. Mogensen CE: Renoprotective role of ace-inhibitors in diabetic nephropathy. *Br Heart J* 72:38–45, 1994

3. Mogensen CE: Glomerular hyperfiltration in human diabetes. *Diabetes Care* 17:770–75, 1994

4. Mogensen CE, Poulsen PL: Epidemiology of microalbuminuria in diabetes and in the background population. *Curr Opin Nephrol Hypertens* 3:248–56, 1994

5. Mogensen CE: Management of early nephropathy in diabetic patients with emphasis on microalbuminuria. *Ann Rev Med* 46:79–94, 1995

6. Hansen KW, Poulsen PL, Mogen-

sen CE: Ambulatory blood pressure and abnormal albuminuria in type 1 diabetic patients. *Kidney Int* 45 (Suppl.):S134–40, 1994

7. Mogensen CE, Vestbo E: Abnormal albuminuria and diabetic renal disease: microalbuminuria and the metabolic-vascular-renal-sydrome in NIDDM patients. In *Pathogenesis and Treatment of NIDDM and Its Related Problems.* Sakamoto N, Alberti KGMM, Hotta N, Eds. Amsterdam, Elsevier, 1994, p. 9–13

8. Mogensen CE: Management of the diabetic patient with elevated blood pressure or renal disease: early screening and treatment programs: albuminuria and blood pressure. In *Hypertension: Pathology, Diagnosis & Management.* 2nd ed. Laragh JH, Brenner BM, Eds. New York, Raven, 1995, p. 2335–65

9. Mogensen CE: Microalbuminuria: an important warning sign from the laboratory. *J Diabetes Complications* 8:135–36, 1994

10. Schmitz A: Renal function changes in middle-aged and elderly Caucasian type 2 (non-insulin-dependent) diabetic patients: a review. *Diabetologia* 36:985–92, 1993

11 Mogensen CE, Vestbo E, Poulsen PL, Christiansen C, Damsgaard E, Eiskjær H, Frøland A, Hansen KW, Nielsen S, Pedersen MM: Microalbuminuria and potential confounders: a review and some observations on variability of urinary albumin excretion. *Diabetes Care* 18:572–81, 1995

17. Nephropathy: Advanced

Highlights
Nephropathy: Advanced

■ Exercise capacity in patients on dialysis is lower than that of age-matched sedentary individuals.

■ Exercise capacity in patients on dialysis can be increased significantly by a graded exercise training program.

■ Exercise capacity in patients on dialysis can be increased significantly by correction of the anemia of chronic renal failure by synthetic erythropoietin.

■ Autonomic neuropathy, anemia, and myopathy limit exercise capacity in diabetic patients on dialysis.

■ Exercise capacity in patients receiving a successful renal transplant is similar to that of sedentary age-matched individuals.

■ A program of exercise and rehabilitation should be incorporated into the outpatient care plan for all patients on dialysis and after renal transplantation.

■ Treadmill exercise testing should be performed in all patients before initiation of an exercise program to help design the appropriate intensity level for the program.

■ The exercise program for patients on dialysis should be performed in the dialysis unit bolstered by the caring and enthusiastic support of the health-care team.

Nephropathy: Advanced

GREGORY L. BRADEN, MD

INTRODUCTION

Exercise capacity in patients on dialysis is significantly lower than it is in normal, age-matched sedentary individuals (1,2). Renal transplantation increases exercise capacity in most patients to the levels found in sedentary individuals with normal renal function (3). Although no studies of exercise capacity in diabetic, dialysis-dependent, or renal transplant patients have been performed, exercise studies in nondiabetic, dialysis, and transplant patients are useful in developing safe and beneficial exercise programs for diabetic individuals with renal disease.

EXERCISE CAPACITY IN DIALYSIS PATIENTS

Cardiorespiratory exercise tolerance is usually measured by exercising patients to exhaustion on either a bicycle ergometer or treadmill. Respiratory gases are analyzed for their volume, and the maximum oxygen uptake (VO_{2max}), expressed as $ml \cdot kg^{-1} \cdot min^{-1}$, is calculated. VO_{2max} is affected both by changes in cardiac output and the ability of peripheral tissues to use oxygen. VO_{2max} in dialysis patients is typically reduced to 50% of the level found in normal, age-matched sedentary individuals (1–3). The usual range of VO_{2max} in dialysis patients is 15–21 $ml \cdot kg^{-1} \cdot min^{-1}$ compared with a range of 30–40 $ml \cdot kg^{-1} \cdot min^{-1}$ in normal sedentary individuals.

In order to improve exercise capacity in dialysis patients, graded exercise training has been studied on nondialysis days (4,5) or during the hemodialysis session using a stationary bicycle ergometer (6,7). A 25% (range 15–42%) increase in VO_{2max} occurs in dialysis patients after completing a graded exercise training program. In addition, exercising patients on hemodialysis is safe and attenuates exercise-induced hyperkalemia (7).

The additional benefits of exercise training noted in Chapter 15 also occur in dialysis patients. Thus, in one study, improved blood pressure control after 26 weeks of exercise training allowed seven out of eight patients to discontinue antihypertensive therapy (8). Improvement in plasma lipids occurred, with triglyceride levels decreasing by 37% and high-density lipoprotein cholesterol increasing by 17%. Finally, exercise training in dialysis patients decreases anxiety and depression and enhances functional status measured by improvement in the performance of the pleasant activities of daily life (see Chapter 5) (1,9).

Although submaximal exercise in diabetic dialysis patients is clearly beneficial, even a 25% increase in VO_{2max} does not increase exercise capacity enough in most dialysis patients to allow for more rigorous daily activities, such as washing windows, painting, or shoveling snow (2).

LIMITATIONS TO EXERCISE CAPACITY IN DIALYSIS PATIENTS

Cardiac dysfunction is common in diabetic patients and limits exercise capacity because of impairment of oxygen delivery to peripheral tissues. Measurements of cardiac output in exercising nondiabetic dialysis patients have demonstrated that the maximum increase in heart rate is only 75% of that in sedentary control subjects (10). In addition, diabetic patients frequently have autonomic neuropathy, which may limit the heart rate response to exercise.

The anemia of chronic renal disease might limit the increase in cardiac output needed to sustain exercise activity. Several studies have measured exercise capacity in dialysis patients before and after the administration of synthetic erythropoietin, which corrects the anemia of chronic renal failure (10). Although erythropoietin increases the hematocrit in patients on dialysis to near-normal levels, VO_{2max} increases by only 20% (range 5–25%). Surprisingly, the maximum cardiac output obtainable during exercise was unchanged even though erythropoietin produced significant increases in hematocrit. In addition, the maximal obtainable cardiac output in patients on dialysis was 16 liters/min, which is well below that seen in normal sedentary individuals (range 25–30 liters/min), presumably due to the reduced heart rate response to exercise in patients on dialysis (10). This observation led these investigators to conclude that other factors, such as uremic myopathy (which might decrease tissue oxygen utilization), must reduce VO_{2max} in dialysis patients.

Myopathy in dialysis patients limits exercise capacity; in fact, measurements of isokinetic power in these patients correlate better with VO_{2max} than do any other measurable parameters (11,12). Muscle biopsies demonstrate abnormalities in Type I and Type II fiber areas in predialysis and dialysis patients (12,13). In addition, studies measuring the arterial-venous O_2 difference during exercise in dialysis patients, either at low or near-normal hematocrits, show that the A-VO_2 difference does not increase as hematocrit increases because of decreased tissue oxygen utilization (10). These abnormalities may be partially reversed by exercise training. Thus, myopathy in dialysis patients, with or without diabetes, is an important limiting factor to exercise capacity.

EXERCISE CAPACITY AFTER RENAL TRANSPLANTATION

Exercise capacity, measured as VO_{2max} in patients receiving a successful renal transplant, is similar to that of sedentary age-matched control subjects (3,14). This improvement in exercise capacity is due, in part, to correction of anemia. However, increases in VO_{2max} in renal transplant patients do not fully correlate with increases in hematocrit, and other factors, such as correction of uremic myopathy, may be important (15). In addition, exercise capacity in renal transplant recipients is further enhanced by graded exercise training (16). One study compared renal transplant patients who complet-

ed a 24-week exercise training program to untrained age-matched control subjects (15). Although the preexercise VO_{2max} in renal transplant patients was 29 ml·kg^{-1}·min^{-1} compared with 48 ml·kg^{-1}·min^{-1} in normal control subjects, VO_{2max} increased to 37.5 ml·kg^{-1}·min^{-1} after exercise training. However, muscle metabolism in the best-conditioned transplant patients in this study showed decreased oxidative enzyme activity compared with untrained control patients, possibly because of the catabolic effects of glucocorticoid agents used to prevent rejection (15). In summary, renal transplantation appears to be the most effective way to improve exercise capacity in patients with end-stage renal disease. Most patients reach near-normal levels of exercise capacity after renal transplantation.

RECOMMENDATIONS FOR EXERCISE TRAINING IN DIABETIC PATIENTS WITH RENAL DISEASE

Prevention of Disability

It is important to prevent functional deterioration as patients approach the need for dialysis. Before the initiation of dialysis therapy, the hematocrit can be increased to near-normal levels by subcutaneous erythropoietin. In addition, normal calcium and phosphorus homeostasis should be maintained to prevent secondary hyperparathyroidism by prescribing oral calcium and, if needed, calcitriol. Dialysis should be initiated before patients develop uremia, which may limit their functional status and require a longer period of rehabilitation. New dialysis patients often require frequent hospital admissions, and physical therapy and occupational therapy should be provided early to maintain functional status.

Special Considerations in Dialysis Patients

As dialysis is initiated, a program of exercise and rehabilitation should be incorporated into the outpatient care plan for all patients. In diabetic patients, it is important to assess the level of cardiac function and to screen for subclinical coronary artery disease (see Chapters 6, 15, and 18), since diabetes, hypertension, hyperlipidemia, and the uremic milieu are all associated with accelerated atherosclerosis. Treadmill stress testing is useful to assess the level of physical conditioning, exercise-induced changes in blood pressure, and the appropriate heart rate to prescribe for the exercise program (see Chapters 6, 12, 15, and 18).

Patients on dialysis should also be evaluated for other complications of diabetes that may affect their exercise capability. For example, many diabetic patients have peripheral vascular disease, sensory or motor neuropathy, autonomic neuropathy, and even amputations. A patient who can barely perform daily self-care activities can still benefit from exercise therapy, but appropriate physical and occupational therapy should be provided while the exercise program is being designed.

Design of Exercise Program

Any exercise program should be carefully designed to meet the individual needs of each patient, with particular attention paid to expectations for improvement by determining realistic goals for each patient. This is accomplished by a skilled and coordinated support staff, including enthusiastic and encouraging physicians, nurses, physical therapists, and, when needed, occupational and cardiac rehabilitation therapists. Because there have been no studies of the efficacy and safety of graded exercise in diabetic patients on dialysis, care providers should be cautious and conservative in determining the exercise prescription for each patient, and careful monitoring of each patient must be provided.

The exercise program for a dialysis patient should also take into account where the exercise will take place. If the dialysis facility does not have an in-center exercise program, then the patient will need to be referred to community programs, such as those associated with work, the Young Men's Christian Association (YMCA), the Jewish Community Center, or health clubs. Ideally, the dialysis center should provide a graded exercise program during hemodialysis using a modified bicycle ergometer that allows the patient to perform stationary cycling from the dialysis chair (6,7). This method of exercise is safe, decreases the boredom of chronic hemodialysis, and attenuates hyperkalemia induced by exercise (7). The nurses in the dialysis unit can be trained to provide graded exercise training to the patients, an activity that enhances the patient/nursing relationship. An encouraging, supportive team approach by all personnel involved will help patients attain their goals. Patients on home dialysis must have their program designed for use either at home or at community facilities. Since the heart rate response of dialysis patients is diminished, especially in diabetic patients with autonomic neuropathy, the Borg scale of perceived exertion should be used to carefully monitor the level of exercise delivered during any exercise session (see Chapter 18).

After renal transplantation, an exercise program should be initiated as early as possible to attenuate glucocorticoid-induced muscle wasting. This can be accomplished once the patient is stable and free of rejection, which is usually 6–8 weeks after the transplant. The basic approach for transplant recipients is similar to that for diabetic patients on dialysis.

In summary, diabetic patients on dialysis and after renal transplantation can significantly improve their sense of well-being and functional status, reduce cardiovascular risk, and improve their ability to perform the activities of daily living with an exercise training program. An exercise program can be an important component of the effort to maintain a patient's functional status before and at the initiation of dialysis. It can also be an important component of the rehabilitation process after both the initiation of dialysis and renal transplantation.

REFERENCES

1. Painter P, Zimmerman SW: Exercise in end-stage renal disease. *Am J Kidney Dis* 7:386–94, 1986

2. Painter P: The importance of exercise training in rehabilitation of patients with end-stage renal disease. *Am J Kidney Dis* 24:S2–9, 1994

3. Painter P, Messer-Rehak D, Hanson P, Zimmerman SW, Glass NR: Exercise capacity in hemodialysis, CAPD, and renal transplant patients. *Nephron* 42:47–51, 1986

4. Goldberg AP, Geltman EM, Hagberg JM, Gavin JR III, Delmez JA, Carney RM, Naumowica A, Oldfield MH, Harter HR: Therapeutic benefits of exercise training for hemodialysis patients. *Kidney Int* 24:S303–309, 1983

5. Shalom R, Blumenthal JA, Williams RS, McMurray RG, Dennis VW: Feasibility and benefits of exercise training in patients on maintenance dialysis. *Kidney Int* 25:958–63, 1984

6. Painter PL, Nelson-Worel JN, Hill MM, Thornbery DR, Shelp WR, Harrington AR, Weinstein AB: Effects of exercise training during hemodialysis. *Nephron* 43:87–92, 1986

7. Burke EJ, Germain MJ, Fitzgibbons JP, Braden GL, Hartzog RA: A comparison of the physiologic effects of submaximal exercise during and off hemodialysis treatment. *J Cardiopulm Rehab* 7:68–72, 1987

8. Goldberg AP, Geltman EM, Gavin JR III, Carney RM, Hagberg JM, Delmez JA, Naumovich A, Oldfield MH, Harter HR: Exercise training reduces coronary risk and effectively rehabilitates hemodialysis patients. *Nephron* 42:311–16, 1986

9. Carney RM, Templeton B, Hong BA, Harter HR, Hagberg JM, Schechtman KB, Goldberg AP: Exercise training reduces depression and increases the performance of pleasant activities in hemodialysis patients. *Nephron* 47:194–98, 1987

10. Painter P, Moore GE: The impact of recombinant human erythropoietin on exercise capacity in hemodialysis patients. *Adv Renal Replacement Ther* 1:55–65, 1994

11. Diesel W, Noakes TD, Swanepoel C, Lambert M: Isokinetic muscle strength predicts maximum exercise tolerance in renal patients on chronic hemodialysis. *Am J Kidney Dis* 16:109–14, 1990

12. Moore GE, Parsons DB, Stray-Gundersen J, Painter PL, Brinker KR, Mitchell JH: Uremic myopathy limits aerobic capacity in hemodialysis patients. *Am J Kidney Dis* 22:277–87, 1993

13. Clyne N, Esbjornsson M, Jansson E, Jogestrand T, Lins L-E, Pehrsson SK: Effects of renal failure on skeletal muscle. *Nephron* 63:395–99, 1993

14. Painter P, Hanson P, Messer-Rehak D, Zimmerman SW, Glass NR: Exercise tolerance changes following renal transplantation. *Am J Kidney Dis* 10:452–56, 1987

15. Kempeneers BSc, Noakes TD, van Zyl-Smit R, Myburgh KH, Lambert M, Adams B, Wiggins T: Skeletal muscle limits the exercise tolerance of renal transplant recipients: effects of a graded exercise training program. *Am J Kidney Dis* 16:57–65, 1990

16. Miller TD, Squires RW, Gau GT, Ilstrup DM, Prohnert PP, Sterioff S: Graded exercise testing and training after renal transplantation: a preliminary study. *Mayo Clin Proc* 62:773–77, 1987

18. Neuropathy

Highlights
Neuropathy

- Neuropathy complicates the management of diabetes.
- Somatic neuropathy (calluses and warm insensate feet) with loss of reflexes or vibration perception increases susceptibility to ulcers, Charcot joint destruction, and limb loss.
- Autonomic nerve dysfunction impairs ability to exercise because of *1)* decreased systolic and diastolic cardiac function, *2)* orthostasis (insulin hypotension and edema) and nocturnal hypertension, *3)* impaired cutaneous blood flow and sweating, *4)* impaired pupillary reaction and night vision, and *5)* gastroparesis with irregular fuel delivery.
- Preferred exercises are non–weight-bearing.
- Rate of perceived exertion is a safer guide for exercise intensity than heart rate.
- A paradigm for exercise in patients with cardiovascular autonomic neuropathy is provided.
- Foot care education reduces risk of ulcers and gangrene by one-third.

Neuropathy

AARON I. VINIK, MD, PhD, FCP, FACP

INTRODUCTION

Diabetic neuropathy may have an impact on the risks and benefits of exercise in a number of untoward ways. Although there is good reason to believe that exercise is beneficial to people with diabetes in general, exercise programs for patients with diabetic neuropathy should be carefully managed to avoid disastrous consequences. It is quite appropriate to acknowledge the fact that exercise complicates diabetes management once neuropathy is present. Before providing specific recommendations for exercise in people with diabetic neuropathy, it is useful to review certain aspects of the different kinds of diabetic neuropathy.

TYPES OF NEUROPATHY

Somatic Neuropathy

Neuropathy is the most frequent complication of both insulin-dependent diabetes mellitus (IDDM) and non-insulin-dependent diabetes mellitus (NIDDM) (1–5). According to the San Antonio Convention (6), the main groups of neurological disturbances in diabetes mellitus include *1*) subclinical neuropathy determined by abnormalities in electrodiagnostic and quantitative sensory testing; *2*) diffuse clinical neuropathy with distal symmetric sensorimotor and autonomic syndromes, and *3*) focal syndromes. The signs, symptoms, and neurological deficits vary depending on the classes of nerve fibers that are involved. Neuropathies may be primarily sensory or motor (7–9) and may involve primarily small or large nerve fibers (10).

Small-Fiber Dysfunction

Small nerve fiber damage usually (though not always) precedes large nerve fiber damage and is manifested first in the lower limbs with pain and hyperalgesia, followed by a loss of thermal sensitivity and reduced light touch and pinprick sensation (11). Pain often occurs when nerve conduction velocity is normal or only minimally reduced (12). Small unmyelinated C-fiber damage is associated with loss of warm temperature perception. Pain is usually diffuse, superficial, burning, and dysesthetic; contact with clothes or objects, as well as disturbance of hair follicles, may be excruciating. Deeper pain may be sharp, like a toothache, or gnawing and is due to small myelinated A-delta fiber dysfunction, often accompanied by impairment of cold thermal perception (12,13).

Large-Fiber Dysfunction

Large-fiber neuropathies are manifested by reduced vibration and position sense, weakness, muscle wasting and depressed tendon reflexes, ataxia, and poor coordination. Exercise that requires coordination skills, such as golf and tennis, may be difficult for the patient with neuropathy. Most diabetic peripheral neuropathy is mixed, with both large nerve and small nerve fiber involvement. In our own outpatient population, only 15% of patients with symptoms of electrophysiologically confirmed neuropathy had no objective signs, and 63.7% of patients with signs had no symptoms (11). Thus, it is important to carry out thorough physical examinations before entering an exercise program. A very small proportion of patients show "pure" small nerve or large nerve fiber deficit (10,11).

Sensory neuropathy can be detected by a variety of sensitive quantitative tests (14), but simple identification of loss of vibration sense using a 256° tuning fork confers a relative risk of ulceration and limb loss of 15.5:1 (15). The population attributable risk (that proportion of the neuropathic population in whom ulceration and limb loss can be attributed to loss of large-fiber function) is very significant because of the frequency (≤78%) of loss of vibration perception in this population of subjects. Sensory neuropathy permits minor repeated trauma to cause skin ulcerations due to unperceived pressure. Absence of ankle reflexes may also predict ulceration and limb loss (16). The finding of calluses in a warm dry foot (autonomic neuropathy) confers a 77-fold increase in likelihood of limb loss.

Failure to educate patients with regard to foot care in the presence of neuropathy increases risk 3.2-fold for ulcers and subsequent limb loss (17). The presence of unilateral foot swelling, redness, heat, or discomfort after exercising or walking, even with minimal apparent neuropathy, should alert one to the possibility of a Charcot foot. These symptoms develop in feet with intact cutaneous blood flow and often with preserved small-fiber function. The rapidity with which Charcot foot can develop can be quite disconcerting. If the X-ray is normal, a bone scan should be considered. People with severe Charcot's joints (neuroarthropathy) should avoid weight-bearing exercises because they can result in multiple fractures and dislocation of the bones of the feet and ankle without the patient's awareness.

Diabetic Amyotrophies

The hallmark of diabetic amyotrophy is a triad of symptoms in older, more frequently male, patients: *1*) pain (often sudden in onset, but occasionally gradual) in proximal limb girdles, often beginning on one side and rapidly spreading to the other; *2*) weakness of the proximal muscles; and *3*) spontaneous or provoked fasciculation. Reflexes are diminished in proportion to the wasting, which can be quite profound. The condition is always associated with a distal symmetric polyneuropathy and may be part of a more generalized diabetic cachexia. Fortunately, it is self-limiting, and the patient usually recovers spontaneously within a year or two. It is the one condition in which the exercise prescription should not demand the use of the proximal muscles. On the other hand, recovery from the amyotrophy can be hastened by a well-designed rehabilitation program incorporating the use of weight training (11). Since the condition occurs in older people with long-standing diabetes, a weight-training program must be evaluated in relation to the presence of retinopathy and other complications that limit the use of weights.

Mononeuropathies

Single nerves are often involved in somatic neuropathy. The usual presentation is one of rapid onset, often with severe pain, mimicking a vascular crisis. For example, isolated third nerve palsies may be confused with a ruptured posterior communicating aneurysm (the key difference is retention of intrinsic nerve supply to muscles of the iris and pupillary reflexes in the mononeuritis). Other nerves often attacked include the 4th, 6th, 7th, ulnar, median, radial, lateral cutaneous of the thigh, femoral, sciatic, and sural nerves. The lesion is thought to be an infarct, and the patient recovers spontaneously, usually within a period of 6–8 weeks. Based on our experience, a passive or active exercise program may facilitate return of motor function of the nerves involved and help to preserve whatever muscle function escaped the initial attack (11).

Entrapment Syndromes

Entrapment syndromes are not usually uncovered by the physician unless they are far advanced or are gross. Common sites of nerve entrapment include the foot, where the medial and lateral plantar nerves are compressed, and the carpal tunnel, which compresses the median nerve. The ulnar nerve may also be compressed at the wrist or elbow and the lateral cutaneous of the thigh under the inguinal ligament. Since these conditions do not respond to any form of metabolic intervention, it is important to recognize the entrapping nature of the condition. Exercise constitutes a hazard, because repeated minor trauma accentuates the nerve compression and aggravates the symptoms.

Most people with diabetes have experienced a form of entrapment at some point in their lives and may seek surgery. The symptoms may be as mild as a little tingling in the fingers in carpal tunnel syndrome; however, the tingling may be deceptive, masking more extreme sensory symptoms that may spread to the remaining fingers and even up the arm into areas not supplied by the median nerve. The clinical picture, coupled with the signs of compression of the appropriate nerve, is usually clear enough to make the diagnosis. Confirmation can be obtained by electromyography. Once recognized, the key to a successful response is the cessation of all activity, especially of the repetitive traumatic type, splinting of the affected limb for support, and salvage of residual function. Surgical decompression may be necessary in cases where the condition is progressing, followed by an exercise program to rehabilitate the affected muscles (11).

Autonomic Neuropathy

The autonomic nervous system regulates all involuntary functions in the body, many of which are central to the consideration of an exercise program in the management of diabetes. Functional impairment of the autonomic nervous system accompanying diabetes mellitus was first described more than 40 years ago (18). Involvement of the autonomic nervous system can occur as early as the first year after diagnosis (2,19,20) and may involve any system in the body. Subclinical abnormalities in cardiovascular (21) and gastrointestinal function (22) may be found at diagnosis (23), even in teenagers with diabetes (24). However, clinical features of this form of neuropathy are often unsuspected and, without careful scrutiny, may go undetected. They include resting tachycardia with exercise intolerance, orthostatic hypotension, impaired sweating and cutaneous blood flow regulation, hypoglycemic unawareness, delayed gastric emptying, diarrhea alternating with constipation, bladder atony, and impotence in males.

The use of established, sensitive, and reproducible cardiovascular reflex tests shows a prevalence of 17–40% in the general diabetic population (24–27) and a prevalence of 31% in teenagers (24). In the latter, the neuropathy may be asymptomatic and not confer upon the individual an increased susceptibility to the dire consequences that accompany symptomatic autonomic neuropathy. The precise coincidence of sensorimotor and autonomic neuropathies is variable, but they commonly coexist. In people with peripheral neuropathy, 50% will have asymptomatic autonomic neuropathy (28). The presence of symptomatic autonomic complications is life-threatening, with estimates of mortality ranging from 25 to 50% within 5–10 years of diagnosis (2–4,28,29). Although this statistic emphasizes the need for early diagnosis and intervention, the causes of death are quite variable. They include sudden death for which no explanation has proved satisfactory, silent myocardial infarction with congestive failure or neuropathic cardiopathy, progressive renal failure, aspiration pneumonias with gastroparesis, and perioperative respiratory problems due to impaired hypoxia-induced respiratory drive. Thus, the detection of autonomic neuropathy should alert physicians to the factors contributing to premature demise. In this way, these patients should be more assiduously assessed for worsening renal function, atypical features of coronary artery disease, and congestive failure. Whether any benefit can be derived from intensification of the vigilance in asymptomatic patients with abnormal autonomic function tests remains to be established.

Cardiovascular Autonomic Neuropathy (CAN)

Abnormalities in autonomic function manifested by abnormal heart rate, blood pressure, or response could limit a patient's capability to perform exercise (30–34). Both hypertension (35) and hypotension (30,32,34,36) have been described during exercise in patients with abnormal autonomic function. Exercise tolerance in the person with clinically significant diabetic autonomic neuropathy may be extremely limited because of the impaired sympathetic and parasympathetic nervous systems that normally augment cardiac output and redistribute blood flow to the working muscle.

Diabetic patients with early CAN have resting tachycardia and decreased beat-to-beat variation at rest and during deep breathing (37). There is a progression from early parasympathetic dysfunction (resting tachycardia and lack of heart-rate variability) to later sympathetic dysfunction (impaired blood pressure responses to standing or sustained hand grip and a decrease in resting heart rate from the prior tachycardia) equivalent to a cardiac denervation syndrome (38–42).

In human beings, the maximal heart rate increase with exercise and the blood pressure responses to sustained hand grip, standing, and other types of exercise are mediated mainly by the sympathetic nervous system. In general, sympathetic loss follows parasympathetic dysfunction (39). However, widespread but uneven areas of sympathetic denervation of the heart, which appears normal in all other respects, have been demonstrated using the sensitive test of [^{125}I]metaiodobenzylguanidine scanning (43,44) and predict premature demise.

A high incidence of sudden or unexplained death, not associated with myocardial infarction or anesthesia induction, has been reported in diabetic patients with CAN (45–48); the mechanisms responsible for this sudden death appear diverse. Prolongation of the QT interval is associated with dysrhythmias. Diabetic patients with CAN and without evidence of ischemic heart disease, hypertension, renal disease, idiopathic long QT syndrome, or ingestion of medications known to affect cardiac repolarization have prolonged QT intervals corrected for heart rate (QT_c) (49). A prolonged QT_c interval is a marker for increased risk of sudden death (46–48). With time, QT/QT_c intervals lengthen significantly in association with deterioration of autonomic function. The longest QT/QT_c intervals were found in 13 patients who died over a 3-year period (8 of them died suddenly). The authors postulated a link between sudden death, possibly due to cardiac arrhythmia, and longer QT/QT_c intervals (48).

Diabetic patients with regional sympathetic imbalance and QT_c interval prolongation also may be at greater risk for arrhythmias because of the imbalance between the sympathetic and parasympathetic limbs of the autonomic nervous system. Although vagal stimulation has little intrinsic effect on the excitability of the myocardium, intact vagal function does oppose the arrhythmogenic effects of sympathetic tone (50). Exercise-induced hypoglycemia may activate the sympathetic nervous system and thus predispose to arrhythmia. Because diabetic patients with CAN have vagal denervation, they may lose the protective vagal slowing influence on adrenergic-mediated tachyarrhythmias. These arrhythmias are nearly impossible to detect because they occur so rarely; protracted monitoring or provocative testing may be required. We use the QT/QT_c interval from the electrocardiogram (EKG) as the "poor man's" test for CAN because it does not require sophisticated or time-consuming testing.

Diabetic patients with CAN have higher resting pressure-rate products than those without CAN (33) and lower maximal increases in heart rate, systolic blood pressure, and pressure-rate product (33). The severity of CAN correlates inversely with the maximal increase in heart rate and pressure-rate product (33). Diminished stroke volume at rest and with exercise has been observed in diabetic patients with CAN (51), and impaired ejection fraction responses have been noted (52).

Early radionuclide ventriculographic studies in diabetic patients who have been asymptomatic for a long period have demonstrated abnormal left ventricle ejection fraction responses to exercise (53,54). However, the interpretation of left ventricle function studies in these patients was hindered by the possibility of underlying ischemic heart disease. Our group studied resting and exercise radionuclide ventriculograms from patients with longstanding IDDM and NIDDM who had no clinical, EKG, or stress and resting tomographic thallium scan evidence of ischemic heart disease (52). Abnormal left ventricular systolic function at rest and during exercise was found in 37% of the diabetic patients. CAN was found in 91% of the diabetic patients with abnormal systolic function, and the incidence of abnormal systolic function was 59% in diabetic patients with CAN as opposed to 8% in those without CAN. Mean ejection fractions at rest and with maximal exercise were reduced in the patients with CAN when compared with those in patients without CAN.

We also examined left ventricular diastolic function in diabetic patients with CAN (55). Computer-assisted analysis of high temporal resolution time-activity curves from gated radionuclide ventriculograms were used to assess diastolic filling rates and time intervals. Of the patients, 21% had abnormal test results. The diabetic patients with abnormal left ventricular diastolic function had more severe CAN than those with normal test results. In addition, the patients with abnormal diastolic function had lower mean plasma levels of norepinephrine, both supine and standing, than those with normal diastolic function. The diabetic patients with CAN had a longer mean time-to-peak filling rate, even when normalized to the cardiac cycle length, than those without CAN. The strongest correlate of impaired diastolic filling was an excessive fall in blood pressure upon standing with decreased norepinephrine secretion (a previously described test of sympathetic neuropathy). The correlation of abnormal diastolic function with abnormalities of norepinephrine levels and sympathetic dysfunction suggests a role for sympathetic neuropathy in the cardiac diastolic dysfunction in patients with long-standing diabetes.

Thus, CAN could contribute to abnormal ventricular function in a variety of ways. For instance, abnormal coordination of peripheral arterial resistance and blood flow into vascular beds, such as the splanchnic, skeletal, and venous capacitance, at rest and exercise, could change the loading conditions of cardiac chambers. This could lead to abnormal changes in left ventricular volumes, pressures, and ejec-

tion fractions during exercise testing. In addition, the uneven sympathetic denervation of the myocardium could limit significantly the ability to enhance inotropic (contractility) and lusitropic (relaxation) function during exercise. Diabetic patients may have diminished cardiac reserves of catecholamines, further diminishing the effects of sympathetic innervation to the heart.

Physicians should be aware that as a group, diabetic patients with long-standing disease, particularly those with CAN, have a high incidence of abnormal exercise radionuclide ventriculographic test results, even in the absence of macrovascular coronary artery disease. Therefore, resting or stress thallium myocardial scintigraphy may be a more appropriate noninvasive diagnostic test for the presence and extent of macrovascular coronary artery disease in these patients (56).

Orthostasis

Orthostasis is defined as a fall in systolic blood pressure >30 mmHg upon standing, accompanied by symptoms of dizziness, feeling faint, pain in the back of the head, and loss of consciousness. Orthostasis occurs in CAN as a result of abnormalities in baroreceptor function, poor cardiovascular reactivity, and impaired peripheral vasoconstrictor responses. The combination of decreased release of catecholamines (57,58) with increased sensitivity to their vasoconstrictive effect (59–61) is a cause for concern during exercise, which activates the autonomic nervous system. Further compounding the problem with blood pressure regulation is loss of the normal diurnal rhythm of blood pressure modulation in diabetic patients with autonomic neuropathy (62). These patients may have paradoxical elevation of nocturnal blood pressure, as well as supine hypertension indicative of central sympathetic dysfunction. Of particular relevance is the observation that many people with the symptom complex become hypotensive with eating or within 10–15 min of taking their insulin injection. The symptoms, which are not unlike those of hypoglycemia, are often incorrectly ascribed to the hypoglycemic action of insulin, but occur too early and are actually due to a fall in blood pressure. Orthostasis poses many treatment problems, especially involving the timing of exercise in relation to meals and insulin shots (63).

Sweating Disturbances

Hyperhidrosis of the upper body, often related to eating and anhidrosis of the lower body, is a characteristic feature of autonomic neuropathy. Loss of lower body sweating can cause dry, brittle skin that cracks easily, predisposing one to ulcer formation that can lead to loss of the limb. Special attention must be paid to foot care, especially when exercising (see Chapter 13).

Alterations in Cutaneous Blood Flow

Microvascular skin blood flow is under the control of the autonomic nervous system and is often compromised by autonomic neuropathy. Diabetic patients have impaired responses to vasoconstrictive stimuli, such as cold. In addition, they have poor responses to vasodilators, such as heat (64). These abnormalities may precede all other evidence of neuropathy (65). The impaired vascular reactivity requires care with heat exposure. Although cutaneous blood flow may be accurately measured noninvasively using laser Doppler flowmetry (66), the clinical findings of dryness of the skin with cracking fissure formation and cold toes with bounding pulses is sufficient warning of underlying poor small vessel reactivity.

Edema

Edema often complicates autonomic neuropathy and can be managed with elevation of the foot in bed at night, use of body stockings by day, and administration of ephedrine (67).

Gastroparesis Diabeticorum

The major features of gastroparesis are early satiety, anorexia, nausea, vomiting, epigastric discomfort, and bloating. Gastroparesis is found in up to 25% of patients with brittle diabetes, including those without any gastroparetic symptoms. Hyperglycemia is a potent cause of paralysis of the stomach, and prolonged gastric emptying may simply reflect the blood glucose and not the condition of the gastric nervous system (68). Ultrasound has been introduced for diagnostic testing whereby the antral cross-section can be estimated at fasting and 180 min after a test meal; this may well replace the need to use isotopes or more invasive techniques (69). The major hazard to people with gastroparesis is the dissociation between the time of eating and the arrival of nutrients in the bloodstream. Every attempt should be made to normalize gastric emptying (68), and each patient should learn the vagaries of his or her own stomach with regard to fuel delivery before embarking on an exercise program. The belief that solid food will buffer the tendency toward exercise-induced hypoglycemia is not acceptable in gastroparesis. Rather, liquid supplements ought to be available during and after the exercise, since the rate of liquid emptying remains within normal limits in most individuals with gastroparesis (68).

Diarrhea

Diarrhea in autonomic neuropathy can be sudden, explosive, paroxysmal, nocturnal, seasonal, uncontrollable, and embarrassing (68). Individuals prone to such episodes should prehydrate and make preparations for adequate hydration before and during exercise. The severe and intermittent nature of diabetic diarrhea makes it difficult to anticipate these events with any degree of certainty. Protective padding may be necessary to avoid embarrassment.

Respiratory Dysfunction

Respiratory reflexes may be impaired in diabetic patients with CAN, resulting in cerebral hypoxia and depressed respiration that could potentially be affected by exercise. A temporal relationship between sudden cardiac arrest and interference with normal respiration by hypoxia, drugs, or anesthesia has been reported. Impaired hypoxic ventilatory drive occurs in diabetic patients with CAN (45). Sudden cardiopulmonary arrest in diabetic patients with CAN may be respiratory in origin, but the effects of exercise are not clear.

Pupillary Abnormalities
The pupil in diabetic autonomic neuropathy reacts poorly to light and does not dilate appropriately in the dark (70). This abnormality interferes with night vision and places subjects at risk of injury if exercise is performed at night. Patients should be warned about this possible hazard.

Autonomic Function Testing
Because the cardiovascular system is a prime target of autonomic dysfunction in diabetic patients, a number of simple, objective tests of cardiovascular function and reflexes have been developed to aid in the diagnosis of CAN (Table 18.1). Increased resting heart rate and loss of heart rate variation in response to deep breathing are primary indicators of parasympathetic dysfunction. Tests for sympathetic dysfunction include measurements of heart rate and blood pressure responses to standing, exercise, and hand grip. Abnormalities in two or more assessments are required for a diagnosis of autonomic neuropathy. However, there is a direct correlation between the number of abnormal autonomic function tests and both impaired cardiac

---

Table 18.1. Special Tests of Cardiovascular Function

TEST	METHOD/PARAMETERS
Resting heart rate	>100 beats/min is abnormal.
Beat-to-beat heart rate variation	With the patient at rest and supine (no overnight coffee or hypoglycemic episodes), breathing 6 breaths/min, heart rate monitored by EKG or Q-Med device, a difference in heart rate of >15 beats/min is normal and <10 beats/min is abnormal, R-R inspiration/R-R expiration >1.17 (abnormal <1.0).
Heart rate response to standing	During continuous EKG monitoring, the R-R interval is measured at beats 15 and 30 after standing. Normally, a tachycardia is followed by reflex bradycardia. The 30:15 ratio is normally >1.03.
Heart rate response to Valsalva maneuver	The subject forcibly exhales into the mouthpiece of a manometer to 40 mmHg for 15 s during EKG monitoring. Healthy subjects develop tachycardia and peripheral vasoconstriction during strain and an overshoot bradycardia and rise in blood pressure with release. The ratio of longest R-R to shortest R-R should be >1.2.
Systolic blood pressure response to standing	Systolic blood pressure is measured in the supine subject. The patient stands and the systolic blood pressure is measured after 2 min. Normal response is a fall of <10 mmHg, borderline is a fall of 10–29 mmHg, and abnormal is a fall of >30 mmHg.
Diastolic blood pressure response to isometric exercise	The subject squeezes a handgrip dynamometer to establish a maximum. Grip is then squeezed at 30% maximum for 5 min. The normal response for diastolic blood pressure is a rise of >16 mmHg in the other arm.
EKG QT/QT_c intervals	The QT_c should be <440 ms.

function and predisposition to premature demise (71) (Table 18.2).

EXERCISE PRESCRIPTION IN PATIENTS WITH NEUROPATHY

If, at the urging of the patient or in the opinion of the managing physician, exercise training is deemed appropriate, certain considerations pertaining to exercise in the diabetic patient with neuropathy must be addressed before the exercise program begins. Occult heart disease is a major concern, and repeated cardiac ischemia or arrhythmias may have serious consequences if not addressed (see Chapter 4). Symptoms of angina are not reliable indicators of important coronary artery disease in patients with diabetic neuropathy because of the higher frequency of silent myocardial ischemia and infarction in such patients (72). A high frequency of abnormal radionuclide ventriculographic responses to exercise in diabetic patients with a low likelihood of coronary artery disease reflects diabetic cardiopathy, which may be due to autonomic neuropathy. Therefore, we advocate exercise thallium scintigraphy as the preferred screening technique for coronary artery disease in this population (52). Evidence of myocardial ischemia or important arrhythmias during supervised stress testing must postpone plans for initiating an exercise program.

CAN must be addressed before embarking on regular exercise training. As mentioned previously, diabetic patients with CAN have blunted maximal heart rate and blood pressure responses to maximal exercise, a finding that must be integrated into the exercise prescription (36). There is a higher incidence of abnormal ventricular responses to exercise in patients with CAN, suggesting that slower progression and more careful monitoring of an exercise prescription are in order (52). CAN is associated with prolongation of the QT interval, and concern over the predisposition to ventricular arrhythmias associated with long QT intervals is prudent (73).

We recommend that exercise programs for diabetic patients with CAN be closely supervised, with consideration given to the poor exercise tolerance associated with resting tachycardia, lower maximal heart rate, and abnormal blood pressure responses: usually decreased maximal blood pressure, but occasionally, severely exaggerated increased blood pressure (71).

Pay special attention to the feet of diabetic patients before starting them on an exercise program. Neuropathy is a frequent accompaniment of diabetes. Proper fitting shoes are of great importance. Nail care, regular removal of calluses, and aggressive treatment of edema become crucial. Careful examination of the feet before and after exercise must become routine. One hour of education reduces by one-third the risk of an ulcer and foot loss. Pain may prevent patients from exercising. Superficial C-fiber pain can be reduced

---

Table 18.2. Effects of Diabetic Autonomic Neuropathy on Exercise Risk

Silent myocardial ischemia
- Resting tachycardia and decreased maximal responsiveness
- Decreased heart rate variability
- Orthostasis/hypotension with exercise
- Exaggerated blood pressure responses with supine position and exercise
- Loss of diurnal blood pressure variation
- Cardiovascular and cardiorespiratory instability
- Abnormal systolic ejection fractions at rest/exercise
- Abnormal diastolic filling rates/times at rest/exercise
- Poor exercise tolerance
- Failure of pupil adaptation to darkness
- Gastroparesis and diabetic diarrhea
- Hypoglycemia
- Decreased hypoglycemia awareness
- Hypoglycemia unresponsiveness
- Heat intolerance due to defective sympathetic thermoregulation and sweating (prone to dehydration)
- Susceptibility to foot ulcers and limb loss due to disordered regulation of cutaneous blood flow
- Incontinence

Adapted from Zola and Vinik (71).

by topical application of capsaicin (0.075% applied 4 times/day), use of body stockings to prevent movement of hair follicles, or clonidine (0.1–0.5 mg just before sleep; an initial dose of 0.1 mg should be titrated up slowly to avoid causing hypotension in a nonhypertensive person). Deep pain can be ameliorated by insulin infusion or mexilitine (an initial dose of 150 mg before the evening meal should be increased over several days to 10 mg·kg^{-1}·day^{-1} in four daily divided doses; mexilitine is contraindicated in patients with conduction abnormalities). If these measures fail, try amitriptyline (25–150 mg just before sleep; an initial dose of 25 mg should be titrated slowly upward to effect) or clonazepam (0.5–3.0 mg/day) with or without fluphenazine (1–6 mg/day) (13). Even minor pains cannot be ignored; we have seen patients continue to exercise for weeks on fractured feet, believing their injuries to be minor because of insensate feet.

Metabolic control must be assessed before exercise is begun. Regulation of fuel supply and demand to exercising muscles is complex; attempts at intensive management of diabetes center around the supply of insulin and glucose. Neuropathy results in major perturbations of the normal pattern of metabolic responses to exercise. In severely neuropathic patients with gastroparesis and with blood glucose values >240 mg/dl, inadequate insulin during exercise may result in decreased muscle uptake of glucose from the blood despite ongoing hepatic glycogenolysis and gluconeogenesis and inappropriate gut delivery of glucose, resulting in extreme elevations in serum glucose levels (6,20). Therefore, if blood glucose is >240 mg/dl, exercise is best left for another day.

Hypoglycemia is more frequently encountered in autonomic neuropathy during and after exercise and must be addressed before a regular exercise program is begun. Although insulin levels are normally suppressed during exercise, patients receiving exogenous insulin may, at times, be exercising in a high-insulin state, which suppresses hepatic glucose output. Couple that with failure of counterregulation and the result may be hypoglycemia during or soon after exercise (74,75). Furthermore, after exercise, the muscle continues to take up increased amounts of glucose for up to 8–12 h, and delayed hypoglycemia may result because of irregular gut fuel delivery and impaired counterregulatory hormone responses. Indeed, as little as 20 min of aerobic exercise in the early morning may be associated with hypoglycemia in the evening, and the association between the two go unrecognized by the unwary patient or physician.

Exercise for Patients With Peripheral Neuropathy

Non–weight-bearing activities that improve tone, poise, balance, and awareness of the lower extremities are appropriate exercise choices for patients with peripheral neuropathy (76). Recommended exercises include T'ai Chi, swimming, bicycling, rowing, and upper extremity (chair and arm) exercises (if they do not cause severe hypertension). For a detailed discussion, see Chapter 13.

Patients should begin with gentle pain-free stretching before exercise. More stretching can be done when the patient is fully warmed up. Patients with improved muscle function should be taught to stretch using props (e.g., a towel or stick).

Although exercise cannot reverse the occurrence of peripheral neuropathy, it can help slow the rate of its development and prevent further loss of fitness associated with disuse. Range of motion activities for the major joints (i.e., the ankle, knee, hip, trunk, shoulder, elbow, and wrist) should be performed to prevent or minimize contractures.

Exercise and Autonomic Neuropathy

Patients with symptomatic autonomic neuropathy are at high risk for developing complications during exercise. Sudden death and silent myocardial infarction have been attributed to autonomic neuropathy in diabetes, in which the heart has become unresponsive to nerve impulses (77). Hypotension and hypertension after vigorous exercise, particularly when starting an exercise program (78), are more likely to develop in patients with autonomic neuropathy. The risk of hypotension is greater in patients with significant autonomic neuropathy who perform high-intensity exercises with rapid changes in body position (79). There is also a strong correlation between autonomic neuropathy and microvascular disease. Patients with advanced retinopathy and nocturnal hypertension should not participate in anaerobic activity at night, especially weight lifting, because of increased risk for retinal hemorrhage.

Individuals with autonomic neuropathy can have difficulty in thermoregulation and are prone to dehydration. Therefore, they should avoid exercise in hot or cold environments and should be vigilant about adequate hydration. Because these patients are prone to hypoglycemia and may also have a reduced ability to detect hypoglycemia, they require more careful glucose monitoring.

Physicians should review the drug treatment list for their patients with orthostasis and eliminate, if possible, those drugs potentially contributing to hypotension with exercise. Also, physicians should encourage the use of full-length supportive garments, such as body stockings, to increase venous return during exercise. Patients with orthostasis should coordinate their exercise with their mealtimes and insulin shots and avoid administration of insulin immediately before beginning their exercise.

For patients with autonomic neuropathy, a conservative approach to exercise is best. For example, if a patient is unable to talk or maintain pedaling frequency, the exercise should be terminated. Whether patients with asymptomatic abnormalities in autonomic function tests are at similar risk is unclear, but a prudent approach to their exercise programs may be in order.

Insulin and Blood Glucose Monitoring

The metabolic response to exercise in patients with diabetic neuropathy is highly variable and cannot be predicted for an individual. Therefore, guidelines can only be viewed as approximate and alterations must be tailored for each patient.

Self-monitoring of blood glucose (SMBG) is the cornerstone of effective management. It is essential that patients master SMBG before exercise training begins (see Chapter 11).

In the insulin-requiring patient, a set time for exercising each day is best to minimize the number of adjustments necessary. Patients should be educated about the duration and peak actions of various insulin preparations in relation to gastric emptying to avoid exercising at peak insulin levels and before the stomach delivers its nutrient contents. In an attempt to gain maximal benefit from the acute glucose-lowering effects of exercise, exercise may be planned each day around a meal to blunt the glycemic fluxes (74,80) or can occur at home when the tardy stomach is emptying.

Patients must be made fully aware of the potential risk of early and delayed hypoglycemia. Patients should wear an I.D. bracelet or necklace that indicates the presence of diabetes and medications for use during exercise in the event of an emergency. Physicians should provide a prescription for syringes prefilled with 1 mg glucagon for emergency intramuscular administration and insist that the patient carry them.

It is important to avoid injecting insulin into the exercising limbs. The abdomen is the preferred injection site, especially in patients with autonomic neuropathy who are more prone to insulin-induced hypotension, which tends to be worse in the morning and improves later in the day (75). Exercise may thus have to be deferred.

Intensity of Exercise

Although gentle exercise for 20 min 3 times/week reduces the likelihood of foot loss, studies indicate that exercise at 50–75% of maximal oxygen uptake is required for improved cardiovascular fitness. The heart rate in non-neuropaths is a conveniently monitored reflection of maximal oxygen uptake and is used to guide management (see Chapter 6). A formula used with success to identify the target heart rate to be attained during exercise is 50–70% of the maximal heart rate minus the resting heart rate added to the resting heart rate: i.e., target heart rate = 0.5–0.7(maximum heart rate – resting heart rate) + resting heart rate. A more simple formula is to subtract the patient's age from 220 and multiply the result by 0.7. However, published tables of maximal expected heart rates must be avoided when preparing an exercise prescription, particularly in patients with CAN whose maximal levels are depressed (36). Rather, the rate of perceived exertion (RPE) scale (Fig. 18.1) should be used for determining exercise intensity for these patients. Patients should aim to achieve moderate-range RPEs gradually over 2–4 weeks. The intensity of the exercise should not be increased to compensate for an abbreviated exercise session. Isometric exercise in the patient with neuropathy may be in order, provided that it does not cause an excessive rise in blood pressure. Figure 18.2 is a suggested paradigm for exercise management of patients with autonomic neuropathy.

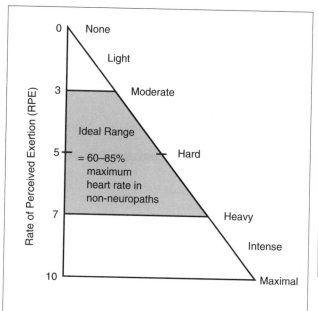

Figure 18.1. Suggested method for subjective evaluation of intensity of exercise in diabetic neuropathy.

REFERENCES

1. Harris M, Eastman R, Cowie C: Symptoms of sensory neuropathy in adults with NIDDM in the U.S. population. *Diabetes Care* 16: 1446–52, 1993
2. Ewing D, Campbell I, Clarke B: The natural history of diabetic autonomic neuropathy. *Q J Med* 49: 95–108, 1980
3. Ewing D, Campbell I, Clarke B: Mortality in diabetic autonomic neuropathy. *Lancet* 1:601–603, 1976
4. Sampson M, Wilson S, Karaginnis P: Progression of diabetic autonomic neuropathy over a decade in insulin-dependent diabetics. *Q J Med* 278:635–46, 1990
5. Boulton A, Knight G, Drury J, Ward J: The prevalence of symptomatic, diabetic neuropathy in an insulin-treated population. *Diabetes Care* 8:125–28, 1985
6. The American Diabetes Association: Report and recommendations of the San Antonio Conference on Diabetic Neuropathy. *Diabetes Care* 11:592–97, 1988
7. Thomas PK, Eliasson SG: Diabetic neuropathy. In *Peripheral Neuropathy.* Dyck PJ, Thomas PK, Lambert EH, Bunge R, Eds. Philadelphia, Saunders, 1984, p. 1773–1810
8. Ellenberg M: Diabetic neuropathy. In *Diabetes Mellitus: Theory and Practice.* Ellenberg M, Rifkin H, Eds. New York, McGraw-Hill, 1982, p. 777–801
9. Greene DA, Pfeifer MA: Diabetic neuropathy. In *Diabetes Mellitus: Management and Complications.* Olefsky JM, Sherwin RS, Eds. New

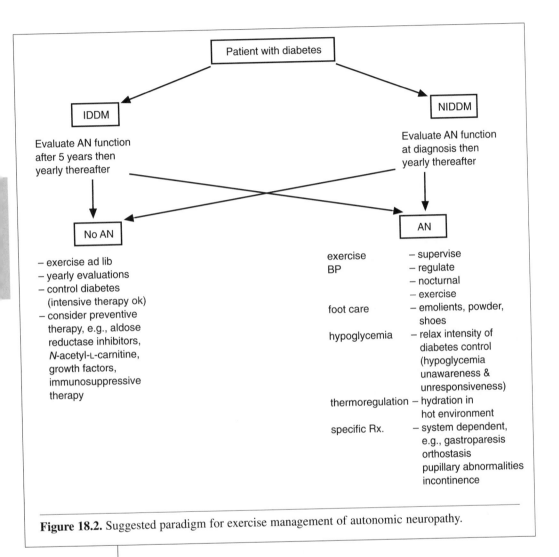

Figure 18.2. Suggested paradigm for exercise management of autonomic neuropathy.

York, Churchill Livingston, 1985, p. 223–54

10. Brown M, Asbury A: Diabetic neuropathy. *Ann Neurol* 15:2–12, 1984

11. Vinik AI, Holland MT, LeBeau JM, Liuzzi FJ, Stansberry KB, Colen LB: Diabetic neuropathies. *Diabetes Care* 15:1–50, 1992

12. Archer A, Watkins P, Thomas P, Sharma A, Payan J: The natural history of acute painful neuropathy in diabetes mellitus. *J Neurol Neurosurg Psychiatry* 46:491–99, 1983

13. Ross MA, Taylor TR, Vinik AI: Strategies for easing diabetic pain. *Patient Care* 27:48–72, 1993

14. Vinik AI, Suwanwalaikorn S, Stansberry KB, Holland MT, McNitt PM, Colen LE: Quantitative measurement of cutaneous perception in diabetic neuropathy. *Muscle & Nerve.* In press

15. Reiber GE, Pecoraro RE, Koepsell TD: Risk factors for amputation in patients with diabetes mellitus. *Ann Intern Med* 117:97–105, 1992

16. Nelson RG, Gohdea DM, Everhart JE, Hartner JA, Zweiner FL, Pettit

DJ: Lower extremity amputations in non-insulin-dependent diabetes: 12-year follow-up study in Pima Indians. *Diabetes Care* 11:8–16, 1988

17. Pecoraro RE, Reiber GE, Burges EM: Pathways to diabetic limb amputation: basis for prevention. *Diabetes Care* 13:513–21, 1990
18. Rundles RW: Diabetic neuropathy. *Medicine* 24:110–60, 1945
19. Pfeifer MA, Weinberg CR, Cook DL, Reenan A, Halter JB, Ensinck JW, Porte D Jr: Autonomic neural dysfunction in recently diagnosed diabetic subjects. *Diabetes Care* 7:447–53, 1984
20. O'Brien IA, O'Hare JP, Lewin IG, Corrall RJ: The prevalence of autonomic neuropathy in insulin-dependent diabetes mellitus: a controlled study based on heart rate variability. *Q J Med* 61:957–67, 1986
21. Ewing DJ, Bellavere F, Espi F, McKibben BM, Buchanan KD, Riemersma RA, Clarke BF: Correlation of cardiovascular and neuroendocrine tests of autonomic function in diabetes. *Metabolism* 35:349–53, 1986
22. Feldman M, Schiller L: Disorders of gastrointestinal motility associated with diabetes mellitus. *Ann Intern Med* 98:378–84, 1983
23. Fraser D, Campbell I, Ewing D: Peripheral and autonomic nerve function in newly diagnosed diabetes mellitus. *Diabetes* 26:546–50, 1977
24. Young R, Ewing D, Clarke B: Nerve function and metabolic control in teenage diabetics. *Diabetes* 32:142–47, 1983
25. Niakan E, Harati Y, Comstock J: Diabetic autonomic neuropathy. *Metabolism* 35:224–34, 1986
26. McLeod J, Tuck R: Disorders of the autonomic nervous system. II. Investigation and treatment. *Ann Neurol* 21:519–29, 1987
27. Ewing D, Clarke B: Diabetic autonomic neuropathy: present insights and future prospects. *Diabetes Care* 9:648–65, 1986
28. Vinik AI, Mitchell BD, Leichter SB, Wagner AL, O'Brian JT, Georges LP: Epidemiology of the complications of diabetes. In *Diabetes: Clinical Science in Practice.* Leslie RDG, Robbins DC, Eds. Cambridge, U.K., Cambridge University Press, 1994, p. 221–87

29. Bennett T: Physiological investigation of diabetic autonomic failure. In *Autonomic Failure: A Textbook of Clinical Disorders of the Autonomic Nervous System.* Bannister R, Ed. Oxford, U.K., Oxford University Press, 1983, p. 406–36
30. Hilsted J, Galbo H, Christensen NJ: Impaired cardiovascular responses to graded exercise in diabetic autonomic neuropathy. *Diabetes* 28: 313–19, 1979
31. Hilsted J, Galbo H, Christensen NJ: Impaired responses of catecholamines, growth hormones and cortisol to graded exercise in diabetic autonomic neuropathy. *Diabetes* 29:257–62, 1980
32. Hilsted J, Galbo H, Christensen NJ, Parving H, Benn J: Haemodynamic changes during graded exercise in patients with diabetic neuropathy. *Diabetologia* 22:318–23, 1982
33. Kahn J, Zola B, Juni J: Decreased exercise heart rate in diabetic subjects with cardiac autonomic neuropathy. *Diabetes Care* 9:389–94, 1986
34. Margonato A, Grundini P, Vicedomini G, Gilardi MC, Pozza G, Fazio F: Abnormal cardiovascular response to exercise in young asymptomatic diabetic patients with retinopathy. *Am Heart J* 112: 554–60, 1986
35. Karlefors T: Exercise test in male diabetes. *Acta Med Scand* 180 (Suppl. 449):3–80, 1966
36. Kahn JK, Zola B, Juni JE, Vinik AI: Decreased exercise heart rate and blood pressure response in diabetic subjects with cardiac autonomic neuropathy. *Diabetes Care* 9: 389–94, 1986
37. Wheeler T, Watkins PJ: Cardiac denervation in diabetes. *Br Med J* 4:584–86, 1973
38. Ewing D, Campbell I, Clarke B: Heart rate changes in diabetes mellitus. *Lancet* 1:183–86, 1981

39. Kempler P, Varadi A, Tamas G: Which battery of cardiovascular autonomic function tests? Suggestion for a rational diagnostic model. *Diabetologia* 33:640, 1990
40. Ewing DJ, Neilson JMM, Travis P: New method for assessing cardiac parasympathetic activity using 24-hour electrocardiograms. *Br Heart J* 52:396–402, 1984
41. Malpas SC, Maling TJB: Heart-rate variability and cardiac autonomic function in diabetes. *Diabetes* 39:1177–81, 1990
42. Bernardi L, Rossi M, Soffiantino F, Marti G, Ricordi L, Finardi G, Fratino P: Cross correlation of heart rate and respiration versus deep breathing. *Diabetes* 38:589–96, 1989
43. Sisson JC, Wieland DM, Sherman P, Mangner TJ, Tobes MC, Jacques JR: Metaiodobenzylguanidine as an index of the adrenergic nervous system integrity and function. *J Nucl Med* 28:1620–24, 1987
44. Sisson JC, Shapiro B, Meyers L, Mallette S, Mangner TJ, Wieland DM, Glowniak JV, Sherman P, Beierwaltes WH: Metaiodobenzylguanidine to map scintigraphically the adrenergic nervous system in man. *J Nucl Med* 28:1625–36, 1987
45. Sobotka P, Liss H, Vinik A: Impaired hypoxic ventilatory drives in diabetics with autonomic neuropathy. *J Clin Endocrinol & Metab* 62:658–63, 1992
46. Kahn JK, Sisson JC, Vinik AI: QT interval prolongation and sudden cardiac death in diabetic autonomic neuropathy. *J Clin Endocrinol & Metab* 64:751–54, 1987
47. Kahn JK, Sisson JC, Vinik AI: Prediction of sudden cardiac death in diabetic autonomic neuropathy. *J Nucl Med* 29:1605–606, 1988
48. Ewing DJ, Boland O, Neilson JM, Cho CG, Clarke BF: Autonomic neuropathy, QT interval lengthening, and unexpected deaths in male diabetic patients. *Diabetologia* 34:182–85, 1991
49. Gonin J, Kadrofske M, Schmaltz S: Corrected Q-T interval prolongation as diagnostic tool for assessment of cardiac autonomic neuropathy in diabetes mellitus. *Diabetes Care* 13:68–71, 1990
50. Kolman BS, Verrier RL, Lown B: Effect of vagus nerve stimulation upon excitability of the canine ventricle. *Am J Cardiol* 37:1041, 1976
51. Cryer PE: Normal and abnormal sympathoadrenal function in patients with insulin-dependent diabetes mellitus. *NY State J Med* 82:886–91, 1982
52. Zola B, Kahn J, Juni J, Vinik A: Abnormal cardiac function in diabetics with autonomic neuropathy in the absence of ischemic heart disease. *J Clin Endocrinol & Metab* 63:208–14, 1986
53. Mildenberger RR, Bar-Shlomo B, Druck MN: Clinically unrecognized ventricular dysfunction in young diabetic patients. *J Am Coll Cardiol* 4:213, 1984
54. Vered Z, Battler A, Sega P: Exercise-induced left ventricular dysfunction in young men with asymptomatic diabetes mellitus (diabetic cardiomyopathy). *Am J Cardiol* 54:633–37, 1984
55. Kahn JK, Zola B, Juni JE, Vinik AI: Radionuclide assessment of left ventricular diastolic filling in diabetes mellitus with and without cardiac autonomic neuropathy. *J Am Coll Cardiol* 7:1303–309, 1986
56. Kahn JK, Vinik AI: Exercise training in the diabetic patient. *Med Interne* 9:117–25, 1988
57. Hilsted J, Parving HH, Christensen NJ, Benn J, Galbo H: Hemodynamics in diabetic orthostatic hypotension. *J Clin Invest* 68:1427–34, 1981
58. Cryer PE, Silverberg AB, Santiago JV, Shah SD: Plasma catecholamines in diabetes: the syndromes of hypoadrenergic and hyperadrenergic postural hypotension. *Am J Med* 64:407–16, 1978
59. Barany FR: Abnormal vascular reactions in diabetes mellitus. *Acta Med Scand* 152 (Suppl. 304):3–129, 1955
60. Moorehouse JA, Carter SA, Doupe J: Vascular responses in diabetic peripheral neuropathy. *Br Med J* 1:883–88, 1966

61. Abrahm DR, Hollingsworth PJ, Smith CB, Jim L, Zucker LB, Sobotka PA, Vinik AI: Decreased alpha 2-adrenergic receptors on platelet membranes from diabetic patients with autonomic neuropathy and orthostatic hypotension. *J Clin Endocrinol & Metab* 63:906–12, 1986

62. Hornung RS, Mahler RS, Raftery EB: Ambulatory blood pressure and heart rate in diabetic patients: an assessment of autonomic function. *Diabetic Med* 6:579–85, 1989

63. Vinik A, Mitchell B: Clinical aspects of diabetic neuropathies. *Diabetes Metab Rev* 4:2233–53, 1988

64. Stansberry KB, Hill M, McNitt PM, Bhatt BH: Cutaneous blood flow reactivity and neuropathy (Abstract). *Diabetes* 43 (Suppl. 1): 107A, 1994

65. McDaid EA, Monaghan B, Parker AI, Hayes JR, Allen JA: Peripheral autonomic impairment in patients newly diagnosed with type II diabetes. *Diabetes Care* 17:1422–27, 1994

66. Neubauer B, Christensen NJ: Norepinephrine, epinephrine, and dopamine contents of the cardiovascular system in long-term diabetics. *Diabetes* 25:6–10, 1976

67. Edmonds M, Archer A, Watkins P: Ephedrine: a new treatment for diabetic neuropathic oedema. *Lancet* 1:548–51, 1983

68. Barnett JL, Vinik AI: Gastrointestinal disturbances. In *Therapy for Diabetes Mellitus and Related Disorders*. Lebovitz HE, Ed. Alexandria, VA, American Diabetes Association, 1994, p. 288–96

69. Burgstaller M, Barthel S, Kasper H: Diabetic gastroparesis and gallbladder disease: ultrasound diagnosis after multiple-component meals. *Dtsch Med Wochenschr* 117: 1868–73, 1992

70. Levy DM, Rowley DA, Abraham RR: Portable infrared pupillometry using Pupilscan: relation to somatic and autonomic nerve function in diabetes mellitus. *Clin Autonom Res* 2:335–41, 1992

71. Zola BE, Vinik AI: Effects of autonomic neuropathy associated with diabetes mellitus on cardiovascular function. *Curr Sci* 3:33–41, 1992

72. Chiariello M, Indolfi C, Cotecchia MR, Sifola C, Romano M, Condorelli M: Asymptomatic transient ST changes during ambulatory ECG monitoring in diabetic patients. *Am Heart J* 110:529, 1985

73. Kahn J, Sisson J, Vinik A: QT interval prolongation and sudden cardiac death in diabetic autonomic neuropathy. *J Clin Endocrinol & Metab* 64:751–54, 1987

74. Zinman B: Comparison of the acute and long-term effects of exercise on glucose control in type I diabetes. *Diabetes Care* 7:515, 1984

75. Berger M: Metabolic and hormonal effects of muscular exercise in juvenile type I diabetes. *Diabetologia* 13:355, 1977

76. Graham C, Lasko-McCarthey P: Exercise options for persons with diabetic complications. *Diabetes Educ* 16:212–20, 1990

77. Ewing D, Clarke B: Diagnosis and management of diabetic autonomic neuropathy. *Br Med J* 285:916–18, 1982

78. Vitug A, Schneider SH, Ruderman NB: Exercise and type I diabetes mellitus. *Exercise Sport Sci Rev* 16:285–304, 1988

79. Campaigne B, Lampman R: The clinical application of exercise in type I diabetes. In *Exercise in the Clinical Management of Diabetes*. Champaign, IL, Human Kinetics Publishers, 1994, p. 139–68

80. Caron D: The effects of postprandial exercise on meal-related glucose intolerance in insulin-dependent diabetes individuals. *Diabetes Care* 5:364, 1982

19. Musculoskeletal Injuries

Highlights
Musculoskeletal Injuries

■ Whether an athlete with diabetes mellitus is at greater risk for musculoskeletal injury than one without this disease is unknown.

■ Precautionary measures that alter or modify training methods, sports equipment, and/or mode of physical activity may reduce risk for athletic injury.

■ Individuals with diabetes should be encouraged to participate in regular exercise involving competitive or recreational sports and/or physical fitness for enjoyment and health.

Musculoskeletal Injuries

RICHARD M. LAMPMAN, PhD

INTRODUCTION

Routine exercise is engaged in for a variety of reasons. Many people exercise for relaxation and social camaraderie. Others participate for health, fitness, and recreation. Age is probably a major determinant for the interest level of physical activity of many individuals (Table 19.1). The young are more inclined to engage in competitive sports, whereas as one ages, recreation and health are usually given as the major reasons to exercise. Enhanced cardiovascular fitness, weight control, and increased muscular strength are typically what draw the interest of the middle-aged and elderly to exercise.

The more competitive the sport and the higher the intensity of the activity, the more likely the chance for injury. The prevalence of musculoskeletal injuries attributable to participation in these activities in individuals with and without diabetes mellitus has not been studied.

EXERCISE AS A THERAPY FOR DIABETIC INDIVIDUALS

Individuals with diabetes are encouraged to exercise routinely because of the well-documented physical, metabolic, and psychological benefits (1,2). As discussed elsewhere in this book, exercise may help normalize glycemia (see Chapter 3), enhance cardiovascular function (see Chapter 15), aid in weight loss for the individual with type II diabetes (see Chapter 10), provide psychological benefits (see Chapter 5), and may prevent or delay many pathologies associated with diabetes (see Chapters 4 and 24). Routine exercise or sports activities may also prevent or delay non-insulin-dependent diabetes mellitus in those at high risk for developing this disease (3-7) (see Chapters 4 and 24).

INJURIES ASSOCIATED WITH EXERCISE AND SPORTS

Individuals Without Diabetes

Musculoskeletal injuries associated with exercise and sports can be minimized by having knowledge of preventive measures and their application. Individuals need to be cognizant of their physical and medical limitations and of their metabolic and physiological responses to exercise. In addition, they should be knowledgeable of appropriate exercise training regimens and injury prevention. Because many injuries result from inappropriate training techniques, poor or faulty equipment, or biomechanical abnormalities, these factors should be closely monitored. Perhaps all athletes, including those with or without diabetes, who violate rules of training may be subject to acute or overuse injuries. A higher incidence of musculoskeletal injuries occurs with competitive sports. The aggressiveness of sports often requires a participant to perform maneuvers involving sudden accelerations and decelerations that can cause extreme biomechanical stresses resulting in musculoskeletal injuries. Trauma injuries happen frequently in contact sports, whereas overuse injuries to soft tissues, ligaments, muscles, and bone occur with repetitive sports such as jogging and running.

Table 19.1. Activity Interests Associated With Age

INTEREST LEVEL	YOUNG	MIDDLE-AGED	ELDERLY
1	Competitive Sports	Health/Fitness	Health/Fitness
2	Recreational Sports	Recreational Sports	Recreational Sports
3	Health/Fitness	Competitive Sports	Competitive Sports

Interest level: 1 > 2 > 3.

Individuals With Diabetes

Whether diabetic individuals exercising routinely or participating in sports have a greater propensity for injury than do people in the general population is unknown. An individual with diabetes may be at a disadvantage for high-intensity sports because of altered glucose production and/or utilization (8,9). However, whether this leads to athletic injuries secondary to abnormal muscle responses is unclear.

An epidemiological study conducted over a 3-year period showed an association between diabetes and obesity with sports-related, trauma-induced ankle fractures in middle-aged and older adults (10). Whether this relationship exists independent of obesity is unknown. Other reports (11-14) have suggested a relationship between diabetes and stress fractures of the lower extremities. These fractures may be associated with neuropathic bone changes (15), vascular disease (11), or reduced bone mass (16). Lower limb fractures may occur even in the young diabetic patient with or without symmetric peripheral neuropathy. Case reports of two diabetic runners in their early twenties suggest that jogging may increase the risk of bilateral calcaneal region stress fractures (14).

Upper extremity injuries, especially of the glenohumeral joint, also may be more prevalent in those with diabetes. Bridgeman (17) described an association of periarthritis (phases of severe pain, increasing stiffness, diminution in joint capacity, and slow recovery to normal) of the shoulder with diabetes. The incidence of this condition in 800 diabetic individuals was 10.8% and was significantly greater ($P < 0.005$) than the incidence of 2.3% found in nondiabetic subjects. Interestingly, 42% of diabetic patients had involvement of both shoulders, but this symmetrical problem appeared unrelated to polyneuropathy.

PREVENTION OF INJURIES

In general, a young person with diabetes should be encouraged to exercise (see Chapter 21) (1). Young athletes in good metabolic control need not be limited in their choice of recreational and competitive sports. The middle-aged to older individual with diabetes should be encouraged to lead a normal active lifestyle. The natural degeneration of muscles, bones, tendons, ligaments, and articular surfaces associated with aging may be accelerated with inactivity, and in the case of diabetes, may be more pronounced. Because they are often sedentary and may suffer from latent or overt metabolic and neurological abnormalities, some individuals with diabetes are potentially at greater risk for cardiac and musculoskeletal complications when exercising. Before beginning an exercise program, especially a high-intensity one, an individual should be thoroughly evaluated for any underlying medical problems that may put them at risk for injury. Aerobic exercise should be performed in ways that do not traumatize the feet. High resistance exercise using free weights or machines may be appropriate for young diabetic individuals but not for those with long-term diabetes. Systolic blood pressure, if monitored, should not go over 180 mmHg during exercise (18). A bracelet or shoe tag indicating an individual has diabetes and other relevant medical information should always be carried while exercising.

Overuse Injuries

Musculoskeletal injuries can result from chronic, repetitive, impact-related stresses rather than acute trauma. These are referred to as overuse injuries. They are common when an individual progresses from one level of training to a higher level too quickly. The beginner is usually enthusiastic, poorly conditioned, and often uses inferior equipment. Training overload by both inexperienced and competitive athletes can lead to musculoskeletal stress sufficient to cause strains, sprains, and fractures. The causes of these injuries can be multifactorial and may involve training errors, biomechanical factors, and poor equipment. Diabetic patients should set realistic exercise training goals with respect to intensity of effort, duration of sustained activity, and frequency of exercise (1). During an exercise session, the individual can help avoid musculoskeletal injuries by warming up thoroughly before the exercise and stretching and cooling down adequately after it is completed. If minor joint or muscle pain persists or becomes more severe, the diabetic individual should rest these areas for a few days. Alternative training modes should be performed until this condition subsides.

Major concerns for diabetic patients with either peripheral vascular occlusive arterial disease and/or peripheral neuropathy are repetitive physical activities that may traumatize the feet, ankles, and lower leg. Patients with diabetic neuropathy may have a reduction in the sensation of pain and be unaware of excessive impact forces (see Chapters 13 and 18). Unchecked forces associated with repetitive stresses in exercises such as brisk walking or jogging could place an individual at increased risk for lower extremity stress fractures. Suitable shoe selection is very important. Shoes should have a built-up heel to absorb impact forces and a good arch support (firm but not rigid) to prevent excessive pronation. The midsoles of athletic shoes, if constructed with air or silica gel pockets, provide additional absorbency of shearing forces generated by impact with the ground. Shoes having this feature can be very beneficial to those with peripheral neuropathy and/or microvascular disease. Rather than wearing tube-type socks that easily fold in the shoe and can cause blisters, a cotton/polyester blend sock with a constructed toe and heel design is best. An individual should carefully inspect his or her feet before and after exercise. In the event of an overuse injury to the foot in a person with diabetes, special care to minimize the danger of more serious complications has been recommended (19).

Trauma Injuries

No major studies have demonstrated that individuals with diabetes are at greater risk for trauma injuries than those without diabetes. In the event of injury in the general population, evidence suggests a higher prevalence of later life complications such as reduced range of motion, bursitis, articular laxity, tendinitis, and synovitis (20). Whether an individual with diabetes has a greater prevalence or severity of later life sequelae associated with a previous athletic injury is unknown.

CONCLUSIONS

Additional scientific and clinical evidence is necessary before it can be determined whether an individual with diabetes is at increased risk for musculoskeletal injuries when exercising. Although accidental trauma injuries occur in many sports, overuse injuries may be more prevalent in individuals with diabetes. This relates to the method of training usually recommended to diabetic individuals, namely, endurance training programs involving activities such as brisk walking and jogging. Inadvertent overuse injuries may be avoided by taking appropriate precautions to minimize potential problems. Treatment and rehabilitation for injuries should be similar to that for people without diabetes, pending further clinical or experimental information.

It is reasonable to recommend caution to a person with diabetes planning to engage in a high-intensity, repetitive-impact activity, such as brisk walking, jogging, or running. In most cases, the risk for complications and injuries can be minimized with adequate medical screening, prudent approaches to exercise training, proper equipment, and coordination of exercise, diet, insulin dosages, and hydration. Existing evidence suggests that the metabolic, physical, and psychological benefits of exercise training far outweigh the potential risks of musculoskeletal injuries in this population. A person with diabetes should not be discouraged or excluded from athletics, sports, or health/fitness-related activities unless the risk-to-benefit ratio suggests otherwise.

REFERENCES

1. Campaigne BN, Lampman RM: *Exercise in the Clinical Management of Diabetes*. Champaign, IL, Human Kinetics Publishers, 1994
2. Wallberg-Henriksson H: Exercise and diabetes mellitus. *Exercise Sport Sci Rev* 20:339–68, 1992
3. Cruickshanks KJ, Moss SE, Klein R, Klein BE: Physical activity and proliferative retinopathy in people diagnosed with diabetes before age 30 yr. *Diabetes Care* 15:1267–72, 1992
4. Frisch RE, Wyshak G, Albright TE, Albright NL, Schiff I: Lower prevalence of diabetes in female former college athletes compared with nonathletes. *Diabetes* 35:1101–105, 1986
5. Kujala UM, Kaprio J, Taimela S, Sarna S: Prevalence of diabetes, hypertension, and ischemic heart disease in former elite athletes. *Metabolism* 43:1255–60, 1994
6. LaPorte RE, Dorman JS, Tajima N, Cruickshanks KJ, Orchard TJ, Cavender DE, Becker DJ, Drash AL: Pittsburgh Insulin-Dependent Diabetes Mellitus Morbidity and Mortality Study: physical activity and diabetic complications. *Pediatrics* 78:1027–33, 1986
7. Perry IJ, Wannamethee SG, Walker MK, Shaper AG: Sporting activity and hyperglycemia in middle-aged men. *Diabetes Care* 16:581–83, 1993
8. Bak JF, Jacobsen UK, Jorgensen FS, Pedersen O: Insulin receptor function and glycogen synthase activity in skeletal muscle biopsies from patients with insulin-dependent diabetes mellitus: effects of physical training. *J Clin Endocrinol Metab* 69:158–64, 1989
9. Menon RK, Grace AA, Burgoyne W, Fonseca VA, James IM, Dandona P: Muscle blood flow in diabetes mellitus: evidence of abnormality after exercise. *Diabetes Care* 15:693–95, 1992
10. Daly PJ, Fitzgerald RH Jr, Melton LJ, Ilstrup DM: Epidemiology of ankle fractures in Rochester, Minnesota. *Acta Orthop Scand* 58:539–44, 1987
11. Conventry MB, Rothacker GW Jr: Bilateral calcaneal fracture in a diabetic patient: a case report. *J Bone Jt Surg* 61A:462–64, 1979
12. Daffner RH: Stress fractures: current concepts. *Skeletal Radiol* 2:221–29, 1978
13. Heath H III, Melton LJ III, Chu CP: Diabetes mellitus and risk of skeletal fracture. *N Engl J Med* 303:567–70, 1990
14. Jones R, Johnson KA: Diagnostic problems: jogging and diabetes mellitus. *Foot Ankle* 1:362–64, 1981
15. El-Khoury GY, Kathol MH: Neuropathic fractures in patients with diabetes mellitus. *Radiology* 134:313–16, 1980
16. Levin ME, Bolsseau VC, Avioll LV: Effects of diabetes mellitus on bone mass in juvenile and adult-onset diabetes. *N Engl J Med* 294:241–45, 1976
17. Bridgeman JF: Periarthritis of the shoulder and diabetes mellitus. *Am Rheum Dis* 31:69–71, 1972
18. Bernbaum M, Albert SG, Cohen JD: Exercise training in individuals with retinopathy and blindness. *Arch Phys Med Rehabil* 70:605–11, 1989
19. Coughoin RR: Common injuries of the foot: often more than "just a sprain." *Postgrad Med* 86:175–79, 182, 185, 1989
20. Raskin RJ, Rebecca GS: Post-traumatic sports-related musculoskeletal abnormalities: prevalence in a normal population. *Am J Sports Med* 11:336–39, 1983

IV. Exercise in Special Patient Groups

20. Women and Exercise

Highlights
Women and Exercise

EXERCISE AND PREGNANCY

- Exercise may not be efficacious for the pregestational woman with type I diabetes who is planning a pregnancy or is currently pregnant.
- Exercise in the form of arm ergometry is a safe and helpful adjunctive therapy to diet for a woman with gestational diabetes.
- Postpartum, if glucose control is maintained, the woman with diabetes should be able to return to an exercise program similar to that of a woman without diabetes.

AMENORRHEA AND EXERCISE

- The adolescent woman with diabetes who is amenorrheic needs intensive therapy to assure that she does not develop accelerated retinopathy when glucose control is achieved. If amenorrhea persists beyond the age of 16 years, treatment with estrogen therapy to protect the bones is advised.

OSTEOPOROSIS AND EXERCISE

- Women with diabetes should be offered a weight-bearing exercise program along with hormonal replacement therapy when they reach menopause. In addition, smoking cessation programs are recommended to improve the bone mass status. Insulin dosing for the exercising menopausal woman who is taking hormonal replacement therapy is complicated; thus, a team that is expert in insulin therapy is needed as part of the exercise program.

Women and Exercise

LOIS JOVANOVIC-PETERSON, MD

EXERCISE FOR THE PREGESTATIONAL WOMAN WITH DIABETES

The state of pregnancy may be considered to be a form of mild exercise: metabolic rate, minute ventilation, and respiratory exchange all increase to a level equal to mild-to-moderate exercise (1). When counseling a woman with type I diabetes who contemplates pregnancy, tight glucose control should be stressed. The risks of exercise to the pregnancy, including its sometimes negative impact on glucose control, should be emphasized. If exercise is undertaken in pregnancies complicated by diabetes (2), the insulin doses need constant surveillance to assure the best possible control under the circumstances (3).

The utility of an exercise program as part of the glucose control protocol for the woman with pregestational diabetes, be it insulin-dependent or non-insulin-dependent, is questionable. The paramount management goal for the best outcome of pregnancy is to achieve and maintain normoglycemia (4). Exercise adds an additional variable that may make glucose control more difficult. The only study to investigate the use of exercise to manage insulin-dependent diabetes in pregnancy used a walking program in women with type I diabetes (5) and found no improvement in after-dinner glucose levels.

Whether exercise in the first trimester increases the risk of a spontaneous abortion is not known. Women with type I diabetes have no increased risk of spontaneous abortion as long as their blood glucose levels are within four standard deviations of the levels of a pregnant woman without diabetes. If the blood glucose levels of a woman with diabetes are above four standard deviations, then her risk of spontaneous abortion rises dramatically in direct relation to her degree of hyperglycemia (6). Thus, exercise would only be a risk for a spontaneous abortion if the exercise program interfered with the maintenance of as near normal glucose levels as are feasible. If a woman with type I diabetes has vascular complications, then the recommendations for any type I patient who has vascular compromise should be followed, including restrictions of certain exercises for the patient with retinopathy. If a woman has preexisting or pregnancy-induced hypertension, then bedrest may be needed to manage the blood pressure and exercise cannot be performed. There are also obstetrical indications for bedrest during pregnancy that independently require that patients avoid exercise, such as vaginal bleeding (due to impending abortion or placental previa) or premature labor.

EXERCISE FOR THE WOMAN WITH GESTATIONAL DIABETES MELLITUS (GDM)

GDM is one form of diabetes occurring in pregnancy in which exercise may be a helpful adjunctive therapy (7–9). Current management of GDM consists of diet and careful monitoring of fasting and postprandial glucose levels. The goal of therapy is maintenance of euglycemia. When euglycemia is not achieved by diet alone, exercise can improve glucose intolerance and may obviate the need for insulin therapy.

GDM is considered to be, in part, a disease of glucose clearance, although it has been shown that this disorder is a heterogeneous entity (10). Initiation of insulin therapy per se is palliative, but does not speak to the primary defects(s), which may include hyperinsulinemia. Rather, treatment modalities that overcome peripheral resistance to insulin, such as sulfonylurea treatment or exercise, might be preferable. Although the sulfonylureas are reported to increase insulin sensitivity (11), these agents are contraindicated for use in patients with GDM in the United States (12).

One form of exercise has emerged as safe and efficacious for the sedentary, obese, unfit, aging, pregnant woman with GDM: arm ergometry. This form of exercise has only recently been applied to women with GDM (13).

Is exercise safe for the pregnant woman and her fetus? Most research in humans has used fetal heart rate as an indicator of fetal distress. While some researchers have observed marked fetal bradycardia during exercise, most have found no significant change (14–23). Some data suggest that exercise may increase uterine activity (24–27). However, Veille et al. (28) studied the effect of exercise on uterine activity in the last 8 weeks of pregnancy and found no effect on the prevalence of uterine contractions. They studied women before and after exercise, which consisted of either walking on an indoor track or riding on a bicycle ergometer. Neither fetal heart rate nor uterine activity were monitored during the 30 min of exercise. In addition, weight-bearing exercise has been shown to be an increased stress to the mother during pregnancy (29).

In summary, the safest form of exercise should not cause 1) fetal distress, 2) low infant birth weight, or 3) uterine contractions. It would also appear logical to avoid exercise that produces maternal hypertension (blood pressure >140/90 mmHg).

In a recent report (30), five types of equipment were used while maternal blood pressure, fetal heart rate, and uterine activity were monitored. Those exercises that use the upper body muscles or place little mechanical stress on the trunk appeared safest. When excessive weight-bearing by the lower body is avoided, workload can be increased safely, permitting a cardiovascular workout without fear of fetal distress. Women can be taught to palpate their uterus during exercise and stop exercising if they detect contractions.

Based on preliminary work to derive a safe mode of exercise for pregnant women, Jovanovic-Peterson et al. (13) applied arm ergometer training to a population of women with GDM and compared their glycemia to women with GDM who were only given diet instruction (31). The two groups' glycemic levels started to diverge by week 4 of the program. By week 6, the women in the exercise group had normalized their HbA_{1c}, fasting plasma glucose, and their response to a glucose challenge test. The women in the diet alone group did not improve their glucose levels. These observations appear contrary to the literature, which asserts that the natural progression of glucose intolerance during gestation is deterioration with increasing gestational age. The implications of these studies for the health care of women with GDM remain to be determined, although these results imply that a cardiovascular conditioning program might obviate insulin treatment in some women with GDM. The economic and health-care implications of these observations warrant further testing.

POSTPARTUM EXERCISE PROGRAMS

Women should be encouraged to resume an exercise program as soon as they feel ready. Most women are able to exercise by 2 weeks after a vaginal delivery. After a cesarean delivery it is recommended that 4–6 weeks pass before an exercise program is undertaken. As long as postpartum glucose levels are well controlled, women with diabetes recover at the same rate as women without diabetes. Thus, women with diabetes can safely return to an exercise program in the same time period as women without diabetes (32).

THE ASSOCIATION OF EXERCISE AND MENSTRUAL DISORDERS IN WOMEN WITH DIABETES

An important measure of pubertal development is an abrupt increase in growth velocity. This growth spurt occurs at a specific bone age rather than at a specific chronological age (33). The rapid growth phase decelerates at mid-puberty and ceases as bony epiphyseal fusion occurs.

A later growth spurt and later sexual maturation are associated with mild chronic illness and undernutrition. Exercise, as well as undernutrition, may have a profound effect on the pituitary-gonadal axis: delayed release of gonadotropins and subsequent delay in ovarian maturation in adolescent women. Numerous studies have shown that menarche occurs later in athletes than in nonathletes (34–36). Gonadotropin and steroid hormone patterns in amenorrheic athletic women show no monthly phasic elevations and no follicular or luteal development (34). Lack of effective gonadotropin stimulation is indicated by a largely quiescent and disorganized pattern of luteinizing hormone secretion (35), most likely the result of decreased activity of gonadotropin-releasing hormone pulse generator in the hypothalamus of the brain. One study clearly showed that exercise per se is a cause of menstrual irregularities (37). Normal cycling women become amenorrheic within 2 months of the initiation of a strenuous exercise program. Despite the effort by these investigators to control for caloric intake and weight, exercise could not be implicated as the only variable causing amenorrhea. Some proposed hypotheses as to the mechanism for exercise-associated amenorrhea include low body fat composition, hyperandrogenism, hyperprolactinemia, psychological and physical stress, and premature menopause (38). Two of these hypotheses seem to be most likely. The hypothalamic gonadotropin-releasing hormone pulse generator may be inhibited by an increase in adrenal hormone. Consistent with this hypothesis, most studies show mildly elevated cortisol levels in amenorrheic athletes (37). The second hypothesis, which is equally likely, is that there is a net energy drain. Caloric intake is not adequate to supply energy needs, and the amenorrhea is starvation-induced (39).

The American Association for Pediatrics (40) has suggested that low-dose oral contraceptives (50 µg estrogen equivalent per day) for amenorrheic girls over the age of 16 be prescribed to protect against skeletal demineralization. In addition, improved nutritional programs are needed to replace the increased energy needs of puberty and the energy costs of strenuous exercise. In the case of an amenorrheic athletic girl with type I diabetes, dietary instruction is paramount as part of the exercise program, not only as treatment of the exercise-induced menstrual disorder, but also to maintain as near normal blood glucose levels as is safe and feasible, for chronic hyperglycemia delays puberty and is associated with short stature. Normalization of blood glucose initiates a growth spurt in pubescent adolescent girls and menarche follows soon after (41). One concern associated with rapid normalization of blood glucose in the population of adolescents with diabetes is the risk of malignant diabetic retinopathy, postulated to be due to exaggerated growth hormone levels that aggravate a predisposed retina (41,42). Thus, the diabetes management program for an amenorrheic, adolescent woman with diabetes whose blood glucose levels are less than optimal should be carried out by a skilled health-care team to improve glucose control without aggravating retinal status.

OSTEOPOROSIS AND THE WOMAN WITH DIABETES: UTILITY OF AN EXERCISE PROGRAM

Currently, it is fashionable to define osteoporosis as a critical reduction in bone mass to the point that fracture vulnerability increases. In this sense, osteoporosis is analogous to anemia defined as a low red blood cell mass. However, this definition is not strictly accurate. Osteoporosis consists not only of a reduction in bone mass, but also of important changes in trabecular structure, such as trabecular perforation and loss of connectivity (43).

Osteoporosis, and the associated fracture risk, are major public health problems, especially for older women. Peak bone mass is attained by the second decade. There is then a marked acceleration of bone loss in women after menopause, especially during the immediate perimenopausal years (44). By the age of 65, women's bone mass falls to a critical point where women are at an increased risk of fracture. Men, too, lose bone mass after their menopause. However, because they reach a higher peak mass, the age at which they reach a critical fracture level is well into the seventh and eighth decades (Fig. 20.1).

The relationship between physical activity and bone mass has been well studied (45). These studies clearly show that bone responds to the physical stress of exercise. The observation that resistance exercise provides a superior stimulus for bone carries important therapeutic implications, because weight-bearing exercise has been traditionally prescribed to maintain skeletal integrity. Regular physical activity is likely to boost peak bone mass in young women, to slow the decline in bone mineral density in middle-aged women, and may increase bone mineral density in patients with established osteoporosis. Although serious resistance training in an elderly, frail population is not feasible, the benefits of high-intensity, progressive resistance training in some older subjects has been demonstrated. The reduction in risk of fracture in active women is highly significant compared with the relative risk in sedentary women (relative risk = 0.76). Furthermore, active individuals have greater muscle mass and are stronger, which also decreases the risk of falling (46,47).

The adaptations in aging skeletal muscle to exercise training may prevent sarcopenia, enhance the ease of carrying out the activities of daily living, and exert a beneficial effect on age-associated diseases to which diabetic women are predisposed: coronary artery disease, hypertension, osteoporosis, and obesity (45,48,49).

There has been an attempt to quantify the effectiveness of different exercises in increasing bone mass. Although these studies are indirect (50), there appears to be the greatest bone response when women run or walk up and down steps. Non–weight-bearing exercises, such as cycling, produced relatively low bone responses (51).

Although estradiol plays an important role in reproduction, this hormone can also exert physiological actions on a variety of nonreproductive tissues. Under certain conditions, estradiol can alter blood glucose levels by effects on gluconeogenesis and glycogenolysis (52). It can also alter plasma lipids by effects on their production and utilization. Thus, estrogens can lower plasma cholesterol levels in postmenopausal women (52). In some women with hypertriglyceridemia, they may increase plasma triglycerides, however.

Many studies have shown that estrogens increase the bone mineral content in menopausal women (53). Estrogen

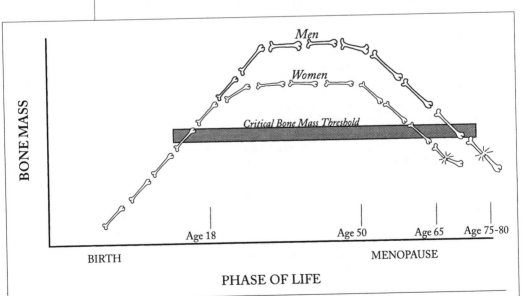

Figure 20.1. Schematic representation of bone mass accrual and bone mass loss to the point of critical levels that predispose to fracture. Men achieve a higher bone mass by early adulthood than women and thus have more reserves to forfeit before the critical level is achieved.

212

therapy also prevents bone loss in post-menopausal women who take it early in the postmenopausal period as well as later in life. If a woman stops taking estrogen after 7 years, however, when she reaches 75, bone density reveals only a minimal residual benefit (54). Therefore, estrogen therapy should be continued for a lifetime. When a menopausal woman is advised about the benefits of hormonal replacement therapy, she should be told that there is a slight increase in the risk of cancer, which must be weighed in each case. Also, women with either hypertension or cardiovascular disease need close monitoring of their status if and when hormonal replacement therapy is started.

Diabetes out of control is an independent risk factor for osteoporosis. In addition, end-stage kidney disease and associated secondary hyperparathyroidism also result in osteoporosis. Demineralization and pathological fractures are well-described complications of diabetes, along with Charcot's joints and osteoarthropathies. These conditions result in disuse atrophy of the muscles and thus a higher risk of falls. Improvement in glycemic control has markedly decreased the prevalence of these problems. Women with diabetes need exercise to maintain well-mineralized bones before menopause. Because estrogens have been reported to prevent bone loss and diminish the risk of cardiovascular disease, they are often recommended as part of the treatment of women with diabetes as long as they do not worsen glycemic control or markedly increase plasma triglycerides. Smoking decreases the effect of estrogen on the maintenance of bone density. Therefore, smoking cessation programs are mandatory for women with diabetes who are predisposed to osteoporosis.

Postmenopausal women with diabetes not on hormonal replacement therapy will need to decrease their insulin requirement about 20%. Guidance from the health-care team concerning the appropriate insulin adjustments is especially important. When an exercise program is combined with hormonal replacement therapy, the insulin regimen becomes especially challenging.

Menopause changes the diabetes program for women with non-insulin-dependent diabetes mellitus, also. Unfortunately, because menopause is associated with a decrease in metabolic rate, fewer calories are needed to maintain body weight. If caloric intake is not reduced by at least 20% after menopause, weight gain is inevitable (55). Adding exercise to the daily routine of a postmenopausal women allows her to ingest more calories and avoid weight gain. An exercise program for women with non-insulin-dependent diabetes mellitus not only prevents additional weight gain associated with menopause, but also independently decreases insulin resistance. Thus, the hyperglycemia associated with the weight gain of menopause is minimized.

REFERENCES

1. Bonen A, Campagna P, Gilchrist L, Young DC, Beresford P: Suhtrate and endocrine responses during exercise at selected stages of pregnancy. *J Appl Physiol* 73:134–42, 1992
2. Artal R: Exercise in gestational diabetes. In *Controversies in Diabetes and Pregnancy.* Jovanovic L, Ed. New York, Springer-Verlag, 1988, p. 101–11
3. Artal R, Wiswell RA, Drinkwater BL, St. John-Repovich WE: Exercise guidelines in pregnancy. In *Exercise in Pregnancy.* 2nd ed. Artal R, Wiswell RA, Drinkwater BL, Eds. Baltimore, Williams & Wilkins, 1991, p. 87–99
4. Jovanovic L, Druzin M, Peterson CM: The effect of euglycemia on the outcome of pregnancy in insulin-dependent diabetics as compared to normal controls. *Am J Med* 71:92–27, 1981
5. Hollingsworth DR, Moore TR: Postprandial walking exercise in pregnant insulin-dependent (type I) diabetic women: reduction of plasma lipid levels but absence of a significant effect on glycemic control. *Am J Obstet Gynecol* 157:1359–63, 1987

6. Mills JL, Simpson JL, Driscoll SG, Jovanovic-Peterson L, Van Allen M, Aarons JH, Metzger BE, Bieber FR, Knopp RH, Holms LB, Peterson CM, Witham-Wilson M, Brown Z, Ober C, Harley E, Macpherson TA, Duckles AE, Mueller-Heubach E, The National Institutes of Child Health and Human Development: Diabetes In Early Pregnancy Study: Incidence of spontaneous abortion among normal women and insulin-dependent diabetic women whose pregnancies were identified within 21 days of conception. *N Engl J Med* 319:1617–23, 1988

7. Horton ES: Exercise in the treatment of NIDDM: applications for GDM? *Diabetes* 40 (Suppl. 2): 175–78, 1991

8. Bung P, Artal R, Khodufuian N, Kjos S: Exercise in gestational diabetes: an optional therapeutic approach? *Diabetes* 40 (Suppl. 2): 182–85, 1991

9. Jovanovic-Peterson L, Peterson CM: Is exercise safe or useful for gestational diabetic women? *Diabetes* 40 (Suppl. 2):179–81, 1991

10. Summary and Recommendations of the Second International Workshop-Conference on Gestational Diabetes Mellitus. *Diabetes* 34 (Suppl. 2):123, 1985

11. Peterson CM, Sims RV, Jones RL, Rieders F: Bioavailability of glipizide and its effect on blood glucose and insulin levels in patients with non-insulin-dependent diabetes. *Diabetes Care* 5:497–500, 1982

12. Jovanovic L: Preface to *Controversies in Diabetes and Pregnancy*. Jovanovic L, Ed. New York, Springer-Verlag, 1988, p. vii

13. Jovanovic-Peterson L, Durak EP, Peterson CM: Randomized trial of diet versus diet plus cardiovascular conditioning on glucose levels in gestational diabetes. *Am J Obstet Gynecol* 161:415–19, 1989

14. Emmanouilides GC, Jobel CJ, Yashiro K: Fetal responses to maternal exercise in the sheep. *Am J Obstet Gynecol* 112:13–37, 1972

15. Jovanovic L, Kessler A, Peterson CM: Human maternal and fetal response to graded exercise. *J Appl Physiol* 58:1719–22, 1985

16. Dressendorfer E, Goodlin R: Fetal heart rate response to maternal exercise testing. *Physician Sportsmed* 8:91–94, 1980

17. Edwards M, Metcalfe J, Dunham M, Paul M: Accelerated respiratory response to moderate exercise in late pregnancy. *Respir Physiol* 45:229–41, 1981

18. Hauth JC, Gilstrap LC, Widmer CK: Fetal heart rate reactivity before and after maternal jogging during the third trimester. *Am J Obstet Gynecol* 142:545–47, 1982

19. Collings C, Curet LB: Fetal heart rate response to maternal exercise. *Am J Obstet Gynecol* 151:498–50l, 1985

20. Dale E, Mullinax K, Bryan D: Exercise during pregnancy: effect on the fetus. *Can J Appl Sport Sci* 7:98–103, 1982

21. Pomerance JJ, Gluck L, Lynch VA: Maternal exercise as a screening test for uteroplacental insufficiency. *Obstet Gynecol* 44:383–87, 1974

22. Hon EH, Wohlgemuth R: The electronic evaluation of fetal heart rate: the effect of maternal exercise. *Am J Obstet Gynecol* 81: 361–71, 1961

23. Artal R, Romem Y, Wiswell R: Fetal bradycardia induced by maternal exercise. *Lancet* 2:258–60, 1984

24. Pernoll ML, Metcalfe J, Paul M: Fetal cardiac response to maternal exercise. In *Fetal and Newborn Cardiovascular Physiology: Fetal and Newborn Circulation.* Vol. 2. Longo LD, Reneau DD, Eds. New York, Garland STPM Press, 1978, p. 67–84

25. Morris N, Osborn SB, Wright HP: Effective uterine blood flow during exercise in normal and preeclamptic pregnancies. *Lancet* 2:481–84, 1956

26. Erkkola R: The physical work capacity of the expectant mother and its effect on pregnancy, labor

and the newborn. *Int J Gynaecol Obstet* 14:153–59, 1976

27. Balfour M: The effect of occupation on pregnancy and neonatal mortality. *Publ Health* 51:106–10, 1938

28. Veille JC, Hohimer RA, Burry K, Speroff L: The effect of exercise on uterine activity in the last eight weeks of pregnancy. *Am J Obstet Gynecol* 151:727–30, l985

29. Artal R, Masaki KI, Khodi-quian N, Romen Y, Rutherford SE, Wiswell RS: Exercise prescription in pregnancy: weight-bearing versus non-weight-bearing exercise. *Am J Obstet Gynecol* 161:464–69, 1989

30. Durak EP, Jovanovic-Peterson L, Peterson CM: Comparative evaluation of uterine response to exercise on five aerobic machines. *Am J Obstet Gynecol* 162:754–56, 1990

31. Jovanovic-Peterson L, Peterson CM: Dietary manipulation as a primary treatment strategy for pregnancies complicated by diabetes. *J Am Coll Nutr* 9:320–25, 1990

32. American College of Obstetricians and Gynecologists: *Home Exercise Programs.* Washington, D.C., l986

33. Bullen BA, Skrinar GS, Beitins IZ, Von Mering G, Turnbull BA, MacArthur JW: Induction of menstrual disorders by strenuous exercise in untrained women. *N Engl J Med* 312:1349–53, 1985

34. Ding JH, Sheckter CB, Drinkwater BL, Soules MR, Bremner WJ, Shainholtz S, Southworth MB: High cortisol levels in exercise-associated amenorrhea. *Ann Intern Med* 108:530–34, 1988

35. Loucks AB, Mortola JF, Girton L, Yen SSC: Alterations in the hypothalamic-pituitary-ovarian and the hypothalamic-pituitary-adrenal axes in athletic women. *J Clin Endocrinol Metab* 68:402–11, 1989

36. Marcus R, Cann C, Madvig P: Menstrual function and bone mass in elite women distance runners: endocrine and metabolic features. *Ann Intern Med* 102:158–63, 1985

37. Louks AB, Vaitukaitis, Cameron JL, Rogol AD, Skrinar G, Warren MP, Kendrick J, Limacher MC: The reproductive system and exercise in women. *Med Sci Sports Exercise* 24:S288–93, 1992

38. Warren MP: The effect of exercise on pubertal progression and reproductive function in girls. *J Clin Endocrinol Metab* 51:1150–57, 1980

39. Tanner JM, Davies SWD: Clinical longitudinal standards for height and height velocity for North American children. *J Pediatr* 107:317–29, 1985

40. Committee on Sports Medicine of the American Academy of Pediatrics: Amenorrhea in adolescent athletes. *Pediatrics* 84:394–95, 1989

41. Drash AL, Daneman D, Travis L: Progressive retinopathy with improved metabolic control in diabetic dwarfism (Mauriac's syndrome). *Diabetes* 29 (Suppl. 2.): 1A, 1980

42. Tamborlane WV, Puklin JE, Bergman M, Verdonk C, Rudolf MC, Felig P, Genel M, Sherwin R: Long-term improvement of metabolic control with the insulin pump does not reverse diabetic microangiopathy. *Diabetes Care* 5 (Suppl. 1):58–64, 1982

43. Marcus R, Drinkwater B, Dalsky G, Dufek J, Raab D, Slemenda C, Snow-Harter C: Osteoporosis and exercise in women. *Med Sci Sports Exercise* 24:S301–307, 1992

44. Snow-Harter C, Marcus R: Exercise, bone mineral density, and osteoporosis. In *Exercise and Sports Medicine Reviews.* JO Holloszy, Ed. Baltimore, Williams & Wilkins, 1991, p. 606–18

45. Sorock GS, Bush TL, Golden AL, Fried LP, DeFronzo R: Increased insulin sensitivity and insulin binding to monocytes after physical training. *N Engl J Med* 301:1200–204, 1979

46. Talmage RV, Stinnett SS, Landwehr JT, Vincent LM, McCartney

WH: Age-related loss of bone mineral density in non-athletic women. *Bone Miner* 1:115–25, 1986

47. Pocock NJ, Eisman J, Gwinn T: Muscle strength, physical fitness and weight but not age predict femoral neck bone mass. *J Bone Miner Res* 4:441–47, 1989

48. Tipton CM, Vailas AC: Bouchard C, Shephard RJ, Stephens T, Sutton H, McPherson B (Eds.): *Exercise, Fitness and Health: A Consensus of Current Knowledge.* Champaign, IL, Human Kinetics Publishers, 1990, p. 331–34

49. Dalsky GK, Stocke KS, Ehsani RG: Weight-bearing exercise training and lumbar bone mineral content in post-menopausal women. *Ann Intern Med* 108:824–28, 1988

50. Rodgers MA, Evans WJ: Changes in skeletal muscle with aging: effects of exercise training. *Exercise Sport Sci Rev* 21:65–102, 1993

51. Woodward MI, Cunningham JL: Skeletal accelerations measured during different exercises. *J Engineer Med* 2017:79–85, 1993

52. van der Mooren MJ, de Graaf J, Demacker PN, de Haan AF, Rolland R: Changes in the low-density lipoprotein profile during 17 beta-estradiol-dydrogesterone therapy in post-menopausal women. *Metab Clin Exp* 43:799–802, 1994

53. Bunt JC: Metabolic actions of estradiol: significance for acute and chronic exercise responses. *Med Sci Sports Exercise* 22:286–90, 1990

54. Felson DT, Zhang Y, Hannan MT, Kiel DP, Wilson PWF, Anderson J: The effect of post-menopausal estrogen therapy on bone density in elderly women. *N Engl J Med* 329:1141–46, 1993

55. Reilly JJ, Lord A, Bunker VW, Prentice AM, Coward WA, Thomas AJ, Briggs RS: Energy balance in healthy elderly women. *Br J Nutr* 69:21–27, 1993

21. Children and Adolescents

Highlights
Children and Adolescents

With proper guidance and counseling, exercise participation can be a safe and successful experience for children and adolescents with insulin-dependent diabetes mellitus (IDDM).

■ Participating in exercise for a child with IDDM is complicated by the need for self-management in the areas of blood glucose monitoring, supplemental snacking, insulin adjustments, and coping with hypoglycemia.
■ The normalcy of play is challenged by the demands of maintaining glycemic control.

■ Physiological and psychosocial benefits of exercise mandate its inclusion in an activity program.
■ The general principles for adjusting insulin during and after exercise in adults may be similarly applied to children and adolescents with IDDM.
■ Parents must educate coaches, teachers, camp counselors, and teammates to the signs/symptoms of hypoglycemia.
■ Mandatory for safe participation in exercise is a well-conceived and rehearsed plan for treating hypoglycemia.

Children and Adolescents

JOY KISTLER, MS, CDE

INTRODUCTION

Managing diabetes mellitus creates many special situations for children with the disease. Not least among them are the considerations that surround physical activity—whether it be a far-ranging game of hide-and-seek with neighborhood friends or a more structured activity like Little League baseball or soccer. Getting to a Little League game becomes more than just putting on a uniform and grabbing a glove. The player and his or her parents must consider the timing of the game in relation to meals, insulin action, and snack requirements. A hypoglycemic treatment plan must be developed before leaving the house. The child with diabetes may be concerned not only about how well he or she will play but also about the potential embarrassment of being hypoglycemic in front of friends, coaches, and game spectators. This chapter provides a rationale for prescribing exercise and the guidelines necessary for ensuring safe and successful exercise of all kinds for children and their families.

BENEFITS

The benefits of physical activity, general play, and team sports for children, in terms of healthy childhood development, occur on many levels. The immediately apparent benefits, such as improved fitness and coordination, interact with the less obvious, but equally important, developmental areas like self-esteem and self-confidence. Along the way, it is likely that the child will learn something about important social skills, such as cooperation, teamwork, and group participation, as well.

While such experiences are an important and enjoyable part of the growing process for all children, exercise has yet another dimension for people with diabetes. In adults with the disease, the benefits of regular exercise include improved insulin sensitivity, cardiovascular fitness, and blood lipids, as well as decreased blood pressure. These are also important considerations for children with diabetes (1). Some scientific evidence demonstrates that regular exercise improves overall glucose levels in these children (2,3). This and the other physical and psychosocial gains merit recommending exercise for its therapeutic value.

CHALLENGES

There are several challenges in managing exercise participation in the child or adolescent with diabetes. For many, the most difficult of these may be balancing glycemic control with the normalcy of play. In social situations, attention directed toward diabetes is seldom welcomed by young people with the disease. Interrupting a game or play while it is in progress—if it is even possible—is bound to draw unwanted attention to the child with diabetes. Maintaining the flow of normal play may be further complicated by frequent episodes of hypoglycemia and hyperglycemia.

Exercise-Related Hypoglycemia

Hypoglycemia is frequently brought on by physical exertion and is a result of increased insulin sensitivity and depletion of glycogen stores. Some children may mistake the symptoms of hypoglycemia for the physical effects of exercise. Ignoring the symptoms may result in severe hypoglycemia immediately after exercise. Conversely, fear of a hypoglycemic reaction may lead to excessive ingestion of snacks or avoidance of activity altogether.

Hypoglycemia can be prevented by supplemental snacking before, during, or after activity, depending on the nature of the activity and its timing relative to the young person's meal and insulin schedule (4) (see Chapters 6 and 11). When considering the type and size of the snack, it is important to keep in mind the quantity of insulin acting during and after exercise, the length of time since the last meal, and the duration and intensity of the activity (see Chapter 9). Snack planning, and indeed the meal plan in general, should also reflect daily play and spontaneous activity typical of children and adolescents.

A well-conceived treatment plan for hypoglycemia should be in place for those who interact with the child on a regular basis. As part of the plan, parents should be encouraged to educate coaches, camp counselors, teammates, friends, or any supervisor of their childrens' activities about the signs and symptoms of hypoglycemia in their child and the necessary steps for its treatment. Hypoglycemia supplies should be provided and always available on the sidelines.

While it is easy to say that coaches, teachers, or friends must be alert to possible hypoglycemia and be prepared to treat it, this is not always practical or possible. For this reason, it may be a good idea for parents to attend or be available during sporting events or play activities whenever possible.

In addition, the health-care provider must assure children and parents that a low blood glucose reaction does not automatically mean a child should sit out for the remainder of the game; once treatment is provided, it is often safe and appropriate to return to the game.

Hyperglycemia

Hyperglycemia after exercise occurs as a result of insulin deficiency. Blood glucose values >250 mg/dl warrant testing for ketone bodies. If ketone bodies are present, exercise should be delayed until they are no longer present or control has been reestablished. If no ketone bodies are present, exercise participation may occur up to a blood glucose value of 300 mg/dl (5). Occasionally, glucose levels may be elevated immediately after competitive sports or intense exercise. In this situation, if no ketone bodies are present (which suggests significant levels of insulin in the circulation), an effective strategy might be to significantly reduce the preexercise snack. Alternatively, one might reduce the snack only slightly and reevaluate the child's insulin dose.

If sports or other participatory athletic activities are planned, then it is almost certain that snacks to supplement the meal plan should be provided. When activity is scheduled within 1–2 h following a meal, additional carbohydrate may not be necessary at the onset but will be needed during and after the activity. Snacking guidelines for sports or athletic activities are summarized in Table 21.1 and should be adjusted accordingly.

Adjustment of Snacks and Insulin Dose

Providing "treats" not usually permitted in the meal plan as exercise snacks has been a traditional practice. A chocolate bar is one such common treat. While it will do no harm, and many have used this kind of treat with good results, keep in mind that the fat content of the chocolate bar may retard absorption of the carbohydrate, and

Table 21.1. Supplemental Snacks

SPORTS/ATHLETIC PARTICIPATION	BLOOD GLUCOSE VALUE	SUPPLEMENTAL SNACK
Examples: Recreational or community activities, soccer, baseball, basketball, swimming, gymnastics, ice/roller hockey, football, dance class	<120 mg/dl	30 g CHO and 14 g protein. Monitor blood glucose carefully
	120–180 mg/dl	15 g CHO and 7–8 g protein
	180–240 mg/dl	15 g CHO
	≥240 mg/dl	No supplemental snack needed

CHO, carbohydrate. For each additional hour of exercise, 15 g CHO should be supplemented. Adapted from Holleroth (3).

Table 21.2. Developmental Exercise and Sports Participation Guidelines for Children and Adolescents

	EARLY CHILDHOOD 3–5 YEARS	CHILDHOOD 6–9 YEARS	ADOLESCENT 10–12 YEARS
Exercise guidelines	No competition, instruct through demonstration, emphasize fun	Minimize competition, de-emphasize scorekeeping, rules should remain flexible, limit time of instruction, complex sports are difficult	Monitor competition to keep focus on motor and sport skills
Recommended activities	Free play, gross motor skills; walking, running, swimming, throwing, catching, tumbling	Fundamental skill development; swimming, running, gymnastics	Complex skill and contact sports; wrestling, basketball, football, tennis, field hockey
		Entry-level sports; soccer, baseball	

this could be counterproductive. For this reason, a more appropriate snack, such as graham crackers, may ultimately be more effective. It is also possible that the snack addition may cause an elevated blood glucose value after exercise. When this happens, it is advisable to reduce the size of the snack. Finally, insulin should be adjusted as needed for regularly scheduled and planned physical activity or athletic participation.

Most parents and care providers depend on verbal reports from children for clues to changes in their blood glucose levels. As noted earlier, some children may confuse the feelings created by physical activity with those of hypoglycemia. For this reason, testing blood glucose levels after physical activity is recommended to evaluate the effect of individual exercise patterns and make needed adjustments. If blood glucose values are <120 mg/dl after activity, 15–30 g of carbohydrate should be provided immediately and a reevaluation of the preexercise snack or insulin adjustment should occur (4). Children and adolescents, like adults, are prone to postexercise late-onset hypoglycemia. An additional snack immediately after exercise is a good idea in most cases. This is an instance when the nontraditional treat as a snack may actually be a better choice.

An exercise plan for children with diabetes should aim to achieve two goals: *1*) physical needs must be evaluated beforehand, and necessary adjustments of food intake or insulin requirements must be made; *2*) the plan must take into account the children's feelings about diabetes—are they embarrassed by their disease or are they comfortable with it? Is it reasonable to expect them to perform diabetes management in front of friends or in a public location? The fear of experiencing a hypoglycemic episode in front of peers can be a source of anxiety and may inadvertently affect a child's acceptance of performing adjustments. In fact, children often develop strategies that keep them from appearing different from their peers. When assessing problems related to glycemic management, it should be kept in mind that education about appropriate adjustments for exercise does not ensure adherence.

EXERCISE PRESCRIPTION

The specific objectives of an exercise program for children with IDDM should focus on maintaining normal developmental growth and preventing exercise-induced hypoglycemia. The American Alliance for Health, Physical Education, Recreation and Dance recommends that children receive 30 min of daily exercise (6). This does not change when children have diabetes. But what is best for the individual child? The actual exercise prescription for a child is less formal than usually created for adults. It takes into account the child's and adolescent's personal preferences, developmental skill level, and physical abilities (Table 21.2). It is then up to the professional or parent to determine appropriate insulin and snack requirements.

Parents play a key role in their child's success in balancing the demands of exercise and glycemic control. A parent's ability to transport children to their activities (7), to perform the necessary insulin or snack adjustments, and to assist in the overall program for their child or adolescent with diabetes is critical for successful exercise participation.

REFERENCES

1. Rowland TW: *Exercise and Children's Health.* Champaign, IL, Human Kinetics Books, 1990, p. 215–33
2. Landt KW, Campaigne BN, James FW, Sperling MA: Effects of exercise training on insulin sensitivity in adolescents with type I diabetes. *Diabetes Care* 8:461–65, 1985
3. Stratton R, Wilson DP, Endres RK, Goldstein DE: Improved glycemic control after supervised 8-week exercise program in insulin-dependent diabetic adolescents. *Diabetes Care* 10:589–93, 1987
4. Holleroth H: *A Guide for Children and Youth With Diabetes.* Boston, MA, Joslin Diabetes Center, 1988
5. Santiago J (Ed.): *Medical Management of Insulin-Dependent (Type I) Diabetes.* Alexandria, VA, American Diabetes Association, 1994, p. 69–70
6. Green L, Adeyanju M: Exercise and fitness guidelines for elementary and middle school children. *The Elementary School Journal* 91:437–44, 1991
7. Sallis JF, Simons Morton BG, Stone EJ, Corbin CB, Epstein LH, Faucette N, Iannotti RJ, Killen JD, Klesges RC, Petray CK, Rowland TW, Taylor WC: Determinants of physical activity and interventions in youth medicine and science in sports and medicine. *Med Sci Sports Exercise* 24:5248– 57, 1992
8. Bhatia V, Wolfsdorf JI: Severe hypoglycemia in youth with insulin-dependent diabetes mellitus frequency and causative factors. *Pediatrics* 88:1187–93, 1991

22. Exercise and Aging

Highlights
Exercise and Aging

- Exercise causes improvements in fitness in the elderly that are similar to those seen in young people.
- Aging is associated with dramatic decreases in muscle mass and with an increase in body fat.
- Differences in the levels of physical activity explain much of the variability in body fat stores between individuals at any age.

- High-intensity strength training is a safe and very effective way to improve functional capacity.
- This type of training has been shown to be effective in increasing muscle size and strength through the 10th decade of life.
- Resistance training improves glucose tolerance, increases overall levels of physical activity, and decreases the risk of osteoporotic fractures in the elderly.

Exercise and Aging

WILLIAM J. EVANS, PhD

INTRODUCTION

Exercise has served as a cornerstone for the treatment of type II diabetes and may be useful in its prevention. Despite this, and the fact that the incidence of type II diabetes increases dramatically with advancing age, clinicians and their patients often have outmoded attitudes toward the capacity of elderly to participate in a vigorous exercise training program. This brief review will describe age-associated changes in body composition and the capacity of the elderly to respond to regularly performed exercise.

BODY COMPOSITION AND AGING

Recent research has demonstrated that men and women over the age of 60 years respond to both aerobic and strength training with greater relative increases in fitness, strength, functional status, and glucose tolerance than a comparable group of younger men and women. Advancing age is associated with a remarkable number of changes in body composition. Reductions in lean body mass have been well characterized. This decreased lean body mass occurs primarily as a result of a loss in skeletal muscle mass, which has been termed sarcopenia (1,2). Loss in muscle mass accounts for the age-associated decreases in basal metabolic rate, muscle strength, and activity levels, which, in turn, cause the decreased energy requirements of the elderly. In sedentary individuals, the main determinant of energy expenditure is fat-free mass, which declines by about 15% between the 3rd and 8th decades of life. It also appears that declining caloric needs are not matched by an appropriate decline in caloric intake, the result being an age-associated increased body fat content. Increased body fatness, along with increased abdominal obesity, are thought to be directly linked to the greatly increased incidence of type II diabetes among the elderly (3,4).

Age-related reductions in muscle mass are a direct cause of the age-related decrease in muscle strength in older people. Our laboratory (1) recently examined muscle strength and mass in 200 healthy 45- to 78-year-old men and women and concluded that muscle mass, not function, is the major determinant of age and sex-related differences in strength. This relationship is independent of muscle location (upper versus lower extremities) and function (extension versus flexion). With advancing age and the very low physical activity levels seen in the very old, muscle strength and power become a critical component of walking ability (5). The high prevalence of falls among the institutionalized elderly may be a consequence of the decrease in their lower muscle strength.

The question that we have been attempting to address: to what extent are these changes inevitable consequences of aging? Our data suggest that changes in body composition and aerobic capacity that are associated with increasing age may not be age-related at all. By examining endurance-trained men, we saw that body fat stores and maximal aerobic capacity were not related to age, but rather to the total number of hours these men were exercising per week (6). Even among sedentary individuals, energy spent in daily activities explains more than 75% of the variability in body fatness among young and older men (7). These data and the results of other investigators indicate that levels of physical activity are important in determining energy expenditure and, ultimately, body fat accumulation.

AEROBIC EXERCISE

Aerobic exercise has long been recommended for patients with impaired glucose tolerance or type II diabetes. Regularly performed aerobic exercise increases VO_{2max} and enhances insulin action. The responses of initially sedentary young (age 20–30 years) and older (age 60–70 years) men and women to 3 months of aerobic conditioning (70% of maximal heart rate, 45 min/day, 3 days/week) were examined by Meredith et al. (8). They found that the absolute gains in aerobic capacity were similar between the two age-groups. However, the mechanism for adaptation to regular submaximal exercise may be different between old and young people. Muscle biopsies taken before and after training showed a more than twofold increase in oxidative capacity in the muscles of the older subjects, whereas muscles of the young subjects showed a smaller increase. In addition, skeletal muscle glycogen stores in the older subjects, which were initially lower than those of the young men and women, increased significantly.

The degree to which the elderly demonstrate an increase in maximal cardiac output in response to endurance training is unclear. Seals et al. (9) found no increase in cardiac output after 1 year of endurance training, whereas Spina et al. (10) observed an increased maximal cardiac output in older men, but not in older women. However, the techniques used to measure cardiac output varied with each of these studies. If these gender-related differences in cardiovascular response are real, it may explain the lack of response of maximal cardiac output when older men and women are included in the same study population.

The fact that aerobic exercise has significant effects on insulin action in skeletal muscle may help explain its value in the treatment of glucose intolerance and type II diabetes. Hughes et al. (11) demonstrated that regularly performed aerobic exercise without weight loss results in improved glucose tolerance and rate of insulin-stimulated glucose disposal and increased skeletal muscle GLUT4 levels in older glucose-intolerant subjects (mean age 64 ± 2 years). In this investigation, a moderate-intensity aerobic exercise program was compared with a higher intensity program (50 vs. 75% of maximal heart rate reserve, 55 min/day, 4 days/week, for 12 weeks). No differences were seen between subjects on the two programs with respect to glucose tolerance, insulin sensitivity, or muscle GLUT4 levels. This suggests that a prescription of moderate aerobic exercise should be recommended for older men or women with type II diabetes,

since it should ensure better compliance and cause fewer musculoskeletal injuries and cardiovascular complications than a more intense exercise program. In contrast to this study, Seals et al. (12) found that a high-intensity training program produces a greater improvement in the insulin response to an oral glucose load than a lower intensity aerobic exercise program. Their subjects began the study with normal glucose tolerance. However, Kirwan et al. (13) found that 9 months of endurance training at 80% of the maximal heart rate (4 days/week) results in reduced glucose-stimulated insulin levels. No comparison was made to a lower intensity exercise group.

Endurance training is generally recommended as an adjunct to dietary modifications in the primary treatment of many patients with type II diabetes. Cross-sectional analysis of dietary intake supports the hypothesis that a low-carbohydrate/high-fat diet is associated with the onset of type II diabetes (14); however, prospective studies have not shown such a correlation in dietary habits (3,14). The effects of a high-carbohydrate diet on glucose tolerance have been equivocal (15,16). Hughes et al. (17) compared the effects of a high-carbohydrate (60% carbohydrate and 20% fat)/high-fiber (25 g dietary fiber/1,000 kcal) diet with and without 3 months of high-intensity (75% maximal heart rate reserve, 50 min/day, 4 days/week) endurance exercise in older, glucose-intolerant men and women. Subjects were fed all of their food on a metabolic ward during the 3 months of the study and were not allowed to lose weight. Neither the diet nor the diet plus exercise group improved their glucose tolerance or insulin-stimulated glucose uptake, suggesting that the high-carbohydrate, high-calorie diet countered the effect of the exercise on insulin action.

In summary, the response of elderly men and women to regularly performed aerobic exercise is similar to that of young subjects. Increased fitness levels are associated with reduced mortality and increased life expectancy. In addition, regular exercise may prevent the development of type II diabetes in individuals who are at the greatest risk for developing this disease (18). Thus, regularly performed aerobic exercise is an important way for older people to improve their glucose tolerance.

INCREASING LEVELS OF PHYSICAL ACTIVITY IN THE ELDERLY

It is never too late to begin to exercise. It is prudent, however, for people with diabetes to consult with their physicians before beginning an exercise program. The following questionnaire and informational comments were written for those individuals about to begin a moderate- or low-intensity exercise program. Patients should be advised to consult a physician before beginning training if they answer "yes" to any of these questions.

Pretraining Program Questionnaire

The American College of Sports Medicine recommends a physician-supervised stress test for anyone over the age of 35 (even without diabetes) who wants to begin a training program. For an individual who will engage only in a mild-intensity exercise, such as walking, this test is not necessary. If you answer "yes" to any of the following questions, you should be carefully examined by a physician.

■ Do you get chest pains while at rest and/or during exertion?

  If you answered "yes" to the above question, have you seen a physician to diagnose the cause of the pains?

■ Have you ever had a heart attack?

  If you answered "yes" to the above question, was your heart attack within the last year?

■ Do you have high blood pressure?

  If you do not know the answer to the above question, was your last blood pressure reading more than 150/100?

■ Are you short of breath after extremely mild exertion, at rest, or at night in bed?

■ Do you have any ulcerated wounds or cuts on your feet that do not seem to heal?

■ Have you lost 10 lb or more in the past 6 months without trying to diet?

■ Do you get pains in your buttocks or the back of your legs (thighs or calves) when you walk?

■ While at rest, do you frequently experience fast, irregular heartbeats or, at the other extreme, very slow beats?

■ Are you currently being treated for any heart or circulatory condition, such as vascular disease, stroke, angina, hypertension, congestive heart failure, poor circulation to the legs, valvular heart disease, blood clots, or pulmonary disease?

■ As an adult, have you ever had a fracture of the hip, spine, or wrist?

■ Did you fall more than twice in the past year, no matter what the cause?

Advancing age results in increased muscle stiffness and reduced elasticity of connective tissue. For this reason, proper warm-up and stretching can have a greater effect in reducing the risk of an orthopedic injury in the elderly than in young men and women. A 5-min warm-up (exercise at a reduced intensity) followed by 5–10 min of slow stretching is highly recommended.

Cooling down after exercise is important in older individuals. You should never finish a workout by immediately jumping into a hot shower. End your exercise session with a slow walk and more stretching. Your postexercise stretching will be more effective than the stretching you did before the exercise. This is because your muscles have warmed up and, along with tendons and ligaments, are much more elastic.

Find a friend to exercise with. The more people you exercise with, the more likely you are to stay with the exercise. This is a perfect opportunity for sons and daughters to spend time with their older parents, to the benefit of both generations.

STRENGTH TRAINING

While endurance exercise has been the more traditional means of increasing cardiovascular fitness, strength or resistance training is currently recommended by the American College of Sports Medicine as an important component of an overall fitness program. This is particularly important in the elderly, in whom loss of muscle mass and weakness are prominent deficits.

In strength conditioning or progressive resistance training, the resistance against which a muscle generates force is progressively increased over time. Progressive resistance training involves few contractions against a heavy load. This type of exercise is distinctly different from endurance exercise, which involves repetitive contractions against little resistance. The metabolic and morphological adaptations to these two different types of exercise are very different. Muscle strength has been shown to increase in response to training between 60 and 100% of the 1 repetition maximum (1 RM), defined as the maximum amount of weight that can be lifted with one contraction. Strength conditioning will result in an increase in muscle size; this increase in size is largely the result of an increase in contractile proteins. The mechanisms by which the mechanical events stimulate an increase in RNA synthesis and subsequently protein synthesis are not well understood. Lifting a weight requires that a muscle shortens as it produces force. This is called a concentric contraction. Lowering a weight, on the other hand, requires that the muscle lengthens as it produces force. This is an eccentric muscle contraction. These lengthening muscle contractions have been shown to produce ultrastructural damage that may stimulate increased muscle protein turnover.

Our laboratory has examined the effects of high-intensity resistance (80% of 1 RM, 3 days/week) training of the knee extensors and flexors in older men (age 60–72 years) (19). The average increases in knee flexor and extensor strength were 227 and 107%, respectively. We used computer tomography (CT) scans and muscle biopsies to determine muscle size. Total muscle area by CT analysis increased by 11.4%, and the muscle biopsies showed an increase of 33.5% in Type I fiber area and 27.5% in Type II fiber area. In addition, lower body VO_{2max} increased significantly, whereas upper body VO_{2max} did not, indicating that increased muscle mass can increase maximal aerobic power. It appears that the age-related loss in muscle mass may be an important determinant in the reduced maximal aerobic capacity seen in elderly men and women (20). Improving muscle strength can enhance the capacity of many older men and women to perform such activities as climbing stairs, carrying packages, and even walking.

We have applied this same training program to a group of frail, institutionalized elderly men and women (mean age 90 ± 3 years, range 87–96) (21). After 8 weeks of training, the 10 subjects in this study increased muscle strength by almost 180% (Fig. 22.1) and muscle size by 11%. This intervention on frail nursing home residents demonstrated not only increases in muscle strength and size, but also increased gait speed, stair-climbing power, and balance. In addition, spontaneous activity levels increased significantly. In contrast, the activity of a nonexercised control group was unchanged. It should be pointed out that the subjects in the latter study were very old and very frail, and many of them had multiple chronic diseases. The increase in overall levels of physical activity caused by strength training in the elderly has been a common observation in our studies (19,21,22). Since muscle weakness is a primary deficit in many older individuals, increased strength presumably stimulates them to perform more aerobic activities, such as walking and cycling.

In addition to its effect on increasing muscle mass and function, resistance training can have an important effect on energy balance in elderly men and women (23). Men and women participating in a resistance training program of the upper and lower body muscles require 15% more calories to maintain body weight after 12 weeks of training than they did before training (Fig. 22.2). This increase in energy requirement appears to result from a combination of factors, including an increased resting metabolic rate (RMR), the small energy cost of the exercise, and a presumed increase in the energy cost of muscle protein metabolism.

Because resistance training can preserve or even increase muscle mass during weight loss, this type of exercise for older men and women who must lose weight may be of genuine benefit. Endurance training has been demonstrated to be an important adjunct to weight-loss programs in young men and women, in part by increasing their daily energy expenditure. Its utility in treating obesity in the elderly may not be great. This is because many sedentary older men and women do not expend many calories when they perform endurance exercise, because of their low fitness levels. Thirty to forty minutes of aerobic exercise may increase energy expenditure by only 100–200 kcal, with very little residual effect on calorie expenditure. Recently, strength training has been demonstrated to cause improved glucose tolerance in elderly subjects (24). In addition, by improving bone density, muscle mass and strength, balance, and overall level of physical activity, resistance training may be an important means to decrease the risk of osteoporotic bone fractures in postmenopausal women and elderly men.

Muscle Strength Training in the Elderly

Muscle strength training can be accomplished by virtually anyone. Many health-care professionals have directed their patients away from strength training in the mistaken belief that it can cause undesirable elevations in blood pressure. With proper technique and extreme intensity, excessive systolic blood pressure elevations during resistance training can be minimized. Muscle strengthening exercises are rapidly becoming a critical component to cardiac rehabilitation programs as clinicians realize the need for strength as well as endurance in many activities of daily living.

Candidates

- Adults of all ages are candidates for this type of exercise.

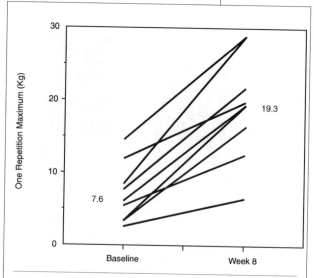

Figure 22.1. Percentage gains in knee extensor strength (1 RM) after 8 weeks of high-intensity resistance training in a group of nine very old men and women (87–96 years).

Redrawn from Fiatarone MA, Marks EC, Ryan ND, Meredith CN, Lipsitz LA, Evans WJ: High-intensity strength training in nonagenarians: effects on skeletal muscle. *JAMA* 263:3029–34, 1990.

- Elderly, hypertensive patients should be carefully evaluated before beginning a strength training program.

- Instead of a treadmill stress test, we use a weight-lifting stress test. Have the patient perform three sets of 8 repetitions at 80% of the 1 RM. Monitor electrocardiogram and blood pressure responses during the exercise.

- Patients with rheumatoid or osteoarthritis may also participate. Patients with a limited range of motion should train within the range of motion that is relatively pain-free. Most patients will see a dramatic improvement in the pain-free range of motion as a result of resistance training.

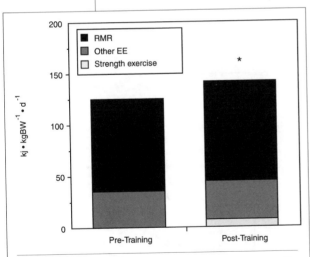

Figure 22.2. Increased total energy intake and expenditure in older men and women as a result of 12 weeks of resistance training ($n = 10$). RMRs were measured in each subject by indirect calorimetry. The other energy expenditure represents the portion of the energy expenditure that was not due to RMR or resistance exercise and includes the additional thermic effect of feeding and the energy cost of nonresistance exercise and daily activity ($P < 0.05$).

Redrawn from Campbell WW, Crim MC, Young VR, Evans WJ: Increased energy requirements and body composition changes with resistance training in older adults. *Am J Clin Nutr* 60:167–75, 1994.

Exercises

- Resistance training should be directed at the large muscle groups that are important in everyday activities, including the shoulders, arms, spine, hips, and legs.

- Each repetition is performed slowly through a full range of motion, allowing 2–3 s to lift the weight (concentric contraction) and 4–6 s to lower the weight (eccentric contraction). Performing the exercise more quickly will not enhance strength gains and may increase the risk of an injury.

Training Intensity and Duration

- A high-intensity resistance training program has been shown to have dramatic effects at all ages. This is a training intensity that will approach or result in muscular fatigue after 8–12 complete repetitions of the movement. A weight that can be lifted 20 or more times without fatigue will increase muscular endurance, but will cause little gain in muscle strength or mass.

- The amount of weight that is lifted should increase as strength builds. This should take place about every 2–3 weeks. In our research studies, we have observed a 10–15% increase in strength per week during the first 8 weeks of training.

- We have seen significant gains in muscle strength and mass as well as an improvement in bone density after 1 year of only 2 days/week of training.

Breathing Technique

- Advise patients to inhale before a lift, exhale during the lift, and inhale as the weight is lowered to the beginning position.

- Make sure patients avoid performing the Valsalva maneuver (holding their breath during force production).

- With proper breathing technique, the cardiovascular stress of resistance exercise is markedly diminished.

- Heart rate and blood pressure should rise only slightly above resting values in the elderly who follow these guidelines.

Equipment

- Any device that provides sufficient resistance to stress muscles beyond levels usually encountered may be used.

- Weight-stack or compressed-air resistance machines may be found at many community fitness facilities or purchased for home use.

- Simple weight-lifting devices might include Velcro-strapped wrist and ankle bags filled with sand or lead shot; heavy household objects, such as plastic milk jugs filled with water or gravel; or food cans of various sizes.

CONCLUSIONS

There is no other group in our society that can benefit more from regularly performed exercise than the elderly. While both aerobic and strength conditioning are highly recommended, only strength training can stop or reverse sarcopenia. Increased muscle strength and mass in the elderly can be the first step toward a lifetime of increased physical activity and a means for maintaining functional status and independence.

REFERENCES

1. Frontera WR, Hughes VA, Evans WJ: A cross-sectional study of upper and lower extremity muscle strength in 45- to 78-year-old men and women. *J Appl Physiol* 71:644–50, 1991
2. Tzankoff SP, Norris AH: Longitudinal changes in basal metabolic rate in man. *J Appl Physiol* 33:536–39, 1978
3. Lundgren H, Bengstsson C, Blohme G, Isaksson B, Lapidus L, Lenner RA, Saaek A, Winther E: Dietary habits and incidence of non-insulin-dependent diabetes mellitus in a population study of women in Gothenburg, Sweden. *Am J Clin Nutr* 49:708–12, 1989
4. Marshall JA, Hamman RF, Baxter J: High-fat, low-carbohydrate diet and the etiology of non-insulin-dependent diabetes mellitus: the San Luis Valley Diabetes Study. *Am J Epidemiol* 134:590–603, 1991
5. Bassey EJ, Fiatarone MA, O'Neill EF, Kelly M, Evans WJ, Lipsitz LA: Leg extensor power and functional performance in very old men and women. *Clin Sci* 82:321–27, 1992
6. Meredith CN, Zackin MJ, Frontera WR, Evans WJ: Body composition and aerobic capacity in young and middle-aged endurance-trained men *Med Sci Sports Exercise* 19:557–63, 1987
7. Roberts SB, Young VR, Fuss P, Heyman MB, Fiatarone MA, Dallal GE, Cortiella J, Evans WJ: What are the dietary energy needs of elderly adults? *Int J Obes* 16:969–76, 1992
8. Meredith CN, Frontera WR, Fisher EC, Hughes VA, Herland JC, Edwards J, Evans WJ: Peripheral effects of endurance training in young and old subjects. *J Appl Physiol* 66:2844–49, 1989
9. Seals DR, Hagberg JM, Hurley BF, Ehsani AA, Holloszy JO: Endurance training in older men and women: cardiovascular responses to exercise. *J Appl Physiol: Respir Environ Exercise Physiol* 57:1024–29, 1984
10. Spina RJ, Ogawa T, Kohrt WM, Martin WH III, Holloszy JO, Ehsani AA: Differences in cardiovascular adaptation to endurance exercise training between older men and women. *J Appl Physiol* 75:849–55, 1993
11. Hughes VA, Fiatarone MA, Fielding RA, Kahn BB, Ferrara CM, Shepherd P, Fisher EC, Wolfe RR, Elahi D, Evans WJ: Exercise increases

muscle GLUT4 levels and insulin action in subjects with impaired glucose tolerance. *Am J Physiol* 264: E855–62, 1993

12. Seals DR, Hagberg JM, Hurley BF, Ehsani AA, Holloszy JO: Effects of endurance training on glucose tolerance and plasma lipid levels in older men and women. *JAMA* 252:645–49, 1984

13. Kirwan JP, Kohrt WM, Wojta DM, Bourey RE, Holloszy JO: Endurance exercise training reduces glucose-stimulated insulin levels in 60- to 70-year-old men and women. *J Gerontol* 48:M84–90, 1993

14. Feskens EJM, Kromhout D: Cardiovascular risk factors and the 25-year incidence of diabetes mellitus in middle-aged men. *Am J Epidemiol* 130:1101–108, 1989

15. Borkman M, Campbell LV, Chisholm DJ, Storlien LH: Comparison of the effects on insulin sensitivity of high carbohydrate and high fat diets in normal subjects. *J Clin Endocrinol Metab* 72:432–37, 1991

16. Garg A, Grundy SM, Unger RH: Comparison of effects of high and low carbohydrate diets on plasma lipoprotein and insulin sensitivity in patients with mild NIDDM. *Diabetes* 41:1278–85, 1992

17. Hughes VA, Fiatarone MA, Fielding RA, Ferrara CM, Elahi D, Evans WJ: Long-term effects of a high carbohydrate diet and exercise on insulin action in older subjects with impaired glucose tolerance. *Am J Clin Nutr*. In press

18. Helmrich SP, Ragland DR, Leung RW, Paffenbarger RS Jr: Physical activity and reduced occurrence of non-insulin-dependent diabetes mellitus. *N Engl J Med* 325:147–52, 1991

19. Frontera WR, Meredith CN, O'Reilly KP, Evans WJ: Strength training and determinants of VO_{2max} in older men. *J Appl Physiol* 68: 329–33, 1990

20. Flegg JL, Lakatta EG: Role of muscle loss in the age-associated reduction in VO_{2max}. *J Appl Physiol* 65:1147–51, 1988

21. Fiatarone MA, O'Neill EF, Ryan ND, Clements KM, Solares GR, Nelson ME, Roberts SB, Kehayias JJ, Lipsitz LA, Evans WJ: Exercise training and nutritional supplementation for physical frailty in very elderly people. *N Engl J Med* 330:1769–75, 1994

22. Nelson ME, Fiatarone MA, Morganti CM, Trice I, Greenberg RA, Evans WJ: Effects of high-intensity strength training on multiple risk factors for osteoporotic fractures: a randomized controlled trial. *JAMA* 272:1909–14

23. Campbell WW, Crim MC, Young VR, Evans WJ: Increased energy requirements and body composition changes with resistance training in older adults. *Am J Clin Nutr* 60:167–75, 1994

24. Miller JP, Pratley RE, Goldberg AP, Gordon P, Rubin M, Treuth MS, Ryan AS, Hurley BF: Strength training increases insulin action in healthy 50- to 65-yr-old men. *J Appl Physiol* 77:1122–27, 1994

23. Patients on Various Drug Therapies

Highlights
Patients on Various Drug Therapies

- Patients with diabetes frequently take medications or other chemical agents in addition to insulin or oral hypoglycemic agents.
- Many commonly used drugs may cause significant alterations in the metabolic and nonmetabolic responses to exercise, sometimes affecting exercise performance.
- More commonly used drugs with potential significance in patients with diabetes include diuretics, ß-adrenergic blockers, calcium channel blockers, angiotensin-converting enzyme inhibitors, glucocorticoids, anabolic steroids, lipid-lowering agents, salicylates, and nonsteroidal analgesics.
- Patients with chronic complications, such as cardiovascular disease, hypertension, autonomic neuropathy, peripheral vascular disease, and nephropathy, are particularly vulnerable to the adverse effects of pharmacological agents.
- Prudent choice of drugs in individual situations can minimize their adverse effects in regularly exercising diabetic patients.

Patients on Various Drug Therapies

OM P. GANDA, MD

INTRODUCTION

Patients engaged in exercise or endurance training programs should be aware that certain drugs or chemical agents may cause significant alterations in the metabolic, cardiovascular, or hemodynamic responses to exercise. In such patients, therefore, the anticipated clinical effects of exercise on blood glucose, glucose counterregulation, and lipid levels may be appreciably different. Of these, the effects of various commonly used drugs on carbohydrate metabolism (1,2) are perhaps the most pertinent and are summarized in Table 23.1. In patients with certain chronic complications, such as cardiovascular disease, peripheral vascular disease, autonomic neuropathy, and renal disease, many pharmacological agents can potentially modify and limit physical performance during exercise. The following is a brief discussion of the multiple sites of action of commonly used agents in patients with diabetes or impaired glucose tolerance. The interaction of exercise with actions of insulin and glucose regulation in insulin-treated patients will not be discussed here (see Chapter 11). Similarly, note that exercise can enhance the hypoglycemic effects of sulfonylureas (3).

DIURETICS

The hyperglycemia induced by diuretic agents, particularly thiazides and chlorthalidone, is well known. This effect is produced via multiple mechanisms, including decreased insulin secretion as well as impaired insulin sensitivity. Hypokalemia, caused by these agents, is at least partially responsible for this effect. Patients engaging in regular exercise may be more at risk if fluid and electrolyte balance is not maintained. Other metabolic effects of thiazides and related diuretics include decreased sodium and magnesium levels, increased uric acid levels, modest increases in low-density lipoprotein (LDL) cholesterol and triglyceride levels, and lower high-

density lipoprotein (HDL) cholesterol levels (4,5). In general, all of the adverse effects are more prominent after prolonged use at a higher dosage.

ß-ADRENERGIC ANTAGONISTS

ß-adrenergic antagonists are frequently used in patients with angina or after myocardial infarction. They may decrease exercise capacity, lower peak heart rate and blood pressure, and may improve myocardial ischemic changes on stress tests. Some patients with angina may experience better work capacity due to relief of symptoms.

ß-adrenergic antagonists have complex effects on metabolic pathways involving insulin secretion, hepatic and peripheral glucose disposal, lipolysis, and lipoprotein metabolism (5,6). In all of these respects, noncardioselective agents, e.g. propranolol, nadolol, and timolol, have greater activity compared with cardioselective agents, e.g., atenolol and metoprolol. By inhibiting insulin secretion and glucose disposal, ß-blockers may occasionally worsen hyperglycemia (1,2). More frequently, in patients with insulin-dependent diabetes mellitus (IDDM), ß-blockers may induce hypoglycemia by inhibiting muscle and hepatic glycogenolysis. Furthermore, ß-blockers are known to impair the recovery from hypoglycemia that is critically dependent on β_2-adrenergic hepatic effects of epinephrine. In addition, these agents mask the adrenergic symptoms of hypoglycemia by altering the glycemic threshold for symptoms (7). In this regard, it is of interest that one adrenergic symptom, sweating, is increased rather than decreased because it is mediated by a cholinergic mechanism.

ß-adrenergic antagonists might have adverse effects on one's lipid profile, i.e., elevation of triglycerides and lowering of HDL cholesterol. However, these effects are also more frequent with nonselective agents (6). In relation to exercise and diabetes, other pertinent adverse effects include worsening of symptoms of peripheral vascular disease, increased fatigue, and impair-

Table 23.1 Commonly Used Drugs or Agents Capable of Inducing Changes in Glucose Homeostasis

	MECHANISM OF ACTION		COMMENTS
	Insulin secretion	Glucose disposal	
Potentially raise blood glucose			
Diuretics (thiazides, chlorthalidone, furosemide, metolazone)	↓	↓	K$^+$ depletion, other effects
ß-adrenergic antagonists (propranolol, nadolol, timolol)	0, ↓	0, ↓	More likely with non-cardioselective agents
Ca^{2+} channel blockers (dihydropyridine derivatives)	0	0, ↓	Effect rarely significant
Glucocorticoids	↑	↓	Cause marked insulin resistance
Anabolic steroids	0	↓	Cause major lipid effects
Growth hormone	↑	↓	A major insulin antagonist
Niacin	↑	↓	Particularly with high dosage
Cyclosporine	↓	↓	Often used with glucocorticoids
Potentially lower blood glucose			
α-adrenergic antagonists (prazosin, doxazosin, terazosin)	0, ↑	0, ↑	Rarely significant
ACE inhibitors	0	0, ↑	
ß-adrenergic antagonists (propranolol, nadolol, timolol)			May impair recovery from hypoglycemia
Salicylates	0, ↑	0	With high dosage
Alcohol	0, ↑	↑	May cause hyperglycemia in the long term
Pentamidine	↑	0	May cause hyperglycemia in the long term
Quinine	↑	0, ↑	May cause severe hypoglycemia

ment of exercise tolerance. Finally, ß-blockers, by impairing cellular potassium uptake, may promote exercise-induced hyperkalemia, particularly in patients with underlying renal insufficiency or patients on nonsteroidal analgesics. It would therefore be prudent to avoid noncardioselective ß-blockers in patients with either IDDM or non-insulin-dependent diabetes mellitus (NIDDM).

CALCIUM CHANNEL BLOCKERS, α-ADRENERGIC ANTAGONISTS, AND ANGIOTENSIN-CONVERTING ENZYME (ACE) INHIBITORS

The newer classes of antihypertensive agents, including calcium channel blockers, α-adrenergic antagonists, and ACE inhibitors, have more favorable metabolic effects in general and have recently been recommended by the American Diabetes Association as the preferred agents for control of hypertension in diabetic patients (8). Calcium channel blockers improve exercise capacity and ischemia in patients with coronary artery disease. From the glycemic point of view, there appears to be some heterogeneity of responses with different types of calcium channel blockers. Drugs like verapamil and diltiazem have no significant effect on glycemic control, but some members of the dihydropyridine class, such as nifedipine, may impair insulin sensitivity (9), and others, such as amlodipine, may improve glucose tolerance and enhance insulin sensitivity (10). On the other hand, α-adrenergic antagonists and ACE inhibitors have been shown to improve insulin sensitivity (9). The improvement of insulin sensitivity in response to an ACE inhibitor may persist after addition of low-dose thiazides (9). These favorable responses in insulin sensitivity have now been shown for several agents belonging to the α-blocker or ACE inhibitor families, suggesting a class effect. However, certain adverse effects, such as dyspnea and postural hypotension leading to light-headedness, are not uncommon when α-blockers are used for hypertension or benign prostatic hypertrophy. Regarding their effects on lipids, calcium channel blockers and the ACE inhibitors have no significant adverse effects, whereas α-blockers, in several studies, have been shown to moderately raise HDL cholesterol levels and lower triglycerides (4,11). The long-term renoprotective effects of ACE inhibitors in patients with IDDM and either microalbuminuria or clinical proteinuria have been recently demonstrated in prospective, randomized studies (12,13). Finally, several recent, long-term trials have shown enhanced exercise capacity and prolonged survival rates after myocardial infarction, despite congestive heart failure, in patients on ACE inhibitors (14).

GLUCOCORTICOIDS AND ANABOLIC STEROIDS

Glucocorticoids, in supraphysiological and pharmacological doses, are well known to cause insulin resistance and compensatory hyperinsulinemia in nondiabetic individuals or in subjects with impaired glucose tolerance. Increasing the dosage of glucocorticoids progressively worsens preexisting hyperglycemia via multiple effects on liver, adipose tissue, and muscle (1,2). Glucocorticoids, after prolonged use, also alter adipose tissue distribution and cause skin changes, leading to the typical cushingoid appearance, as well as to proximal muscle weakness due to steroid myopathy. These diverse effects may considerably impair physical performance. By inducing insulin resistance and increased lipogenesis, glucocorticoids can cause significant lipid changes, typically hypertriglyceridemia. Even more striking adverse changes in lipids may result from prolonged use of oral anabolic steroids, usually seen in young athletes. In a review of multiple studies evaluating the effects of various oral anabolic steroids, an average reduction of 52% in HDL cholesterol and an average rise of 36% in LDL cholesterol were consistently observed (15). Because these effects were not observed by parenteral administration, it appears quite likely that the lipid alterations are mediated via hepatic effects of these agents. A marked increase in premature atherogenesis can be anticipated from the striking lipid effects of these agents. Moreover, other serious adverse effects, particularly with the use of 17-α alkylated androgens (e.g., methyl-testosterone, oxandrolone, and stanozol), include hepatotoxicity, impaired spermatogenesis leading to infertility, and hirsutism and virilization in women (16). There is no convincing evidence that anabolic steroids significantly improve muscle strength or athletic performance.

GROWTH HORMONE

Growth hormone, like glucocorticoids, is a classic diabetogenic hormone with diverse effects on carbohydrate, lipid, and protein metabolism. The levels of growth hormone and insulin-like growth factor I gradually decline with age and may be related to the decreases in muscle and bone mass and the increased adiposity in older individuals. Growth hormone treatment has been proposed in debilitated elderly people, those with osteoporosis or sepsis, and in posttraumatic or postsurgical states (17,18). However, the safety and efficacy of growth hormone have not yet been proven. Similarly, the efficacy of growth hormone in improving athletic performance has not yet been documented. Potential adverse effects of long-term growth hormone treatment, besides cost, include accelerated atherosclerosis, hypertension, insulin resistance, degenerative arthropathy, and possibly increased incidence of tumors.

LIPID-LOWERING DRUGS

Fibric acid derivatives, such as clofibrate and, less often, gemfibrozil, may, on rare occasions, cause an acute or subacute muscular syndrome characterized by severe muscle pain, tenderness, and weakness generally involving shoulders, hips, and calves (19). Muscle necrosis may result in markedly elevated creatinine phosphokinase, aldolase, and even myoglobinuria. Patients with underlying renal disease, hypothyroidism, and those taking hydroxymethylglutaryl coenzyme A (HMG-CoA) reductase inhibitors (statins) are

more susceptible to this complication, particularly if such patients are also taking erythromycin or cyclosporine.

Niacin (nicotinic acid), another commonly used lipid-lowering agent, can lead to hyperglycemia by inducing insulin resistance, particularly when ß-cells are unable to adapt because of limited reserves, i.e., patients with impaired glucose tolerance or overt type II diabetes (20).

CYCLOSPORINE

Cyclosporine, a widely used immunosuppressant in patients with organ transplants and autoimmune disorders, may precipitate diabetes or glucose intolerance by direct effects on ß-cells as well as on peripheral insulin sensitivity (1,2,21). This effect is probably independent of the glucocorticoids (21) often used simultaneously in such patients. Black individuals may be more susceptible to the hyperglycemic effect of cyclosporine (22). Patients on cyclosporine and engaging in strenuous physical activity should be aware that they may be more susceptible to myositis and even rhabdomyolysis and acute renal failure if they are concurrently taking HMG-CoA reductase inhibitors (statins). In view of the very high incidence of this adverse effect (up to 30% of patients on lovastatin) (23), the statins should be very cautiously used in patients on cyclosporine. Recent evidence suggests that pravastatin (pravachol) may be associated with lower incidence of toxicity in patients on cyclosporine.

SALICYLATES AND NONSTEROIDAL ANTI-INFLAMMATORY DRUGS (NSAIDs)

Salicylates and aspirin, in higher dosages (4–6 g/day), may induce hypoglycemia (1). However, in usual dosages, there are no significant effects on glucose or insulin secretion.

NSAIDs (e.g., acetaminophen, ibuprofen, naproxen, piroxicam, etc.) have the potential of causing renal injury and inducing hyperkalemia in older patients with NIDDM or any patient with underlying renal disease.

ALCOHOL

Long-term, moderate intake of alcohol (1–3 drinks daily) has been reported to be cardioprotective in several epidemiological studies (24). Recent studies suggest an enhanced insulin sensitivity in light-to-moderate drinkers (1–3 drinks/day) compared with nondrinkers (24). However, these salutary effects of alcohol need to be considered in light of other long-term effects of heavy alcohol intake, which include weight gain, elevated triglycerides, and liver toxicity.

PENTAMIDINE

Pentamidine is frequently used in the prophylaxis or treatment of Pneumocystis pneumonia in patients with acquired immunodeficiency syndrome (AIDS). Its chemical structure is similar to the well-known diabetogenic agents alloxan and streptozotocin. A survey of patients with AIDS receiving intravenous pentamidine revealed a 14% incidence of acute hypoglycemic episodes (blood glucose <55 mg/dl) (26). A few of these episodes were fatal. An increased incidence of IDDM has been reported after prolonged therapy. However, aerosolized pentamidine, which has virtually replaced the intravenous route, has minimal effects on carbohydrate metabolism.

QUININE

Quinine is frequently used for the relief of muscle cramps. In patients with severe falciparum malaria, quinine was shown to induce severe hypoglycemia by multiple mechanisms, including an enhanced insulin release. Quinine, even in a modest dosage, may occasionally precipitate symptomatic hypoglycemia in healthy individuals (27). Patients on endurance exercise programs and on sulfonylurea therapy may conceivably be more susceptible to quinine-induced hypoglycemia.

REFERENCES

1. Pandit MK, Burke J, Gustafson AB, Minocha A, Peiris AN: Drug-induced disorders of glucose tolerance. *Ann Intern Med* 118:529–39, 1993
2. Ganda OP: Secondary forms of diabetes. In *Joslin's Diabetes Mellitus*. 13th ed. Kahn CR, Weir GC, Eds. Philadelphia, PA, Lea & Febiger, 1994, p. 300–16
3. Kemmer FW, Tacken M, Berger M: Mechanism of exercise-induced hypoglycemia during sulfonylurea treatment. *Diabetes* 36:1178–82, 1987
4. Lardinois CK, Neuman SL: The effects of antihypertensive agents on serum lipids and lipoproteins. *Arch Intern Med* 148:1280–88, 1988
5. Joint National Committee on Detection, Evaluation, and Treatment of High Blood Pressure: The fifth report of the Joint National Committee on Detection, Evaluation, and Treatment of High Blood Pressure. *Arch Intern Med* 153:154–83, 1993
6. Burris JF: ß-blockers, dyslipidemia, and coronary artery disease: a reassessment. *Arch Intern Med* 153:2085–92, 1993
7. Hirsch IB, Boyle PJ, Craft S, Cryer PE: Higher glycemic thresholds for symptoms during ß-adrenergic blockade in IDDM. *Diabetes* 40:1177–86, 1991
8. American Diabetes Association: Treatment of hypertension in diabetes (Consensus Statement). *Diabetes Care* 16:1394–1401, 1993
9. Berne C, Pollare T, Lithell H: Effects of antihypertensive treatment on insulin sensitivity with special reference to ACE inhibitors. *Diabetes Care* 14 (Suppl. 4): 39–47, 1991
10. Beer NA, Jakubowicz DJ, Beer RM, Nestler JE: The calcium channel blocker amlodipine raises serum dehydroepiandrosterone sulfate and androstenedione, but lowers serum cortisol, in insulin-resistant obese and hypertensive men. *J Clin Endocrinol Metab* 76:1464–69, 1993

11. Kasiske BL, Ma JZ, Kalil RSN, Louis TA: Effects of antihypertensive therapy on serum lipids. *Ann Intern Med* 122:133–41, 1995

12. Lewis EJ, Hunsicker LG, Bain RP, Rhode RD: The effect of angiotensin-converting enzyme inhibition on diabetic nephropathy. *N Engl J Med* 329:1456–62, 1993

13. Viberti G, Mogensen CE, Groop LC, Pauls JF, the European Microalbuminuria Captopril Study Group: Effect of captopril on progression to clinical proteinuria in patients with insulin-dependent diabetes mellitus and microalbuminuria. *JAMA* 271:275–79, 1994

14. Cody RJ: Comparing angiotensin-converting enzyme inhibitor trial results in patients with acute myocardial infarction. *Arch Intern Med* 154:202–36, 1994

15. Glazer G: Atherogenic effects of anabolic steroids on serum lipid levels: a literature review. *Arch Intern Med* 151:1925–33, 1991

16. Wilson JD: Androgen abuse by athletes. *Endocr Rev* 9:181–99, 1988

17. Kaplan SL: The newer uses of growth hormone in adults. *Adv Intern Med* 38:287–301, 1993

18. Vance ML: Growth hormone for the elderly. *N Engl J Med* 323:52–54, 1990

19. Lane RJM, Mastaglia FL: Drug-induced myopathies in man. *Lancet* 2:562–65, 1978

20. Garg A, Grundy SM: Nicotinic acid as therapy for dyslipidemia in non-insulin-dependent diabetes. *JAMA* 264:723–26, 1990

21. Teuscher AU, Seaquist ER, Robertson RP: Diminished insulin secretory reserve in diabetic pancreas transplant and nondiabetic kidney transplant recipients. *Diabetes* 43:593–98, 1994

22. Sumarini NB, Delaney V, Daskalaxis P, Davis R, Friedman EA, Hong JH, Sommer BG: Retrospective analysis of posttransplantation diabetes mellitus in black renal allograft recipients. *Diabetes Care* 14:760–62, 1991

23. Tobert JA: Rhabdomyolysis in patients receiving lovastatin after cardiac transplantation. *N Engl J Med* 318:47–48, 1988

24. Suh I, Shaten BJ, Cutler JA, Kuller LH: Alcohol use and mortality from coronary heart disease: the role of high-density cholesterol. *Ann Intern Med* 116:881–87, 1992

25. Facchini F, Chen Y-DI, Reaven GM: Light-to-moderate alcohol intake is associated with enhanced insulin sensitivity. *Diabetes Care* 17:115–19, 1994

26. Waskin H, Stehr-Green JK, Helmick CG, Sattler FR: Risk factors for hypoglycemia associated with pentamidine therapy for Pneumocystis pneumonia. *JAMA* 260:345–47, 1988

27. Limburg PJ, Katz H, Grant CS, Service FJ: Quinine-induced hypoglycemia. *Ann Intern Med* 119:218–19, 1993

24. Prediabetes and the Insulin Resistance Syndrome

Highlights
Prediabetes and the Insulin
Resistance Syndrome

- Epidemiological evidence suggests that regular physical activity prevents or at least retards the development of non-insulin-dependent diabetes mellitus (NIDDM) and coronary heart disease.
- This benefit of exercise is likely to be most prominent in individuals predisposed to the insulin resistance syndrome.
- Individuals with this syndrome often have generalized or central obesity; however, they also may not be obese by present standards.

- Exercise may be therapeutically more efficacious in these individuals than in patients with established NIDDM.
- Individuals at risk for NIDDM and the insulin resistance syndrome may be identifiable early by such factors as family history, birth weight, gestational diabetes, and increased adiposity.
- Programs of diet and exercise that prevent excess adiposity and insulin resistance seem warranted for these individuals and probably for the general population.

Prediabetes and the Insulin Resistance Syndrome

NEIL RUDERMAN, MD, DPhil

EXERCISE AND THE REDUCTION IN RISK OF NON-INSULIN-DEPENDENT DIABETES MELLITUS (NIDDM)

Epidemiological evidence suggests that physical activity prevents, or at least retards, the development of NIDDM and coronary heart disease (see Chapter 4). Thus, several studies have shown that the prevalence of NIDDM and heart attacks is 30–55% lower in men and women who exercise regularly than in their sedentary counterparts. Such data raise two important questions: *1*) By what mechanism does exercise exert these effects and *2*) how can patients who are most likely to benefit from physical activity be identified?

HYPERINSULINEMIA AND INSULIN RESISTANCE

It has long been appreciated that physical activity acutely (1) and chronically (Table 24.1) (2) diminishes plasma insulin levels and enhances insulin sensitivity in peripheral tissues: indeed, it was for this reason that exercise was first utilized in the treatment of glucose intolerance (3) and NIDDM (4). As reviewed elsewhere in this book (see Chapter 3), hyperinsulinemia and insulin resistance are more prevalent in patients with NIDDM, hypertension, certain dyslipoproteinemias (increased plasma very-low-density lipoprotein triglycerides and decreased high-density lipoprotein [HDL] cholesterol), central obesity, and premature coronary heart disease (5–7). They appear to be part of an insulin resistance syndrome, sometimes referred to as syndrome X (6), which antedates these disorders and may contribute to their pathogenesis. Thus, hyperinsulinemia and insulin resistance have been observed in offspring and/or other first-degree relatives of patients with NIDDM (8,9), hypertension (10), and hypertriglyceridemia (10,11). In addition, hyperinsulinemia and insulin resistance are present in people who are at increased risk for coronary heart disease in the absence of NIDDM, hypertension, and dyslipidemia (5). As shown in Fig. 24.1, current theory holds that the hyperinsulinemia and insulin resistance may result from genetic factors (e.g., susceptibility genes) acting in concert with obesity and/or physical inactivity. In turn, dependent on the genetic makeup of the individual, the hyperinsulinemia and insulin resistance may lead to NIDDM, hypertension, dyslipoproteinemias, or all three in combination (6). It has been proposed that the high prevalence of hyperinsulinemia and insulin resistance in individuals leading a Western lifestyle accounts for the reported benefits of physical activity in decreasing the incidence of NIDDM and heart attack in epidemiological studies (12). In keeping with this, the most marked benefit of exercise in preventing NIDDM in men has been observed in individuals at high risk because of family history of diabetes or the presence of obesity (13,14). Whether exercise also has a beneficial effect in preventing NIDDM in lean individuals is uncertain because of the small number of cases and low absolute rates of diabetes in this population in published studies. Because of this, the statistical power needed to detect an effect of exercise in these individuals was limited.

RELATION OF INSULIN RESISTANCE SYNDROME TO OBESITY

Hyperinsulinemia and insulin resistance invariably accompany adult-onset obesity and most likely account for the close linkage of obesity, and particularly central obesity, to NIDDM, hypertension, and certain dyslipoproteinemias. Note, however, that insulin resistance is often present in individuals with these disorders who are not overtly obese based on measurements of their height and weight (15–17). Such metabolically obese–normal weight individuals (15) are probably quite common in the gen-

Table 24.1. Characteristics of Athletic and Sedentary Middle-Aged Swedish Men

	SKIERS	NONATHLETES
Age (years)	54	55
Weight (kg)	71	75
Body fat (kg)	10*	16
Triglycerides (mg/dl)	80*	109
Cholesterol (mg/dl)	203*	257
Glucose (mg/dl)		
Fasting	73	64
Postglucose (1 h)	79*	108
Insulin (µU/ml)		
Fasting	2*	10
Postglucose (1 h)	34*	95

Adapted from Bjorntorp et al. (2). *$P < 0.05$, significantly different from nonathletes.

eral population (15–17) (Table 24.2) and may cluster at the upper end of the normal range of body mass index (BMI) (18). Some of them may have a predominantly android (central) fat distribution due to an increase in intra-abdominal fat (19). Such increases in intra-abdominal fat may be evident from measurement of the waist-to-hip ratio or may require more sensitive tests such as computerized axial tomography (CAT) scanning or magnetic resonance imaging for detection. Whether the insulin resistance syndrome occurs in individuals with normal amounts of intra-abdominal fat as judged by CAT scanning is not known. Independent of a high BMI, increases in intra-abdominal fat have been associated with hyperinsulinemia, insulin resistance, and a predisposition to both NIDDM and coronary heart disease (19,21). It has been hypothesized that normal-weight individuals with the insulin resistance syndrome may have been thin when young and that increases in adiposity during

Table 24.2. Characteristics of Italian Factory Workers With Hyperinsulinemia and Normal Glucose Tolerance

	HYPERINSULINEMIA	NORMAL INSULIN
Age (years)	39	39
BMI	24.7	24.7
Glucose (mg/dl)		
Fasting	86	86
Postglucose (1 h)	110*	94
Insulin (µU/ml)		
Fasting	14*	7
Postglucose (1 h)	94*	35
Triglycerides (mM)	1.7*	1.2
Cholesterol (mM)	5.1	4.8
HDL cholesterol (mM)	1.2*	1.4
Blood pressure (mmHg)		95
Systolic	126*	119
Diastolic	85*	78

Adapted from Zavaroni et al. (16). *$P < 0.05$, significantly different from normal insulin group.

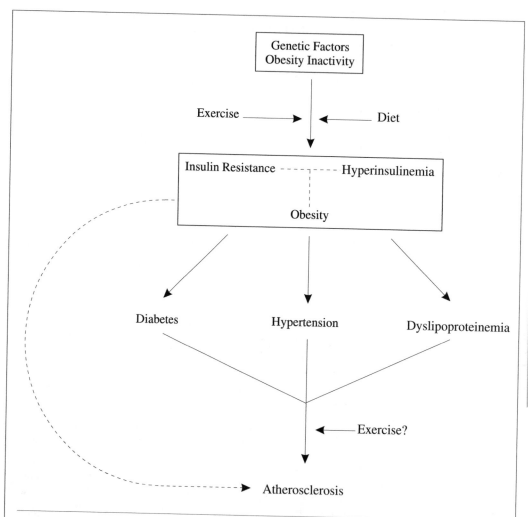

Figure 24.1. Exercise and Atherosclerosis. According to this scheme, exercise and diet decrease hyperinsulinemia and insulin resistance by modifying the effect of genetic factors, diminishing obesity, or preventing the pathogenetic effect of inactivity per se. This, in turn, diminishes the propensity of such individuals to develop type II diabetes, hypertension, and certain dyslipoproteinemias. The antiatherogenic action of exercise could be attributable to any or all of these effects. The report that exercise diminishes the severity of coronary heart disease in monkeys fed an atherogenic diet (29), independent of changes in plasma lipids, glucose, or blood pressure, suggests that it has a more direct antiatherogenic effect. As shown here, whether obesity is a cause and/or a consequence of the hyperinsulinemia and insulin resistance is unclear.

adolescence and adulthood bring them to a normal population mean for body weight (15). Obesity in this group may be characterized by disproportionate increases in intra-abdominal fat and the presence of large adipocytes rather than an increase in adipose mass relative to the general population (20). To a certain extent, such increases in fat cell size, and presumably intra-abdominal visceral fat mass, occur in all individuals in Westernized societies as they pass from young adulthood to middle age (2).

Table 24.3. Predicted Characteristics of Young Individuals Most Likely to Benefit From Exercise and Diet Therapy

- Family history
  - NIDDM
  - Premature atherosclerosis
  - Hypertriglyceridemia
  - Low HDL cholesterol
  - Hypertension

- Presence of
  - Central obesity
  - Manifestations of insulin resistance syndrome
  - Gestational diabetes
  - Low birth weight

- Certain ethnic groups
  - Latinos
  - Blacks
  - Japanese Americans
  - Native Americans

RATIONALE FOR USE OF EXERCISE BEFORE THE ONSET OF DIABETES

Although exercise can improve glucose tolerance, diminish insulin resistance, and improve coronary risk factors in patients with overt NIDDM, its therapeutic efficacy in this population is somewhat limited. Most patients with NIDDM are over age 40 at the time of diagnosis, and they tend to be resistant to the lifestyle changes required by a lifelong exercise (or diet) program (22). Also, many of them (20–40%) already have clinically significant ischemic heart disease (23,24). As stated previously, "these factors do not negate the therapeutic value of exercise in patients with NIDDM; however, they strongly suggest that exercise and other preventive measures (e.g., diet) may be more efficacious if they are instituted earlier in life" (12). A large multicenter NIH prevention trial is currently investigating this possibility.

TARGET POPULATIONS

It has been proposed that a major target population for exercise therapy is people at risk for developing NIDDM and related disorders because of the presence of hyperinsulinemia and insulin resistance. Genetic markers do not as yet allow us to identify these individuals; however, it may be possible to do so on the basis of family history, the presence of components of the insulin resistance syndrome (e.g., hypertriglyceridemia, low HDL cholesterol, or hypertension), and/or central obesity (Table 24.3). One group that is already routinely identified is women with gestational diabetes (see Chapter 20). Yet another may be men or women with a low birth weight for gestational age. Studies in several English populations have shown a dramatically higher prevalence of both NIDDM and syndrome X in middle-aged individuals with a low birth weight (25). Thus, in one population of 64-year-old men whose birth weights were 6.5 lb, 22% had syndrome X, compared with a prevalence of 2% in those with birth weights of >9.5 lb. Likewise, in another group of 64-year-old men, the prevalence of diabetes and impaired glucose tolerance (40%) was nearly threefold greater in the low versus the high birth-weight group. The mechanism for this association is not known, although the observation that such individuals have a low BMI at birth and a somewhat higher BMI than higher birth-weight subjects in middle age suggests they may be more obese. Finally, certain ethnic groups, such as Native Americans, Japanese Americans, Mexican Americans, Australian Aborigines, and blacks (26), are more prone to obesity and NIDDM when living a Western lifestyle. Where studied, these groups have shown an excellent response to exercise and diet therapy (27,28).

EXERCISE PRESCRIPTION

The principles of the exercise prescription described herein (see Chapter 6) also apply to individuals with the insulin resistance syndrome and to those with prediabetes. We would emphasize here that most of the individuals who fit this classification will be young (<40 years old) and will not require an extensive cardiac workup (e.g., stress electrocardiogram). The exceptions will be patients in whom symptoms or specific risk factors for coronary heart disease, such as dyslipoproteinemia or hypertension, are already present. As in patients with overt diabetes, the exercise and diet prescription should take into account the individual's social and cultural background and specific preferences. This is an especially important consideration in the United States, where an extremely high prevalence of diabetes is found in blacks, Native Americans, Latinos, Mexican Americans, and Japanese Americans (see Chapter 25).

CONCLUSIONS

Studies are needed to prove definitively that exercise and diet therapy can be used effectively to prevent (or reverse) the development of NIDDM and other disorders associated with the insulin resistance syndrome. On the other hand, the risk from such a therapeutic approach is low, and the likelihood that it will be beneficial is high. For this reason, we believe that programs of exercise and diet that prevent excess adiposity and diminish insulin resistance are justified in the general population and especially in individuals at high risk for NIDDM and related disorders.

ACKNOWLEDGMENTS

This work was supported in part by National Institutes of Health Grant DK-19514. I thank Maryse Roudier for helpful criticisms and for typing the manuscript.

REFERENCES

1. Richter EA, Garetto LP, Goodman MN, Ruderman NB: Muscle glucose metabolism following exercise in the rat. *J Clin Invest* 69:785–93, 1982
2. Bjorntorp P, De Jounge K, Sjostrom L, Sullivan L: The effect of physical training on insulin production in obesity. *Metabolism* 19:631–38, 1976
3. Saltin B, Lindgarde F, Houston M: Physical training and glucose tolerance in middle-aged men with chemical diabetes. *Diabetes* 28 (Suppl. 1):30–37, 1979
4. Ruderman NB, Ganda OP, Johansen K: The effect of physical training on glucose tolerance and plasma lipids in maturity-onset diabetes. *Diabetes* 28:89–92, 1979
5. Schneider SH, Vitug A, Ruderman N: Atherosclerosis and physical activity. *Diabetes Metab Rev* 1: 513–53, 1986
6. Reaven GM: Role of insulin resistance in human disease. *Diabetes* 37:1595–607, 1988
7. DeFronzo RA, Ferrannini E: Insulin resistance: a multifaceted syndrome responsible for NIDDM, obesity, hypertension, dyslipidemia and atherosclerotic cardiovascular disease. *Diabetes Care* 14:173–94, 1991
8. Eriksson J, Franssila-Kallunki A, Ekstrand A, Groop L: Early metabolic defects in persons at increased risk for non-insulin-dependent diabetes mellitus. *N Engl J Med* 6:337–43, 1989
9. Vaag A, Henriksen JE, Beck-Nielson H: Decreased insulin activation of glycogen synthase in skeletal muscles in young non-obese Caucasian relatives of patients with non-insulin-dependent diabetes mellitus. *J Clin Invest* 89:782–88, 1992
10. Ferrari P, Weidmann P: Insulin, insulin sensitivity and hypertension. *J Hypertens* 8:491–500, 1990
11. Werbin B, Tamir I, Heidenberg D, Ayalen D, Adler M, Lenton O: Immunoreactive insulin response to oral glucose in offspring of patients with endogenous hypertriglyceridemia. *Clin Chim Acta* 76:35–40, 1977
12. Ruderman NB, Schneider SH: Diabetes, exercise, and atherosclerosis. *Diabetes Care* 15 (Suppl. 4): 1787–93, 1992
13. Helmreich SP, Ragland DR, Leung RW, Paffenbarger RS: Physical activity and reduced occurrence of non-insulin-dependent diabetes mellitus. *N Engl J Med* 325:147–52, 1991
14. Manson JE, Nathan DM, Krowlewski AS, Stampfer MJ, Willett WC, Hennekens CH: A prospective

study of exercise and the incidence of diabetes among male physicians. *JAMA* 268:63–67, 1992

15. Ruderman NB, Schneider SH, Berchtold P: The metabolically obese, normal-weight individual. *Am J Clin Nutr* 34:1617–21, 1981

16. Zavaroni I, Bonini L, Fantuzzi M, Dall'Aglio E, Passeri M, Reaven GM: Hyperinsulinemia, obesity and syndrome X. *J Intern Med* 235: 51–56, 1994

17. Zavaroni I, Bonora E, Pagliara M, Dall'Aglio E, Luchetti L, Buonanno G, Bonati PA, Bergonzani M, Gnudi L, Passeri M, Reaven G: Risk factors for coronary artery disease in healthy persons with hyperinsulinemia and normal glucose tolerance. *N Engl J Med* 320:702–706, 1989

18. Chan JM, Rimm EB, Colditz GA, Stampfer MJ, Willett WC: Obesity, fat distribution, and weight gain as risk factors for clinical diabetes in men. *Diabetes Care* 17:961–69, 1994

19. Kissebah AH, Vydelingum N, Murray R, Evans DJ, Hartz AJ, Kalkhoff RK, Adams PW: Relation of body fat distribution to metabolic complications of obesity. *J Clin Endocrinol Metab* 54:254–60, 1980

20. Bernstein RS, Grant N, Kipnis DM: Hyperinsulinemia and enlarged adipocytes in patients with endogenous hyperlipoproteinemia without obesity or diabetes mellitus. *Diabetes* 24:207–13, 1975

21. Bjorntrop P: Metabolic implications of body fat distribution. *Diabetes Care* 14:1132–43, 1991

22. Skarfors ET, Wegener TA, Lithell H, Selinus I: Physical training as treatment for type 2 (non-insulin-dependent) diabetes in elderly men: a feasibility study over 2 years. *Diabetologia* 30:930–33, 1987

23. Nesto RW, Phillips RT, Kett KG, Hill T, Perper E, Young E, Leland S: Angina and exertional myocardial ischemia in diabetic and non-diabetic patients: assessment by exercise thallium scintigraphy. *Ann Intern Med* 108:170–75, 1988

24. Uusitupa M, Siltonen O, Pyorala K, Aro A, Hersio K, Pentilla I, Voutilainen E: The relationship of cardiovascular risk factors to the prevalence of coronary heart disease in recently diagnosed type II (non-insulin-dependent) diabetes. *Diabetologia* 28:653–59, 1985

25. Barker DJP, Hales CN, Fall CHD, Osmond C, Phipps K, Clark PMS: Type 2 (non-insulin-dependent) diabetes mellitus, hypertension and hyperlipidaemia (syndrome X): relation to reduced fetal growth. *Diabetologia* 36:62–67, 1993

26. Ruderman NB, Apelian AZ, Schneider SH: Exercise in the therapy and prevention of type II diabetes: implications for blacks. *Diabetes Care* 13 (Suppl. 4):1163–68, 1990

27. O'Dea K: Marked improvement in carbohydrate and lipid metabolism in diabetic Australian Aborigines after temporary reversion to traditional lifestyle. *Diabetes* 33:596–603, 1984

28. Heath GW, Leonard BE, Wilson RH, Kendrick JS, Powell KE: Community-based exercise intervention: Zuni diabetes project. *Diabetes Care* 10:579–83, 1987

29. Kramsch DM, Aspen AJ, Abramowitz BM, Kreimendahl T, Hood W: Reduction of coronary atherosclerosis by moderate conditioning exercise in monkeys on an atherogenic diet. *N Engl J Med* 305:1483–91, 1981

25. Exercise Programs in Minority Populations

Highlights
Exercise Programs in Minority Populations

- Physical activity levels among minorities are lower than among Caucasians at all stages of life.
- Minorities have higher levels of obesity and increased waist-to-hip ratios compared with Caucasians.
- Minorities are less likely than Caucasians of similar obesity levels to consider themselves obese.
- Diabetes and some of its complications are more prevalent among minorities, yet diabetes may not be perceived as a serious disease.
- Exercise programs should include input from community members during the planning process.
- Participation of family members in the exercise activity may improve success rates.
- Moderate exercise, such as walking, is more readily accepted by some minority groups.
- Other issues that should be addressed in program planning include transportation, child care, cost of equipment, literacy level and language of written materials, and cultural differences in food preferences.

Exercise Programs in Minority Populations

MELANIE J. BRUNT, MD, MPH, AND STUART R. CHIPKIN, MD

INTRODUCTION

The creation of exercise programs for minorities with diabetes mellitus has been a significant and unique challenge because of behavioral, socioeconomic, and cultural issues. Structured programs that encourage aerobic exercise could be of critical importance in such individuals, because physical activity levels are lower among minorities from childhood through adult life (1–7). As with Caucasians, lower levels of exercise appear to contribute to increased weight. The prevalence of obesity among all age-groups in minority populations has been increasing over time, starting as early as kindergarten (8,9). Among African-American women, the prevalence of obesity is double that for whites and is >60% among women over age 45 (10). A higher prevalence of obesity and a greater tendency toward upper body obesity (increased waist-to-hip ratio [WHR]) also have been found in several other ethnic groups, including Native Americans, Mexican Americans, and Puerto Ricans.

Implementing exercise programs in these populations may be difficult, in part, because of a lack of perceived need. African Americans who are at least 20% over ideal body weight are less likely than whites of similar obesity levels to regard themselves as obese (11) or to make efforts to lose weight (1–3). Among Latinos, as well, cultural norms appear to be more tolerant of obesity (12).

At all levels of obesity in the U.S., diabetes is significantly more prevalent and occurs at an earlier age among minorities than among whites. This has been observed in people of African, Central and South American, Native American, and Asian origin (13). In some minority ethnic groups, the risk of diabetes-related morbidity and mortality is also dramatically increased. Among African Americans, micro- and macrovascular complications, such as retinopathy, end-stage renal disease, and amputation, are more prevalent

(14–16), and mortality risk is increased 2.5-fold (16).

Although there are relatively few published reports of exercise interventions in minorities with diabetes, the findings from these as well as other exercise studies among nondiabetic individuals are very instructive. Barriers to successful outcomes and features that enhance success rates among members of different minority groups seem to be relatively consistent across populations.

AFRICAN AMERICANS

Direct involvement of participants is very important when planning an exercise program. Results of the PATH-WAYS program, a diet and exercise intervention for obese inner-city African-American women with non-insulin-dependent diabetes mellitus (NIDDM), indicated that input from these women during the planning process may have contributed to the program's success. The exercise program was of moderate intensity (walking 20–30 min 3 times a week), and printed materials given to participants were reviewed to determine that they did not exceed the 8th grade reading level. The nondidactic instructional program incorporated principles of behavior modification, including stimulus control, self-monitoring, and cognitive modification (18). Participants were guided through a process of learning their own needs and acquiring the knowledge and skills required to meet those needs. Mean weight loss for 10 women at completion of the 18-week program was 4.1 kg, and at 1-year follow-up, weight loss was maintained with an average loss of 4.4 kg. Mean glycated hemoglobin levels were improved at 18 weeks (10.2 vs. 12.8% at baseline), but at 1 year they had regressed to baseline at 12.6%.

In another inner-city African-American community, a 10-week exercise and nutrition intervention program for cardiovascular risk reduction was implemented in obese nondiabetic

Table 25.1. Exercise Programs in Minority Groups

ETHNIC GROUP	PROGRAM	NO. ENROLLED	DURATION (weeks)	NO. COMPLETED	RESULTS
African Americans					
■ Women with NIDDM (18)	Walking 20 min 3 times/week	10	18	10	Weight loss 4.1 kg at 18 weeks; 4.4 kg at 1 year. Glycated hemoglobin decreased by 2.6% at 18 weeks but back to baseline at 1 year
■ Obese men and women, nondiabetic (19)	Exercise and nutrition didactic instruction 2 times/week	Not stated	10	70	Significant reductions in weight and blood pressure persisted at 4 months
■ Healthy families (20)	One educational and two 30-min fitness sessions/week	94 families	14	19 families	No differences in ergometer fitness, weight, or blood pressure
Hispanic Americans					
■ Obese nondiabetic Mexican-American women (23)	Walking program	22	8	21	Significant decreases in BMI, WHR, cholesterol, fitness, and red meat consumption at 8 weeks; WHR and cholesterol returned to baseline at 3 months
■ Obese nondiabetic Mexican-American women; three groups: control, women alone, women with their families (24)	Exercise and nutrition didactic instruction 1 time/week	168 women among the three groups	24	86	Significant weight loss in two intervention groups versus control; no change in fasting blood glucose or lipids
Native Americans					
■ Zuni Pueblo with NIDDM (25)	Aerobics classes 1.7 times/week on average	Not applicable	37	Retrospective study of 30 subjects	Weight decreased 4.09 kg, BMI decreased by 1.5 kg/m², fasting blood glucose decreased by 2.38 mmol/l at 2 years

adults living in Atlanta, Georgia. The study was designed and directed by a community coalition (19). Incentives to participate in exercise classes included free transportation, child care, and a system of rewards. Among a total of 70 participants who completed the program, significant reductions in weight and blood pressure persisted for 4 months after the intervention. In contrast, in a similarly designed program that targeted healthy urban African-American families with children in the 5th through 7th grades, the participation rate was only 20% by the end of 14 weeks (20). The program included one educational and two fitness sessions/week, was based at a community center, and provided free transportation and child care. Input was sought from community leaders and participants, and the program incorporated individualized counseling using behavior modification strategies. However, in contrast to the PATHWAYS program, the participants were actively recruited from a random sample rather than volunteering, which may have significantly affected retention. Additionally, the most frequent barrier to participation cited by participants was conflict with work schedules. Family incomes were extremely low (92% under $15,000/year), and there was a high frequency of job change or job schedule change. The authors postulated that a certain level of family economic stability may be necessary for regular participation in such programs. An alternate solution may involve low-cost exercise programs that incorporate significant flexibility or are located at worksites.

Thus, effective exercise programs must consider economic factors, educational levels, transportation, and child care needs. Other significant factors among African Americans include 1) cultural differences in diet composition; African-American diets have been shown to be higher in cholesterol and saturated fat and lower in fiber than those of Caucasians, 2) a higher prevalence of comorbidity and disability among older African-American patients with NIDDM; this limits the ability to exercise, and 3) the need for plac-

ing a higher emphasis on peer and family attitudes and support, because diet and exercise behaviors are heavily influenced by whether other individuals share the activity and appreciate its value. All of these factors affect compliance with recommended exercise and dietary changes (21).

HISPANIC AMERICANS

Similar issues have been identified among Hispanic Americans. Urban Caribbean Latinos (of Puerto Rican or Dominican origin) with NIDDM who were interviewed regarding diabetes practices cited barriers to exercise, such as fear of walking in unsafe neighborhoods, lack of access to exercise facilities, and lack of supervision (22). Also, although participants understood that exercise was important for people with diabetes, they did not know that exercise might actually improve their prognosis. Strenuous aerobic exercise was not favored by this group. Rather, they indicated a willingness to perform less strenuous exercises, such as walking or dancing.

One group of investigators demonstrated the success of a walking program among obese nondiabetic Mexican-American women. The program involved 22 participants and used behavior modification techniques and a peer support ("buddy") system. Individuals contracted with a peer, as well as with a family member, to complete the program (23). Retention rates were high, with 21 of 22 participants completing the 8-week program. At the end of the program, significant reductions were shown for body mass index (BMI), WHR, total serum cholesterol, fitness level, and red meat consumption in participants compared with control subjects. At 3 months, 47% of participants and 44% of control subjects were reexamined: BMI had decreased further, WHR and total cholesterol had returned to baseline. Results of another program performed for Mexican Americans ("Cuidando el Corazon") were much less impressive, showing much lower retention rates (only 50%) and insignificant amounts of weight loss. Weight loss was higher, however, among those in whom a family-centered approach was used, such that partners and children were included in the intervention (24).

NATIVE AMERICANS

Native Americans, who have an extremely high prevalence of NIDDM, may also derive substantial benefit from modest exercise. In a study of Zuni Pueblo Indians with NIDDM, 30 who exercised were compared with 50 who did not exercise. Exercisers participated in aerobics classes on the average of 1.7 times/week for 37 weeks and showed significant improvements in weight (-4.09 vs. -0.91 kg), BMI (-1.5 vs. -0.40 kg/m^2), and fasting glucose (-2.38 vs. -0.11 mmol/l) at 2 years (25). Factors that promoted longer term participation included organization and supervision of the intervention by community members and location within the community. Among Pima Indians, who have the highest documented NIDDM incidence rates in the world, the level of current physical activity was shown in a cross-sectional analysis to be inversely related to glucose intolerance, obesity, and central distribution of fat, suggesting that activity may protect against NIDDM development even in those with extremely high NIDDM risk (26). Also of note, the level of current physical activity was lower among diabetic than nondiabetic individuals.

OTHER GROUPS

Among a small group of Australian aborigines, reversion to an ancestral hunter-gatherer lifestyle for 7 weeks, with concomitant changes in diet composition and activity level, substantially improved insulin sensitivity and weight (27). Similar findings have been published for native Hawaiians (28), demonstrating that diet and exercise tailored to specific populations can be successful.

CONCLUSIONS

Minority exercise programs character-ized by higher success rates have addressed issues of physical and financial access, child care, appropriateness of exercise activity, and community and family support. The use of behavioral modification techniques adapted from social learning theory has also been effective. Such techniques are based on the concept that new exercise and eating behaviors must be learned through a multistep process. Wing et al. (29) have detailed such a process that was successful in obese NIDDM patients.

Thus, success of physical activity as therapy for minorities with diabetes appears to be determined by several factors beyond intensity and duration. Many barriers to exercise participation exist: some are secondary to the lower socioeconomic status of some members of minority groups in the U.S., others may reflect cultural differences. Barriers include diminished access to safe exercise facilities, lack of financial resources for exercise equipment, negative attitudes regarding the potential benefits of exercise or weight control, lack of peer support, and perceptions that diabetes mellitus is not a serious disease. These factors must be taken into consideration to achieve a successful outcome, whether one is prescribing individual exercise regimens or developing group programs.

Several programs have documented difficulties sustaining compliance and weight change after formal programs have ended. Future work will need to address ways to maintain behavioral changes. Programs that only temporarily remove economic, social, and cultural barriers are likely to have temporary effects. Group programs that are community based and gain family support appear to be more likely to achieve long-term success. (see Chapter 26).

RECOMMENDATIONS

- Program planning should be done in consultation with members of the targeted community.
- Family involvement and support can be incorporated by inclusion of family members in some or all of

the exercise activities or related social gatherings.

- Scheduling must be flexible to accommodate changing work schedules and child care needs.
- Affordability issues can be addressed by the use of public facilities, such as school gymnasiums or malls for walking programs; corporate sponsors may also be sought to provide walking shoes or other exercise equipment as a community service.
- Educational materials should be pretested among target group members; they should be of appropriate literacy level and cultural content.
- Long-term supervised maintenance programs may be necessary to sustain the beneficial effects of the exercise activities.

REFERENCES

1. Bennett EM: Weight-loss practices of overweight adults. *Am J Clin Nutr* 53 (Suppl. 6):S1519–21, 1991
2. Sidney S, Jacobs DR Jr, Haskell WL, Armstrong MA, Dimicco A, Oberman A, Savage PJ, Slattery ML, Sternfeld B, Van Horn L: Comparison of two methods of assessing physical activity in the Coronary Artery Risk Development in Young Adults (CARDIA) Study. *Am J Epidemiol* 133:1231–45, 1991
3. Burke GL, Savage PJ, Manolio TA, Sprafka JM, Wagenknecht LE, Sidney S, Perkins LL, Liu K, Jacobs DR Jr: Correlates of obesity in young black and white women: the CARDIA Study. *Am J Public Health* 82:1621–25, 1992
4. Emmons L: Dieting and purging behavior in black and white high school students. *J Am Diet Assoc* 3:306–12, 1992
5. Duelberg SI: Preventive health behavior among black and white women in urban and rural areas. *Soc Sci Med* 34:191–98, 1992
6. Ainsworth BE, Berry CB, Schnyder VN, Vickers SR: Leisure-time physical activity and aerobic fitness in African-American young adults. *J Adolesc Health* 13:606–11, 1992
7. Folsom AR, Cook TC, Sprafka JM, Burke GL, Norsted SW, Jacobs DR Jr: Differences in leisure-time physical activity levels between blacks and whites in population-based samples: the Minnesota Heart Survey. *J Behav Med* 14:1–9, 1991
8. Kumanyika SK, Huffman SL, Bradshaw ME, Waller H, Ross A, Serdula M, Paige D: Stature and weight status of children in an urban kindergarten population. *Pediatrics* 85:783–90, 1990
9. The Research Group: Obesity and cardiovascular disease risk factors in black and white girls: NHLBI Growth and Health Study. *Am J Public Health* 82:1613–20, 1992
10. Pi-Sunyer FX: Obesity and diabetes in blacks. *Diabetes Care* 113:1144–49, 1990
11. Desmond SM, Price JH, Hallinan C, Smith D: Black and white adolescents' perceptions of their weight. *J Sch Health* 59:353–58, 1989
12. Massara EB: *Que Gordita! A Study of Weight Among Women in a Puerto Rican Community*. New York, AMS Press, 1989
13. Harris MI, Hadden WC, Knowler WC, Bennett PH: Prevalence of diabetes and impaired glucose tolerance and plasma glucose levels in U.S. population aged 10–74 yr. *Diabetes* 36:523–34, 1987
14. Harris MI: Non-insulin-dependent diabetes in black and white Americans. *Diabetes Metab Rev* 6:71–90, 1990
15. Cowie CC, Port FK, Wolfe RA, Savage PJ, Moll PP, Hawthorne VM: Disparities in incidence of diabetes end-stage renal disease according to race and type of diabetes. *N Engl J Med* 321:1074–79, 1989
16. Most RS, Sinnock P: The epidemiology of lower extremity amputations in diabetic individuals. *Diabetes Care* 6:87–91, 1983
17. Kumanyika S: Obesity in black women. *Epidemiol Rev* 9:31–50, 1987
18. McNabb WL, Quinn MT, Rosing L: Weight-loss program for inner-city

black women with non-insulin-dependent diabetes mellitus: PATH-WAYS. *J Am Diet Assoc* 93:75–77, 1993

19. Lasco RA, Curry RH, Dickson VJ, Powers J, Menes S, Merritt RK: Participation rates, weight loss, and blood pressure changes among obese women in a nutrition-exercise program. *Public Health Rep* 104:640–46, 1989

20. Baranowski T, Simons-Morton B, Hooks P, Henske J, Tiernan K, Dunn JK, Burkhalter H, Harper J, Palmer J: A center-based program for exercise change among Black-American families. *Health Educ Q* 17:179–96, 1990

21. Kumanyika SK, Ewart CK: Theoretical and baseline considerations for diet and weight control of diabetes among blacks. *Diabetes Care* 13:1154–62, 1990

22. Quatromoni PA, Milbauer M, Posner BM, Carballeira NP, Brunt MJ, Chipkin SR: Use of focus groups to explore nutrition practices and health beliefs of urban Caribbean Latinos with diabetes. *Diabetes Care* 17:869–73, 1994

23. Avila P, Hovel MF: Physical activity training for weight loss in Latinas: a controlled trial. *Intern J Obes* 18:476–82, 1994

24. Foreyt JP, Ramirez AG, Cousins JH: Cuidando el corazon—a weight-reduction intervention for Mexican Americans. *Am J Clin Nutr* 53: S1639–41, 1991

25. Heath GW, Wilson RH, Smith J, Leonard BE: Community-based exercise and weight control: diabetes risk reduction and glycemic control in Zuni Indians. *Am J Clin Nutr* 53:S1642–46, 1991

26. Kriska AM, LaPorte RE, Pettitt DJ, Charles MA, Nelson RG, Kuller LH, Bennett PH, Knowler WC: The association of physical activity with obesity, fat distribution and glucose intolerance in Pima Indians. *Diabetologia* 36:863–69, 1993

27. O'Dea K: Marked improvement in carbohydrate and lipid metabolism in diabetic Australian aborigines after temporary reversion to traditional lifestyle. *Diabetes* 33:596–603, 1984

28. Shintani TT, Hughes CK, Beckham S, O'Connor HK: Obesity and cardiovascular risk intervention through the ad libitum feeding of traditional Hawaiian diet. *Am J Clin Nutr* 53:S1647–51, 1991

29. Wing RR: Behavioral strategies for weight reduction in obese type II diabetic patients. *Diabetes Care* 12:139–44, 1989

26. Community-Based Exercise Programs

Highlights
Community-Based Exercise Programs

- Motivating individuals to increase their physical activity levels can be difficult.
- A community-based exercise program is one way to promote long-term changes in exercise habits.
- Exercise programs that are culturally acceptable are more likely to be sustainable over the long term.
- Exercise programs that come out of a true "community development" process may improve participation and success rates.
- A community coalition should be the driving force behind an exercise program.
- Community exercise programs that reward participation and completion are most successful.
- A community-based exercise program can be implemented with limited resources.

Community-Based Exercise Programs

EVAN M. BENJAMIN, MD

INTRODUCTION

Diabetes can be controlled and possibly prevented through routine aerobic activity. Regular short-term exercise can improve insulin resistance, but this beneficial effect is transient unless the exercise is continued (1). Long-term changes in exercise patterns are therefore necessary to maintain improved glycemic control, yet motivating individuals to make such permanent lifestyle modifications can be difficult.

Community-based exercise programs are a way to promote wellness and regular physical activity in a given community. Because such programs are created within the context of and supported by the community, they alter the social environment and encourage the community as a whole to accept and reinforce the importance of physical activity for all its members. Exercise initiatives must come out of a genuine "community development" process, by which the efforts of the people themselves are united to improve the health of the community. Community-based exercise programs constitute a significant advantage over individual fitness counseling, which often lacks appropriate and continuous motivation for patients (2–4).

Structured exercise programs have been created in a number of communities, yet there is little data formally documenting the physiological benefits of community-based exercise (5–9). This chapter presents one successful model program and provides suggestions for establishing similar exercise initiatives in other community settings.

A CASE STUDY: THE ZUNI DIABETES PROJECT

The Zuni Indians of New Mexico were once a physically active tribe noted for their running races and farming techniques. In recent years, however, the Zuni, like many other Native Americans, have experienced an epidemic of non-insulin-dependent diabetes mellitus (NIDDM) (10). This epidemic has been attributed to the combination of a contemporary sedentary lifestyle superimposed on a genetically susceptible population (11–14). Among the Zuni, with nearly one-third of the adult population over age 35 afflicted with diabetes (15) and nearly 15% of all pregnancies complicated by diabetes (16), the disease has become a true public health problem. To combat the high rate of diabetes and its complications, the Zuni, in conjunction with the Indian Health Service, initiated a community-based exercise program in the late 1980s (8).

The Zuni Diabetes Project is a structured exercise program created by a community coalition that provides motivation, guidance, and education to patients with diabetes while following them clinically to evaluate their therapeutic response to exercise. The goal of the program is to promote permanent lifestyle changes with regard to physical activity, with a primary focus on individuals with diabetes. Participants are recruited at the Indian Health Service Hospital's diabetes clinic, where exercise specialists from the Zuni Diabetes Project promote exercise classes and events. Additional recruitment occurs through physician referral, community outreach, and advertisement campaigns using radio, newspapers, and posters.

People may participate in the Zuni Diabetes Project in several ways. There are structured exercise classes in aerobics and aerobic circuit training taught by certified instructors who are volunteers from the community. Most of the participants in these classes are women, 18–45 years of age. These women represent 15% of the Zuni population in this age range (according to the 1990 Zuni tribal census). In addition, there are exercise classes designed specifically for people with diabetes. These classes provide education about diabetes management and nutrition, glucose monitoring, and charting of glycemic control in addition to aerobic workouts.

People may also take part in the Zuni Diabetes Project through one of

259

Table 26.1. Mean Changes in Weight, BMI, and FBG for Zuni Indians With NIDDM in a Community Exercise Program

	PARTICIPANTS	NONPARTICIPANTS
n	30	56
Weight (kg)	-4.09 ± 4.90	-0.91 ± 3.90
BMI (kg/m^2)	-1.50 ± 2.20	-0.40 ± 1.30
FBG (mmol/l)	-2.38 ± 4.32	-0.11 ± 3.71

Data are means ± SD; $P < 0.05$ is the statistical significance between groups. FBG, fasting blood glucose.

the incentive programs to promote physical activity and weight loss that are held at different times during the year. Examples include the 100 Mile Club, in which individuals chart their mileage in self-paced walking or running, and the Human Race Fitness Challenge, where participants win prizes based on the number of points earned for physical activity. Prizes are awarded in a public forum. In the annual Holiday Eating Learning Program (HELP), teams compete in weight loss and exercise over a 12-week period in the winter. Finally, the summer-long Zuni Fitness Series of running, biking, walking, and aerobic dancing enrolls over 500 participants each year. The incentives for enrolling in these programs include weekly feedback, community recognition, and personal satisfaction, as well as program T-shirts and other donated awards.

The Zuni Diabetes Project is sustainable and successful because it is a culturally acceptable program that taps into the heritage and pride of the community, resulting in large-scale participation in its exercise programs (17). Zuni Indians with NIDDM who participated in the community exercise program for an average of 37 weeks were compared with 56 Zunis with NIDDM who did not exercise (18). Exercise participants showed improvement in weight and fasting blood glucose (Table 26.1). Additionally, exercise participants were twice as likely as nonparticipants to have decreased their medication. In terms of diabetes risk, a case-control study of Zuni Indians participating in the community-based exercise program revealed that at least once-weekly vigorous physical activity protected individuals from developing diabetes (19). The effect was independent of body mass index (BMI), gender, and family history of diabetes (Table 26.2).

CREATING A COMMUNITY-BASED EXERCISE PROGRAM

The Zuni Diabetes Project is an example of a community-based program that has sustained long-term changes in lifestyle for people who have diabetes or are at risk for developing it (8,18). The Zuni community is unique because of its geographic isolation and historical tradition of exercise, yet the Zuni model can be easily replicated in other communities. Health providers or authorities will need to define the "community" in which they practice. Often this is a geographic area, such as a rural town or county, but more often

Table 26.2. Relative Risk of Development of Diabetes in Zuni Indians According to Regular Exercise Frequency

EXERCISE FREQUENCY	ODDS RATIO
None or less than once a week	1.0 (referent)
Once a week	0.52
More than once a week	0.21

Odds ratios are adjusted for age, gender, BMI, and family history of diabetes. P = 0.001 for trend.

there are predefined communities, such as civic units (e.g., school districts or boroughs), geographic boundaries (e.g., highways or rivers), and historical neighborhoods (e.g., Chinatown or Little Italy). Also, there are practice-defined communities, such as those in which medical practices serve particular groups of patients defined by ethnicity, gender, age, diagnoses, or economic status. It is important to focus on a particular community, however defined, so that resources can be most effectively targeted where the perceived need exists.

Community Empowerment

Health action cannot and should not be an effort imposed from outside and foreign to the people; rather, it must be a response of the community to the problems that the people in the community perceive, carried out in a way that is acceptable to them, and properly supported by an adequate infrastructure.
—Halafdam Mahler,
Director-General
World Health Organization

A successful diabetes exercise program requires that a community be empowered to take action on its own behalf, rather than having someone from the outside attempt to design and implement a health campaign. A community-based program must be created by the members of that community, with technical and organizational support from health agencies and authorities provided as needed and desired.

Establishing A Community Coalition

Ideally, the organizational structure of a community-driven exercise program will take the form of a community coalition that includes community members, neighborhood councils, local agencies, and government agencies, as well as hospital and clinic staff and public health workers. To insure ownership of the campaign, the coalition must seek community input at every phase of the planning process (20). The coalition's responsibilities are to identify specific diabetes-related health problems, to set goals for improving the health of the community, and to design a concrete plan for achieving those goals.

Planning the Program

In order to design an effective exercise program, the coalition must first compile accurate and complete baseline information, such as prevalence, incidence, morbidity, mortality, and behavioral risk factors of diabetes within the community, and must also understand the techniques of data gathering and analysis. Specific questions to be addressed include:
- What are the existing data that document the prevalence and morbidity of diabetes in the community?
- What are the behavioral risk factors for diabetes in the community?
- Is diabetes perceived as a problem by community members?
- What are the resources available in the community, both currently and potentially, to combat diabetes?
- What community barriers exist to prevent an exercise program from being successful?
- What has been successful in other similar communities to combat diabetes?

Once the problem has been defined, the next step is to design an intervention plan that incorporates community resources and obstacles. It is advisable to set short- and long-term goals, to use an incremental approach for changing behavior and attitudes, and to set achievable objectives throughout the process. For example, the coalition's initial focus could be limited to enrolling individuals with known diet-controlled diabetes into an exercise program.

In developing a community-based exercise program, the coalition should not hesitate to explore and draw from other models. Many existing exercise programs are simple to implement and require little expertise to organize and maintain (4,18,21,22). One example from the Zuni Diabetes Project that can easily be replicated in other community settings is the 100 Mile Club. This activity is inexpensive, does not require special facilities, and all age-groups can participate.

Increasing Community Awareness

In order to successfully implement its program, the coalition needs to increase awareness about diabetes as a major community health problem and exercise as an important tool for possible prevention and health management. The awareness campaign should target the specific group that will initially participate in the program, as well as the community as a whole. The media is often a good place to begin through public service announcements, articles, letters, and editorials in local or neighborhood publications. Posters in community centers and health centers are also very effective at letting people know that a problem exists and that there is now a community coalition to fight it. The cost of such publicity is negligible.

The coalition might develop a pamphlet on diabetes that includes information about the resources available in the community and that targets the specific population at risk. Personal communication is also very appropriate for recruiting participants into the program, including one-on-one counseling about diabetes and the importance of exercise.

Encouraging Motivation

Successful management of diabetes requires major lifestyle changes, such as modification of eating habits, weight loss, and exercise. Exercise is particularly beneficial because the variety of activities appeals to many individuals (23) and because, in contrast to weight loss or diet modification alone, the results are evident early on, thus increasing the motivation to continue.

Substantive changes can often be best achieved within a community context where the results are measurable and rewarded. For example, a system of incentives and behavior modifications provided through a multistep process (24) can be integrated into almost every exercise program, serving to motivate individuals from the initiation phase into a sustained exercise routine. Incentives such as program T-shirts, certificates, and community recognition are often all that is necessary to promote completion of the program.

Expanding the Program

Once a small-scale exercise program is off the ground and going well, the coalition may wish to expand its activities. Two possible options are to open the original program to other members of the community or to add a second and complementary program for the initial target group. One good strategy for expanding community awareness and introducing people to the program while also achieving some specific exercise goals is to sponsor an organized running or walking event. A road race or aerobic dance class that includes diabetes awareness and screening booths is also relatively easy to plan. Regardless of the specific activities it uses, the coalition must make a consistent and concerted effort to spread the word that it is trying to reduce the burden of diabetes in the community.

Evaluating the Program

Since experience with community-based exercise programs is still limited, a solid evaluation plan should be a component of the coalition's program (25). An evaluation will help identify the most and least effective methods of improving community health. Additionally, evaluation is central to setting priorities and making the best use of limited resources. Finally, evaluation is necessary to justify expenditures for the program or related research. Academic institutions, government agencies, and local hospitals are often willing to assist in an evaluation project and are open to a solicitation by the coalition.

To assist in program evaluation, the baseline health status of the community as a whole and of the specific individuals participating in the project should be collected at the outset. The program's effectiveness can then be later evaluated in relation to this information. Resultant findings about the health status and the level of participation by community members will be important to share with the program organizers, the community, and potential funding sources.

CONCLUSIONS

Our experience and that of others suggests that exercise programs created through a true community development process have the highest chance for success; community coalitions are especially effective in this regard. With constant community input, the coalition can follow the simple steps outlined in this chapter to identify the problem, set goals for the program, increase community awareness, and provide specific motivation and skills for participation. By altering the social environment and changing attitudes within the context of a community-based initiative, a diabetes exercise program can effectively promote and reinforce physical activity as an acceptable path to disease prevention.

REFERENCES

1. Holloszy JO, Schultz J, Kusnierkiewicz J, Hagberg JM, Ehsani AA: Effects of exercise on glucose tolerance and insulin resistances. *Acta Med Scand Suppl* 711:55–65, 1986
2. Mason JO, Powell KE: Physical activity, behavioral epidemiology and public health. *Public Health Rep* 100:113–15, 1985
3. Powell KE, Paffenbarger RS: Workshop on epidemiologic and public health aspects of physical activity and exercise: a summary. *Public Health Rep* 100:118–26, 1985
4. Health Promotion Research Center: *Promotion of Physical Activity in the Community: A Manual for Community Health Professionals.* Palo Alto, CA, Stanford University Press, 1988
5. Iverson CC, Fielding JE, Crow RS, Christenson GM: The promotion of physical activity in the United States population: the status of programs in medical, worksite, community, and school settings. *Public Health Rep* 100:212–24, 1985
6. Owen N, Dwyer T: Approaches to promoting more widespread participation in physical activity. *Community Health Studies* 12:339–47, 1988
7. Crow R, Blackburn H, Jacobs D, Hannan P, Pirie P, Mittelark M, Murray P, Lyepker R: Population strategies to enhance physical activity: the Minnesota Heart Health Program. *Acta Med Scand* 711: 93–112, 1986
8. Heath GW, Leonard BE, Wilson RH, Kendrick JS, Powell KE: Community-based exercise intervention: Zuni Diabetes Project. *Diabetes Care* 10:579–83, 1987
9. Lasco RA, Curry RH, Dickson VJ, Powers J, Menes S, Merritt RK: Participation rates, weight loss, and blood pressure changes among obese women in a nutrition-exercise program. *Public Health Rep* 104:640–46, 1989
10. Gohdes DM: Diabetes in American Indians: a growing problem. *Diabetes Care* 9:609–13, 1986
11. Knowler WC, Saad MF, Pettitt DJ, Nelson, RG, Bennett PH: Determinants of diabetes mellitus in the Pima Indians. *Diabetes Care* 16: 239–43, 1993
12. Knowler WC, Pettitt DJ, Saad MF, Bennett PH: Diabetes mellitus in the Pima Indians: incidence, risk factors, and pathogenesis. *Diabetes Metab Rev* 6:1–27, 1990
13. Knowler WC, Pettitt DJ, Lillioja S, Nelson RG: Genetic and environmental factors in the development of diabetes mellitus in Pima Indians. In *Genetic Susceptibility to Environmental Factors: A Challenge for Public Intervention.* Smith V, Eriksson S, Lindgarde F, Eds. Stockholm, Sweden, Almquist & Wiskell International, 1987, p. 67–74

14. Knowler WC, Pettitt DJ, Bennett PH, Williams RC: Diabetes mellitus in the Pima Indians: genetic and evolutionary considerations. *Am J Phys Anthropol* 62:107–14, 1983

15. Carter J, Horowitz R, Wilson R, Sava S, Sinnock P, Gohdes G: Tribal differences in diabetes: prevalence among American Indians in New Mexico. *Public Health Rep* 104:665–69, 1989

16. Benjamin EM, Winters D, Mayfield J, Gohdes D: Diabetes in pregnancy in Zuni Indian women: prevalence and subsequent development of clinical diabetes. *Diabetes Care* 16:1231–35, 1993

17. Benjamin EM: The Zuni Diabetes Project: a community-based program for the treatment and prevention of diabetes among Zuni Indians. In *American College of Physician Executives Manual for Contributions to Health Care.* Tampa, FL, American College of Physician Executives, 1993, p. 28–30

18. Heath GW, Wilson RH, Smith J, Leonard BE: Community-based exercise and weight control: diabetes risk reduction and glycemic control in Zuni Indians. *Am J Clin Nutr* 53:1642S–46S, 1991

19. Benjamin E, Mayfield J, Gohdes D: Exercise and incidence of NIDDM among Zuni Indians (Abstract). *Diabetes* 42 (Suppl. 1):203A, 1993

20. Massad RJ: Building a coalition for community-oriented primary care. In *Community-Oriented Primary Care: From Principle to Practice.* Nutting PA, Ed. Washington, D.C., Health Resources and Services Administration Printing Office, 1987, p. 461–69

21. Centers for Disease Control: *Mobilizing a Minority Community to Reduce Risk Factors for Cardiovascular Disease: An Exercise-Nutrition Handbook.* Atlanta, GA, Centers for Disease Control Publications, 1989

22. Centers for Disease Control: *Promoting Physical Activity Among Adults: A CDC Community Intervention Handbook.* Atlanta, GA, Centers for Disease Control Publications, 1991

23. Epstein LH, Wing RR, Koeske R, Valoski A: A comparison of lifestyle exercise, aerobic exercise, and calisthenics on weight loss in obese children. *Behav Ther* 16:345–56, 1985

24. Wing RR: Behavioral strategies for weight reduction in obese type II diabetic patients. *Diabetes Care* 12:139–44, 1989

25. Walker RB: Evaluating impact in community-oriented primary care. In *Community-Oriented Primary Care: From Principle to Practice.* Nutting PA, Ed. Washington, D.C., Health Resources and Services Administration Printing Office, 1987, p. 339–43

V. Sports: Practical Advice and Experience

27. The Diabetic Athlete as a Role Model

The Diabetic Athlete as a Role Model

PAULA HARPER, RN, CDE

INTRODUCTION

For many years, active people with diabetes expressed a common dilemma: they could not find enough information about exercise and diabetes. Some got help from doctors, nurses, books, and magazines, but often this information was too general to be of much value. Over and over people who wanted to exercise had to learn by trial and error.

Today, with increased knowledge of the relationship between diabetes and exercise, participating in regular physical activity is no longer like reinventing the wheel. Now, a bad knee injury is more likely to keep someone sidelined from a professional sport than is diabetes. This chapter highlights a few of the noted professional athletes with diabetes who paved the way. Often the first concern of an athlete faced with a diagnosis of diabetes is "Will I still be able to play?"

BOBBY CLARKE

"Will I be able to continue playing hockey?" was Bobby Clarke's first question to his doctor when he was diagnosed with type I diabetes in 1962 at the age of 13. He had already been playing hockey in his hometown of Flin Flon, Manitoba, Canada for 10 years. His doctor assured him he would be able to continue playing hockey.

Clarke played professional hockey for 15 years, beginning in 1969. As captain of the Philadelphia Flyers hockey team, Clarke led them to two Stanley Cup championships in the mid-1970s. He was named the National Hockey League's (NHL) Most Valuable Player in 1973, 1974, and 1976. After retiring from play, Clarke went into hockey management and is now (since March 1, 1993) general manager and vice president of the Miami Panthers.

Managing his diabetes successfully paid off for Clarke: he never once missed a game because of diabetes-related factors. Diagnosed in the days before blood glucose monitors, he learned to read his body's symptoms to predict episodes of hypoglycemia. Now he uses a meter, carries glucose tablets, and attributes his good control to his exercise program: running 5–10 miles a day, roller-blading 3 times a week, weight-lifting, and golf.

CHRIS DUDLEY

"Will I be able to continue playing ball?" was professional basketball player Chris Dudley's first question to his doctor when he was diagnosed with type I diabetes during his sophomore year in high school. Dudley's physician told him he could continue to play active basketball; his coaches were understanding and supportive.

Dudley, a 29-year-old center for the Portland Trail Blazers, tests his blood glucose levels 4–5 times a day, including during and after games, if necessary. He adjusts his insulin and carbohydrate intake differently for game days, practice days, and travel days. He keeps sweet liquids close by during games. Dudley reads nutrition labels, uses a carbohydrate-counting system, and watches his food intake carefully, especially on the road.

As a role model for active kids with diabetes, Dudley spends time helping them realize they can play any sport they like, as long as they take care of themselves.

CURT FRASER

Curt Fraser grew up playing hockey on the ice rinks of Winnipeg with his two brothers. His father played professional hockey in the U.S. At age 19, Fraser was drafted into the NHL by the Vancouver Canucks. His 12 years as a professional hockey player included stints with Vancouver, Chicago, and Minnesota. It was in his fifth NHL season, in 1983, that Fraser was diagnosed with diabetes.

Fraser was lucky to have Bobby Clarke as a role model. A friend put him in touch with Clarke while he was just starting on insulin. "That was the best thing that ever happened to me," Fraser recalls. "He's had diabetes most of his life, and he told me exactly how he controlled it when he was playing. That eliminated a lot of the experimenting I would have had to do. I basically followed what he did."

Fraser believes strongly in self-monitoring of blood glucose. On practice, travel, and off days, he adjusted his meal and snack times and tested 3 or 4 times a day. On games days, Fraser tested in the morning, after practice, around 4:00 p.m. when he had a snack, before the game, during all the periods of the game, and after the game.

The Chicago Blackhawks hockey team, and especially general manager Bob Pulford, were solidly behind Fraser. Fraser recalls phoning Pulford the day his diabetes was diagnosed, not knowing what the reaction would be. "He said, 'my brother has diabetes. Just make sure you show up in good shape.' It was quite a relief." It's a relief to other professional athletes as well. Fraser's success is part of the reason many more coaches and officials accept and are comfortable with players who have diabetes. Fraser now coaches the Milwaukee Admirals.

JONATHAN HAYES

Jonathan Hayes was diagnosed with type I diabetes in college. In his book, *Necessary Toughness*, he recounts, "I had always valued a healthy body, a strong physique, and I had been willing to pay the price to maintain it. Now the cost was going up. Now the cost included extra care about diet, extra attention during exercise, insulin shots, frequent finger pricks to check my sugar level. I would have to become the doctor of my own body, learning about its processes and fine-tuning my own lifestyle to accommodate it." He goes on to describe how he dealt with diabetes while pursuing a career in professional football.

Now in his 10th year as a tight end for the Kansas City Chiefs, Hayes has been able to maintain excellent control of his diabetes. He spends the off-season on his ranch training quarter horses and riding competitively. It's vigorous work, but Hayes is careful to monitor his blood glucose levels and caloric intake, adjusting his insulin dose accordingly.

JIM "CATFISH" HUNTER

In 1977, during spring training for the NY Yankees, Jim "Catfish" Hunter was diagnosed with type I diabetes. He tried to learn everything he could about the disease and how to listen to his body. Hunter found that the discipline required to stay in shape for baseball greatly helped him in the management of his diabetes. He had always maintained a balanced diet; now he took insulin, monitored his blood glucose, and stayed alert to the signs of hypoglycemia. His teammates and coaches were very supportive; during games, juices were provided in the dugout if he needed them. Because of his control of the disease, diabetes never caused problems with his baseball career.

Hunter retired from baseball in 1979. He stresses that it wasn't because of the diabetes. He had planned all along to stop playing at age 33. Today, the former major-league pitcher finds himself in a different field—coaxing corn, soybeans, and peanuts from the soil as he once lured easy grounders from the bats of opposing hitters. The transition from ballplayer to farmer was easy for Hunter. During the off-season, he had been helping his brother and father on their peanut farm.

In addition to farming, Hunter enjoys hunting deer and birds, fishing, and coaching in the Little League and Babe Ruth Baseball League.

BILL TALBERT

Bill Talbert, age 76, developed type I diabetes at the age of 10. His doctor told his parents that their son would have to avoid activities that demanded lots of energy. Those were the days when exercise was considered dangerous for people with diabetes. But 4 years later, with the family doctor's approval, his father gave him a tennis racket. Talbert became an American tennis legend, winning 38 U.S. titles during the 1940s and 1950s. By 1950, Talbert was rated the number two player at Wimbledon and number one in men's doubles and mixed doubles. He was ranked in the top 10 in the world for 14 years.

However, Talbert believes his greatest accomplishment has been surviving as long as he has. During his years on the tennis circuit, he struggled to maintain control of his diabetes. After experiencing an insulin reaction during a championship match, he began combining his diabetes plan with his game plan. He ended up adjusting his diet, his practice schedule, and his game strategy simultaneously.

Talbert's strong sense of independence and his determination to not let diabetes control his life helped him achieve so much on the tennis court. Now, he spends time with children at diabetes camps, encouraging them to keep their diabetes in control and to continue pursuing their dreams.

WADE WILSON

At age 26, second-string quarterback Wade Wilson was getting ready to pack for the Minnesota Vikings training camp when he was diagnosed with diabetes. With no time to adjust to the demands of his new diagnosis, Wilson had to regain lost weight and learn to manage his diabetes. Of equal importance to him, Wilson had to show his coaches and teammates that diabetes would not alter his performance.

He credits his success to discipline and an attitude that, until his body told him otherwise, he would continue doing everything he used to do. With the right attitude, says Wilson, he was able to take care of himself better than before. In fact, the strenuous requirements of organized sports can help in managing diabetes. As Wilson says, he always had to eat well and stay active; now the only difference was in monitoring blood glucose levels, taking insulin, and avoiding hypoglycemic symptoms.

In the off-season Wilson takes less insulin. He says he works harder then, playing racquetball, golf, and waterskiing. He doesn't believe having diabetes has affected his enjoyment of any competitive sport.

CONCLUSION

Today, many professional athletes successfully manage their diabetes. All maintain that self-monitoring of blood glucose is essential, that teammates and coaches are supportive, and that diabetes does not need to adversely affect their performance. These athletes serve as extraordinary role models; they are examples of the success to which an athlete with diabetes can aspire.

SUGGESTED READINGS

BOBBY CLARKE

1. Dawson LY: Skating at the cutting edge: Bobby Clarke. *Diabetes Forecast*, March 1994, p. 16–19
2. Weiner D: Bobby Clarke: no excuses. *Living Well With Diabetes*, Fall 1987, p. 3–4

CHRIS DUDLEY

3. Wakelee-Lynch J: The man in the middle. *Diabetes Forecast*, November 1994, p. 15–19

CURT FRASER

4. Ortlieb B: Making a power play against diabetes. *Diabetes Forecast*, December 1987, p. 22–25

JONATHAN HAYES

5. Radak JT: Staying in focus. *Diabetes Forecast*, February 1990, p. 30–37
6. Walsh P: Hail to the chief... and author, and rancher: these are the days of Jonathan Hayes. *Diabetes Forecast*, May 1994, p. 65–68

BILL TALBERT

7. Wakelee-Lynch J: A full life of service. *Diabetes Forecast*, August 1991, p. 22–26

WADE WILSON

8. Mazur M: Calling the play against diabetes. *Diabetes Forecast*, November 1988, p. 33–35

28. The Elite Diabetic Athlete

Introduction

Education

Exercise Training Schedule

Insulin and Carbohydrate Adjustments

Blood Glucose Control

Concluding Remarks

The Elite Diabetic Athlete

NEIL J. GOLDBERG, MD

INTRODUCTION

Exercise is a way of life for the elite diabetic athlete. The main limitation to successful exercise performance can be orthopedic rather than metabolic if the athlete has learned to balance the metabolic milieu with appropriate insulin dosage and food ingestion for muscular energy use.

Before the advent of self-monitoring of blood glucose, newer methods of insulin administration, and improved knowledge of metabolism, endurance exercise could not be done in a safe manner. Participation in exercise was truly a trial-and-error experience. Now, with these advances and proper medical screening, a safe approach is possible.

EDUCATION

The first step to successful exercise is education, which a health-care professional can provide. This should include *1*) basic exercise physiology—the insulin and metabolic changes that occur during exercise and the effects of conditioning and deconditioning; *2*) nutrition—general principles applied to diabetes, and energy requirements for specific training; and *3*) insulin use—adjustments of dosage and location of injection for different types of exercises.

EXERCISE TRAINING SCHEDULE

Carefully kept training logs of the types, duration, and intensity of exercise are as essential as records of self-monitoring of blood glucose, food ingestion, insulin dose, and site of injection. All of these data may be correlated to identify patterns and plan a safe exercise training schedule outlining the type, intensity, duration, and timing of exercise. This prearranged exercise training schedule allows for adjustments in diet and insulin in a more predictable manner.

INSULIN AND CARBOHYDRATE ADJUSTMENTS

Because each athlete has his or her own "fingerprint" metabolic response to exercise, only generalizations concerning insulin and carbohydrate adjustments can be made. Insulin requirements are inversely related to intensity and duration of exercise, except at very high exertion levels. Thus, insulin dosage often needs to be diminished in anticipation of intense exercise (see Chapter 11). Carbohydrate ingestion may be necessary despite the reduction in insulin, but rarely will this match the total carbohydrate use of endurance exercise.

BLOOD GLUCOSE CONTROL

Avoidance of significant hyperglycemia (>220 mg/dl) or hypoglycemia (<60 mg/dl) will ensure unhampered exercise performance for most individuals. Exercise should begin with blood glucose levels between 150 and 180 mg/dl to allow for a drop in blood glucose with less chance of hypoglycemia during or after exercise. An educated trial-and-error approach with scheduled repetitive exercises, regular record-keeping, and blood glucose monitoring is the mainstay of blood glucose control during exercise.

CONCLUDING REMARKS

Combining education, scheduled exercise, insulin and carbohydrate adjustments, and blood glucose control with medical screening and interaction with a support team provide the best formula for success for an elite athlete with diabetes.

29. Marathon Running

Marathon Running

ULRIKE THURM, MD, BILL CARLSON, AND ERIK BAEKKLUND, PhD

INTRODUCTION

Running a marathon can be a special challenge, even without diabetes. For runners with diabetes, effective self-management of blood glucose levels is the critical factor. Diabetic athletes determined to compete in this rigorous, but exhilarating, form of exercise need to learn how to balance energy output, energy input, and insulin dosages. This chapter presents some basic suggestions for training for marathon running and describes the use of a running diary as a training tool. In addition, the experience of two successful marathon athletes with diabetes, Bill Carlson and Erik Baekklund, PhD, who have spent years mastering the demands of diabetes management, is described.

BASIC TRAINING FOR MARATHON RUNNING

Runners should see their diabetes specialist for a medical check-up before beginning intensive training. The International Diabetic Athletes Association (IDAA) may provide additional useful information (see RESOURCES). Membership in a local running club can provide companionship and running partners, as well as special advice concerning equipment and other considerations (Table 29.1).

The Running Diary

An important training tool is a running diary. For most marathoners with diabetes, such a diary can be combined with a blood glucose diary. It should include the following information:

- Date and time
- Blood glucose level at the start of exercise
- Adjustment of short-acting and/or long-acting insulin dose (insulin requirements may change with a change in training state)
- Distance or time of run and place it occurred
- Overall evaluation of the run: weather, type of effort (e.g., hard, moderate, easy), feelings, comments
- Pulse rate at rest (taken in the morning while still in bed) and during exercise (record when and where)
- Weight (insulin requirements may change as weight is lost)
- Amount and type of extra carbohydrates taken before, during, and for 8–12 h after exercise
- Blood glucose levels during, shortly after, and 8–12 h after exercise
- Episodes of hypoglycemia: when episode occurred (during or early or late after exercise), symptoms noticed (e.g., feeling weak, dizzy, or unable to run), measurements of blood glucose, treatment, active insulin at time of episode, ideas for prevention (including preferred carbohydrates, snacks, and drinks during exercise)
- Long- and short-term goals: time and distance of training runs and upcoming races (insulin requirements may change as a function of the amount of exercise)

Table 29.1. Information Likely Available at a Running Club

- Running shoes (especially important for those with complications)
- Running apparel (some made of Lycra or Gortex)
- Flexibility exercises (warming up and cooling down)
- Training programs (different levels)
- Nutrition
- Safety rules
- Magazines/books for runners
- Marathon calendars

Warming Up and Cooling Down

Most athletes pay close attention to warming up. Part of warming up for diabetic athletes may involve reducing their insulin dose and taking an extra snack of carbohydrate before a run. In contrast, even experienced athletes often pay little attention to cooling down. Diabetic athletes who don't pay attention to their metabolic adjustments after the run can end up with more than muscle soreness. Late-onset hypoglycemia 8–12 h after exercise is common. Thus, in the interest of safety, athletes need to check their blood glucose levels several hours after training and take extra carbohydrates if needed.

BILL CARLSON

When more sophisticated management techniques are necessary, marathoners with diabetes can learn from the successful experiences of others. Bill Carlson was an active 16-year-old when he came down with what he believed was a bad case of the flu. His symptoms of weight loss, polyphagia, polyuria, and excessive physical weakness did not subside, however, until his diagnosis and treatment for insulin-dependent diabetes mellitus (IDDM).

The Hawaii Ironman Triathalon

Carlson's dream was to compete in Hawaii's 1983 Ironman Triathalon, a grueling event for which only the world's top athletes can qualify. No one with diabetes had ever entered the race. During the year he spent training for the event, he found a physician experienced in diabetes management and sports medicine to design an effective training program for him. Each week, Carlson swam 10 miles, cycled 250–300 miles, and ran 60 miles. After each cycling course, Carlson tested his blood glucose.

During the Ironman race, he tested his blood glucose before and after the swimming event, five times during the cycling event, and each hour of the marathon run. To avoid hypoglycemia and dehydration, Carlson drank a car-bohydrate fluid while cycling and running. He didn't win this competition, but he certainly proved that with diligent training and preparation, as well as the use of effective management techniques, an athlete with diabetes can successfully compete in the most rigorous of athletic events.

Insulin Requirements

During his training year, Carlson experimented with different insulin combinations. He found that the intermediate-acting lente and NPH insulins peaked at inappropriate moments. Carlson was successful using regular insulin exclusively, but he had to inject and monitor frequently. His physician recommended the use of both ultralente and regular insulins (the "poor man's insulin pump"). Carlson found that this regime offered him the greatest freedom to work out without having unplanned insulin peaks.

Carlson uses 35–40% animal ultralente insulin as needed because of its slower onset and lack of peaks. He finds the human ultralente insulin too responsive. He injects a bolus of human regular insulin if he will be sedentary after a meal. Carlson rotates his injection sites daily and seems to have equal absorption and insulin peak activity regardless of injection site.

While training, Carlson keeps a running diary documenting all blood glucose levels before, during, and after exercise and at mealtimes and bedtimes. He records all food eaten; frequency, intensity, and duration of workouts; resting heart rates; and specific physical feelings. Carlson's resting heart rate is 35 beats/min; his blood pressure is 107/72/65, and his body fat is 9.4%. He consumes 3,500 calories a day, consisting of 60% carbohydrate, 20% protein, and 20% fat. His HbA_{1c} is 6.3 when training full-time; otherwise, it is 7.2.

Competing Successfully

Carlson has since competed in over 75 triathlons (including 5 Hawaii Ironman events), 39 marathons, and many smaller athletic endurance contests. In 85% of his races, Carlson placed in the top five in his amateur division. He believes he holds the IDDM marathon record of 2:38, recorded at the Los Angeles Marathon in 1991. He now competes in ultramarathons, which are foot races that are longer than 26.2 miles and typically take place along mountain trails. Carlson has run two 100-milers, with his best time of 23:12 at Angeles Crest 100-Mile Endurance Run, where he placed 12th of 107 starters.

Carlson attributes his success with diabetes management and marathoning to education, bravery, and "fingertips that look like my colander for draining spaghetti." Some people with diabetes are reluctant to commit themselves to the diligent self-monitoring necessary to train seriously, and some physicians do not have the time to teach patients what is required. Coaching a diabetic patient through physical training is difficult, regardless of the patient's experience with managing diabetes. However, for those athletes willing to make the effort, optimal physical health and performance are within reach.

ERIK BAEKKELUND

Erik Baekkelund, PhD, is a 43-year-old marathon runner who has been managing IDDM for 10 years. For a few years after the diagnosis, he ran 5–10 km several times a week with very unpredictable blood glucose results. When he decided to run a marathon, Baekkelund sought advice about more successful management techniques.

Effective Management Techniques

Before Running

Baekkelund reduces the previous shot of fast-acting insulin by 20–40% (he takes fast-acting insulin 5 times a day) before running. He also reduces his carbohydrate intake by 20–40%. Then, he waits 1½-2 h before running to minimize the risk of low blood glucose. About 15–30 min before running,

Baekkelund checks his blood glucose. He needs the reading to be around 180 mg/dl, or at least above 110 and below 230 mg/dl. If his reading is too low, he takes extra carbohydrates; if it is too high, he injects an extra unit of fast-acting insulin. He also checks his urine for ketone bodies; if—as has happened once—his urine contains ketone bodies, he postpones running. For every 15 min of running, Baekkelund takes 10 g of a simple carbohydrate, usually apple juice or bananas.

After Running

Baekkelund usually does not decrease the amount of insulin at the first shot after exercise, and if he does so, it is only by about 20%. A few hours after exercising, Baekkelund usually has to take some extra carbohydrate to raise his blood glucose and to prevent hypoglycemia during the night. He does not change the amount of slow-acting insulin before bedtime. The following morning, Baekkelund reduces his first shot of fast-acting insulin by 20–40%, depending on his prebreakfast blood glucose reading.

Baekkelund finds that exercise usually increases his insulin sensitivity for at least 24 h, and often much longer than that. Regular exercise 4–8 h a week reduces his insulin demand by about 40%. Baekkelund's total daily insulin requirement is about 24 units; if he is on vacation and not exercising, he requires 40 units daily. His HbA_{1c} varies between 4.9 and 7.7, with a mean of 6.7.

Other Factors

Baekkelund does not generally experience problems with hypoglycemia during running. What he finds more unpredictable is whether he develops hypoglycemia afterward and particularly during the night. Consequently, he often takes too many carbohydrates before bedtime.

Baekkelund's attitude about IDDM is that while it certainly affects daily life to an enormous degree, unlike some other chronic conditions, there is much the motivated patient can do to prevent complications, feel well, and lead close to a normal life. For Baekkelund and athletes like him, that always includes strenuous exercise.

CONCLUSION

With the proper training and management techniques, athletes with diabetes can experience the thrill of competing in marathons just as successfully as any runner without diabetes.

30. Weight Lifting

Weight Lifting

W. GUYTON HORNSBY, Jr, PhD, CDE

INTRODUCTION

Although resistance exercise is predominantly used in diabetes management to attain health benefits such as increased muscular strength and flexibility, enhanced body composition, or reduced cardiovascular disease risk, exceptional patients may have goals that go far beyond general health and fitness.

Athletes with diabetes have achieved remarkable success in the competitive sports of weight lifting, power lifting, and body building. Isaac Berger was a two-time Olympic champion in weight lifting, and Tim Belknap won the Mr. America title and went on to become a highly regarded professional body builder.

Physicians and other health-care professionals should be familiar with concepts associated with prescribing resistance exercises for athletes and should be able to advise patient-athletes on training practices that may interfere with glycemic control or that may place these patients at unnecessary risk.

PRESCRIBING TRAINING PROGRAMS

Training programs used by competitive weight lifters are very different from those used by other athletes or by recreational lifters. Program design depends on manipulation of resistance training variables: choice of exercise, order of exercise, resistance (intensity or load used), volume of exercise (number of sets and repetitions performed), and length of rest between exercises (see Chapter 7). Comprehensive explanations of resistance exercise prescriptions for general athletes have been previously provided by Fleck and Kraemer (1,2), and Hornsby (3) has described specific training programs for athletes with diabetes.

HIGH-INTENSITY WEIGHT LIFTING

Development of maximal strength and power requires the use of high-intensity resistance training. Very intense weight lifting has been associated with large acute increases in blood pressure. While this may be potentially harmful for patients with cardiac or vascular complications, researchers have reported using high-intensity resistance training in geriatric patients (4) (see Chapter 22), cardiac patients (5), and in one patient following laser surgery for diabetic retinopathy (6) without detrimental effects. There is no evidence that training with heavy or maximal loads is contraindicated in fit diabetic patients without long-term complications. Thorough preexercise screening would appear to be appropriate for any patient involved in intense resistance training.

GLYCEMIC CONTROL

Research on the glycemic response to intense resistance exercise has been limited when compared with the same type of research involving aerobic activity. Investigations of chronic resistance training have demonstrated improvements in insulin sensitivity and/or glucose tolerance in both diabetic and nondiabetic subjects. The acute response to intense resistance exercise is typically a moderate increase in blood glucose (~20–60 mg/dl) during the exercise session, with reduced insulin requirements or delayed-onset hypoglycemia appearing many hours (6–48 h) after the session ends. Athletes should be advised to make appropriate adjustments in food intake or insulin dosage based on frequent self-monitoring of blood glucose.

TRAINING RISKS

Properly designed training programs can improve physical appearance and athletic performance, but quantity and quality of improvement are largely determined by genetic potential. Unreasonable expectations and a win-at-all-cost philosophy can force some athletes to experiment with fraudulent, hazardous, and/or illegal training aids. Health-care professionals should be able to advise athletes on proper nutrition (7), the risks of using illegal anabolic-androgenic steroids (8), and deceptive tactics used in marketing purported ergogenic aids and dietary supplements (9).

REFERENCES

1. Fleck SJ, Kraemer WJ: Resistance training—basic principles (part 1 of 4). *Physician Sportsmed* 16(3): 160–71, 1988
2. Fleck SJ, Kraemer WJ: Resistance training—exercise prescription (part 4 of 4). *Physician Sportsmed* 16 (6):69–81, 1988
3. Hornsby WG: Strength training basics. *The Challenge: Newsletter of the International Diabetic Athletes Assoc* 7:1–4, 1993
4. Fiatarone MA, Marks EC, Ryan ND, Meredith CN, Lipsitz LA, Evans WJ: High-intensity strength training in nonagenarians. *JAMA* 263:3029–34, 1990
5. Ghilarducci LE, Holly RG, Amsterdam EA: Effects of high resistance training in coronary artery disease. *Am J Cardiol* 64:866–70, 1989
6. Durak EP, Jovanovic-Peterson L, Peterson CM: Randomized crossover study of effect of resistance training on glycemic control, muscular strength, and cholesterol in type I diabetic men. *Diabetes Care* 13:1039–43, 1990
7. Sargent RG, Hohn E: Protein needs for the athlete. *Natl Strength Cond Assoc J* 15(1):54–56, 1993
8. National Strength and Conditioning Association: Position statement and literature review for the NSCA: Anabolic-androgenic steroid use by athletes. *Natl Strength Cond Assoc J* 15(2):9–28, 1993
9. Lightsey DM, Attaway JR: Deceptive tactics used in marketing purported ergogenic aids. *Natl Strength Cond Assoc J* 14(2):26–31, 1992

31. Tennis

Tennis

GARY I. WADLER, MD, FACP, FACSM, FACPM

INTRODUCTION

Tennis is a sport for people of all ages and ability levels. The professional tennis player, who demonstrates extraordinary skill, intensity, and athleticism in such tournaments as the U.S. Open and Wimbledon, faces exceptional metabolic demands and physiological adaptations. Overweight weekend warriors of the tennis court may be less proficient, but their bodies must adapt to the metabolic demands of strenuous exercise as well.

Recognizing the wide variations that exist in ability levels, the United States Tennis Association uses a National Tennis Rating Program, a simple self-placement method to ensure appropriate groupings for league play, tournaments, group lessons, social competitions, and club or community programs. These ratings classify skill levels that may, in part, be viewed as a guide to the exercise intensity required in each range. The ratings rank players on a scale of 1.0 to 7.0. A level 1.0 player is just beginning to play tennis; a level 3.0 player can place shots with moderate success and sustain a rally of slow pace; and a level 7.0 player is world-class.

Skill ratings aside, other parameters affecting the metabolic consequences associated with tennis are the fitness level of the participant; the playing style of the opponent (more active serve-and-volley versus the relatively passive baseline return); the frequency and duration of play; singles or doubles play; the court surface (hard surface, clay, or grass); and very important, different environmental factors. Depending on these variables, the proportion of exercise that is aerobic as opposed to anaerobic (sprinting for the ball versus waiting for the serve) will vary.

PHYSIOLOGICAL DEMANDS OF TENNIS

The specific physiological demands of tennis on people with or without diabetes have received little attention in research. However, a 1991 study by Bergeron et al. (1) of 10 members of an NCAA Division I university tennis team has shed light on some of the physiological alterations associated with a high skill level. Variables measured included heart rate, hematocrit, hemoglobin, blood glucose, plasma lactates, cortisol, and testosterone. Analyses suggested that although tennis is characterized by periods of high-intensity exercise, the overall metabolic response resembles that of prolonged, moderate-intensity exercise.

In the Bergeron study, the duration of play was 85 min, with time allotted for side changeovers and blood sampling. During play, the mean heart rate was 145 beats/min, representing 61% of the maximal heart rate as determined by treadmill testing. Blood glucose concentrations did not significantly change over the duration of the match or during the recovery period compared with pre-exercise levels. Although a slight fall in blood glucose was observed during the 10-min warm-up before actual play, there was a 23% increase in blood glucose after the second 15 min of play. After that, blood glucose concentrations remained steady at levels that were slightly higher than the preexercise levels.

Energy Expenditure

How does the energy expenditure of tennis compare with that of other sports and activities? This question was addressed by Ainsworth et al. (2) in their compendium classifying the energy costs of an array of human physical activities. Activities were compared on the basis of metabolic equivalents (METS), with one MET defined as the energy expended while sitting quietly, which, for the average adult, is ~3.5 ml of oxygen·kg^{-1}·min^{-1} (1 kcal·kg^{-1}·h^{-1}). Table 31.1 illustrates the METS values for various activities.

TENNIS AND DIABETES

As with any exercise prescription for a chronic medical condition, patients with diabetes need to understand their disease and how it relates to an exercise

Table 31.1. METS Values for Various Activities

ACTIVITY	METS VALUE
Tennis (singles)	8.0
Tennis (doubles)	6.0
Bicycling (leisure)	6.0
Golf	4.5
Jogging	7.0
Basketball	8.0
Handball	12.0
Ice Hockey	8.0
Swimming (leisure)	6.0
Ice Skating (leisure)	7.0

Adapted from Ainsworth et al. (2).

or sports program. Diabetic patients should be made aware of several factors affecting diabetes management.

Establishing Preliminary Fitness Levels

As reviewed elsewhere in this book (see Chapter 2), VO_{2max} is a measurement of the maximum ability of the body to absorb and use oxygen, and thus indicates overall fitness level. It is noteworthy, for reasons that are not clear, that the VO_{2max} of people with non-insulin-dependent diabetes mellitus (NIDDM) is lower than the VO_{2max} of sedentary people without diabetes (3). However, if NIDDM patients maintain a consistent exercise training program, their VO_{2max} will increase, and their overall fitness level will improve to reach the fitness levels of sedentary people without diabetes (4). These observations underscore the need for diabetic patients to be exercising regularly to some degree before embarking on a tennis program.

Screening for Coronary Heart Disease (CHD) Risk

As discussed in previous chapters, both insulin-dependent diabetes mellitus (IDDM) and NIDDM are significant risk factors for the development of ischemic heart disease (4). Therefore, an exercise electrocardiogram is rec-

ommended for all diabetic patients who are >35 years of age or have other risk factors for CHD (see Chapters 6 and 15) before they begin a tennis program. Such testing would also detect NIDDM patients who have exaggerated hypertensive responses to exercise (5). In one study of 66 asymptomatic NIDDM patients who underwent ^{210}Tl myocardial scintigraphy to detect silent myocardial ischemia, 18.2% showed ischemic changes, as contrasted with 5.3% of the control subjects (6).

Preventing Hypoglycemia

Usually in a nondiabetic person exercising at moderate intensities (30–60% of VO_{2max}), blood glucose levels remain within a relatively normal range, although both hyperglycemia and hypoglycemia can occur. As VO_{2max} is approached, relative hyperglycemia occurs, with the blood glucose response reflecting both the intensity of the exercise as well as the fitness level of the person exercising. As with other forms of exercise, the IDDM patient's glycemic response to tennis can be quite variable, depending on factors such as insulin type and dosage, time of administration, dietary practices, the duration and intensity of the match, and the time of day (see Chapter 11). The most frequent disturbance is hypoglycemia due to overinsulinization. Hypoglycemia may occur not only during the match, but 4–6 h afterward in some individuals. Maintaining blood glucose levels in a physiological range will require frequent patient monitoring and, in some instances, adjustment of diet and/or insulin dose (see below). Although hypoglycemic episodes are rare in NIDDM patients who are taking oral hypoglycemic medications and following an appropriate diet, similar monitoring of blood glucose levels is still recommended.

Special Considerations

Diet
Tennis players with insulin-requiring diabetes may need to make dietary

adjustments when playing tennis. The most important considerations are probably the length and intensity level of the match. If patients anticipate a long or particularly strenuous match, they should eat adequate complex carbohydrates beforehand. Rapidly absorbable carbohydrates, such as fruit juice, should be available in case of hypoglycemic symptoms.

Dehydration

Because a great deal of water can be lost as sweat during a match, particularly one played in hot, humid weather, diabetic patients should drink large quantities of water long before the match. The amount of water ingested should be sufficient to cause clear urine. Preferably, if the match is to be played in the morning, a generous fluid intake should be initiated the night before and water should be consumed at changeovers during the match. Since thirst lags behind fluid needs, thirst should not be a guide to adequate fluid replacement. At high skill levels, dehydration is often the major cause of leg cramps during prolonged matches in hot, humid weather.

Weather Conditions

Tennis is often played in climatic conditions, such as high temperatures and humidity, low wind velocities, and radiant sunlight, that can result in heat illness. Thus, it is important that diabetic patients not confuse symptoms of heat illness, particularly heat exhaustion (fatigue, weakness, nausea, vomiting, profuse sweating, and tachycardia) with those of hypoglycemia. Furthermore, under such adverse weather conditions, IDDM patients with evidence of autonomic neuropathy risk thermoregulation problems as well as orthostatic hypotension occurring with dehydration. To minimize health risks associated with playing tennis, it is advisable for diabetic patients to avoid playing matches from 10:00 A.M. to 2:00 P.M. when the sun is most intense. Since people with diabetes are at risk of developing a variety of eye problems, including cataracts, they should wear nonbreakable sunglasses properly

rated to block out ultraviolet B rays. Patients should use sunscreens with an SPF (sun protection factor) of at least 15 when playing in the sun and should reapply them as necessary to reduce skin damage. It is helpful to wear lightweight and light-colored tennis clothes and take every opportunity to stay in the shade.

Beta Blockers

Problems due to hypoglycemia can potentially be compounded if a diabetic patient with underlying ischemic heart disease or hypertension is being treated with nonselective beta blockers (see Chapter 23). These drugs might enhance the likelihood of developing hypoglycemia as a result of impaired hepatic glycogenolysis. A cardioselective agent is preferable for a diabetic patient prone to hypoglycemia and requiring a beta blocker. Furthermore, patients should be mindful that beta blockers may mask the symptoms of hypoglycemia during a match.

Foot Care

Since the foot is perhaps the most commonly injured body part in tennis—with injuries ranging from corns, calluses, and ingrown toenails to blisters, bruises, and abrasions—it is imperative that patients wear properly fitting tennis shoes, well-padded socks, and keep their feet as dry as possible. The combination of diabetic peripheral neuropathy and small vessel disease may result in relatively mild foot problems becoming major ones. Patients need to regularly inspect their feet and care for them appropriately (see Chapter 13).

ONE PATIENT'S EXPERIENCE

The anecdotal experience of a 30-year-old man with IDDM highlights some of the points discussed above. David Fischbach (personal communication, 1994) had been ranked number one in the East for men over age 25 for 3 consecutive years. By 1994, he was ranked in the top 10 nationally for men over 30. Normally, David takes 17 units of NPH insulin with 3 units of regular insulin each morning. At 8:00 P.M. he takes 6 units of regular insulin, and at bedtime he takes 15 units of NPH. To play competitively, he has been required to make adjustments both in his precompetition meal and in his regular insulin dosages. These adjustments depend on variables such as court surface, time of day, and the playing style and skill level of his competitors.

David has learned to adjust his dietary habits and insulin doses by closely monitoring his blood glucose during match play. At changeovers, when he is unsure about his blood glucose level, he quickly measures it without delaying the match. He has learned to recognize quite predictably when his blood glucose is too low or too high, and he can distinguish euglycemic exhaustion associated with a long match from exercise-induced hypoglycemia. Similarly, he recognizes when his blood glucose levels are very high because of excessive prematch sweets or when he has underestimated his insulin requirements. For him, poor concentration, a loss of confidence, and tentativeness are a sure sign of very high blood glucose.

From these experiences, and from the monitoring of his blood glucose, David has found that, in general, when he plays a tough match, he likes to start with a blood glucose of 250 mg/dl, having taken some regular insulin 2 h before the match. He then adjusts his carbohydrate intake depending on the course of the match. In short, David has learned to read his body's signals when playing tennis, and when he is uncertain, he checks his blood glucose.

It is important to realize that ideal prematch blood glucose levels should be individually determined, based on both the metabolic demands associated with the patient's level of tennis play and the individual's metabolic response to exercise.

REFERENCES

1. Bergeron MF, Maresh CM, Kraemer WJ, Abraham A, Conroy B, Gabaree C: Tennis: physiological profile during match play. *Int J Sports Med* 12:474–79, 1991
2. Ainsworth BE, Haskell WL, Leon AS, Jacobs DR Jr, Montoye H, Sallis JF, Paffenbarger RS Jr: Compendium of physical activities: classification of energy costs of human physical activities. *Med Sci Sports Exercise* 25:71–80, 1993
3. Schneider SH, Khachadurian AK, Amorosa LF, Clemow L, Ruderman ND: Ten-year experience with an exercise-based outpatient lifestyle modification program in the treatment of diabetes mellitus. *Diabetes Care* 15:1800–10, 1992
4. Wallberg-Henriksson H: Exercise and diabetes mellitus. *Exercise Sports Sci Rev* 20:339–68, 1992
5. Mogenson CE: Reduced progression of diabetic nephropathy by controlling hypertension. *Pract Cardiol* 9:156–80, 1983
6. Yamada J, Tanaka S, Sato T, Suzuki R, Fujii S: The medical evaluation of patients with diabetes mellitus in exercise therapy. *J Nutr Sci Vitaminol* 37 (Suppl.):S17–24, 1991
7. Sutton JR: Hormonal and metabolic responses to exercise in subjects of high and low work capacities. *Med Sci Sports Exercise* 10:1, 1978

32. Swimming

Introduction

Elements of a Successful Exercise Program

Monitoring and Keeping Records
Adjusting to Energy Output
Modifications for Cross-Training

Outcome

Swimming

BETTY FINNEGAN

INTRODUCTION

Swimming can be an excellent exercise for people with diabetes. One long-time swimmer, Betty Finnegan, a 52-year-old grandmother who has had type I diabetes for 38 years, shares her tips for incorporating this sport into her effective diabetes management program.

Betty began swimming at age 35 when she had difficulty performing some prescribed back exercises because of hemorrhaging in her eyes. After checking with her eye surgeon, she enrolled in swimming lessons at the YMCA. Unable to swim the length of the pool, it was a year before she could swim the mile a day that became her daily goal.

After attending her first International Diabetic Athletes Association meeting 5 years ago, Betty decided it was time to cross-train. She gradually added Nautilus, swimnastics classes, low-impact aerobics, treadmill walking, stretching, and yoga to her exercise program. She now swims with a competitive Master's Swim Team for 1.5 h about 4 times a week and works out at a fitness club twice a week.

ELEMENTS OF A SUCCESSFUL EXERCISE PROGRAM

Monitoring and Keeping Records

Betty uses an insulin pump. She tests her blood glucose about 8 times a day. She keeps a daily chart and graphs her blood glucose results and records bolus and basal insulin dosages. She also uses a bar graph to keep track of the time, type, and amounts of exercise she does. She writes down the portion size and carbohydrate count of the meals and snacks she eats. She finds it helpful to read labels and use a digital scale that provides carbohydrate information. Currently, she is trying to use fiber to blunt blood glucose responses and to eat a nutritious vegetarian diet low in fat.

Adjusting to Energy Output

Checking blood glucose levels before, during, and after exercise is a necessity. If her blood glucose is under 200, she'll drink a small can of apple juice before swimming. If it's over 200, she'll wait. She checks her blood glucose levels during the workout to make sure the value is going down rather than up. Even though she doesn't begin her workout until 11:00 A.M., her blood glucose will rise if she had a low blood glucose level while sleeping.

Betty keeps careful track of how much insulin she has taken. If she thinks she needs more, she'll use her pump to take an additional 0.5 to 1.0 unit and continue swimming. Usually, her blood glucose is going down, so she drinks a second can of apple juice (20 g of carbohydrate), and if her workout is unusually long or strenuous, a third can. She puts her blood glucose machine in a plastic bag at the end of the lane, along with her apple juice and a water bottle to keep hydrated before, during, and after exercise.

She is especially careful about keeping hydrated during the summer when she swims outdoors at air temperatures of 90°F and above. The water keeps blood volume stable and reduces lactic acid buildup, which people with diabetes seem to experience more than other athletes. Betty may also swim a longer cooldown period, if necessary, and stretch in the pool to prevent aching muscles.

Modifications for Cross-Training

Two hours before her fitness club routine, Betty reduces her basal insulin dose from 0.3 units/h to 0.1 units/h and continues that rate for 1 h postexercise. She begins with 30 min on a stair-climbing machine at 7 or 8 watts. This activity will drop her blood glucose more rapidly than walking 2 miles in 30 min on the treadmill. After her muscles are warmed up, she works out on strength training machines and then spends 30 min stretching. Betty feels that people with diabetes should do stretching exercises more frequently, because they can develop limited joint mobility due to glycosylation. Betty stretches after each exercise session even if it means reducing the time spent on aerobic activities.

If her exercise is aerobic, Betty usually eats enough carbohydrate in the 4 h after exercise to prevent large decreases in her blood glucose level. After anaerobic strength training, which often requires a long time to replete glycogen stores, she may also eat a bedtime snack. When traveling, Betty plans exercise without any equipment, such as noontime walks.

OUTCOME

When exercising intensively, as she often does, Betty—at 5'1", 110 lb—takes only 60% (14–16 units) of her expected insulin dose using an insulin pump. She gets better HbA_{1c} values by keeping her insulin dose down and her caloric intake on the low side. If she eats more carbohydrates and covers them with insulin, her control is not as good. She also finds that if she waits ~45 min between the bolus of insulin and mealtime, she gets far better results.

As Betty's experience demonstrates, with careful monitoring and reasonable choices about activity type, people with diabetes can find many ways to incorporate an exercise program into effective diabetes management.

33. Scuba Diving

Scuba Diving

CLAUDIA GRAHAM, CDE, PhD, MPH, AND ADDENDUM BY
STEVE PROSTERMAN

INTRODUCTION

Recreational scuba diving has become tremendously popular in the United States, even among people with diabetes. Safety considerations for people with diabetes go beyond those inherent to scuba diving. At this time, there are no firmly established safety guidelines for recreational scuba divers with diabetes. Although individual scuba diving agencies often have their own guidelines for certifying people with diabetes, these may not be based on a thorough understanding of all of the risks involved. This chapter will present potential risks associated with recreational scuba diving and provide preliminary recommendations for safety from the scuba diving committee of the American Diabetes Association Council on Exercise and representatives of the Undersea Hyperbaric Medical Society.

DIVING PHYSIOLOGY

There are chronic and acute physiological effects associated with diving and hyperbaric exposure. Some of the more common acute effects of diving will be discussed here. Being underwater exposes one to risks associated with ambient pressure changes, cold temperatures, physical exertion, mental stress, increased oxygen partial pressure, and the possibility of carbon dioxide and carbon monoxide toxicity. More in-depth discussions of these topics may be found in the references at the end of this chapter.

The risks of scuba diving are largely due to the breathing of gases as ambient pressure increases during descent or decreases during ascent in the water. Pressure effects include:

- **Pulmonary barotrauma.** Although middle ear "squeeze" is a very common diving illness, the most serious is pulmonary barotrauma with subsequent cerebral or cardiac air embolism. Pulmonary barotrauma is an overdistension and/or rupture of the lungs that results from gas expansion during ascent.

Cerebral or cardiac air embolism results from entry of air into the arterial system. Pulmonary barotrauma with arterial air embolism requires immediate treatment. Diving medical expertise and recompression in a hyperbaric chamber are usually needed.

- **Decompression sickness (DCS or "bends").** DCS is the effervescence of dissolved inert gas (nitrogen) into the vasculature and tissues of the diver. DCS occurs when a diver stays too long at depth and his or her body becomes saturated with nitrogen. Symptoms of DCS range from mild limb/joint pain, skin itching, and fatigue to central nervous system disorder and systemic shock. Treatment almost invariably involves diving medical expertise and recompression in a hyperbaric chamber.

- **Inert gas narcosis ("nitrogen narcosis").** Nitrogen narcosis is compressed air intoxication. It results from breathing air at increased depths (i.e., >100 feet). Symptoms resemble alcohol inebriation, with similar resultant loss of motor control and intellectual capabilities. Treatment involves bringing the diver up from depth.

DIABETES AND SCUBA DIVING

The effects of scuba diving on those with diabetes have not been well established. Diabetes is listed as a contraindication by many scuba diving certification agencies. This is apparently based on the risk, and subsequent consequences, of hypoglycemia while diving. The interplay of diabetic complications, e.g., micro/macrovascular diseases, with diving physiology has not been considered the major limiting factor to diving. However, the absence of research in this area does not imply that diving is safe for all people with diabetic complications. Participation in scuba diving should be individually determined with one's physician.

People with diabetes need to be primarily concerned with the prevention of hypoglycemia while scuba diving (and be prepared for in-water treatment of hypoglycemia); the possible relationship between diabetic complications and diving physiology (pressure, circulatory and respiratory); and adequate training to anticipate and treat diabetes-related problems during diving.

Hypoglycemia

Hypoglycemic episodes during diving can lead to accidental drowning. Therefore, a rapid intervention is necessary at the first sign of hypoglycemic symptoms. Because the recognition and occurrence of hypoglycemic symptoms can be confounded by the effects of physical exertion, cold, and anxiety, the major emphasis should be on the prevention of hypoglycemia rather than in-water treatment of hypoglycemia.

Prevention of Hypoglycemia

Occurrence of hypoglycemia with diving can be minimized by frequent self-monitoring of blood glucose (SMBG). Frequent SMBG before a dive can help determine the direction of a blood glucose change. For example, if blood glucose is 200 mg/dl at 90 min before the dive, 135 mg/dl at 45 min before the dive, and 85 mg/dl at 10 min before dive, the blood glucose is dropping, and additional snacks will be necessary for a 30-min dive (see Box 33.1). SMBG should be performed immediately after a dive. Hence, review of the blood glucose pattern, food intake, and exercise will help the diver to determine insulin and carbohydrate adjustment for future dives. To be successful in managing the dive, frequent SMBG, dietary (carbohydrate) intake, and expected physical exertion (i.e., depth and duration of dive, and diving conditions) will need to be determined ahead of time.

In-Water Treatment of Hypoglycemia

Treatment of hypoglycemia in the water can avert a diving emergency. Typically, confusion and symptoms arising from nitrogen narcosis will not occur at depths <~90 feet. Divers with diabetes at depths >90 feet may develop nitrogen narcosis, and it may be mistaken for hypoglycemia and vice versa. In the preclusion of nitrogen narcosis, divers must keep in mind that early recognition may be difficult; decision-making ability is altered. A buddy may be noti-

---

Box 33.1. Steve Prosterman: The Man Behind The Mask

Steve Prosterman, who teaches scuba diving in the Marine Science Department at the University of the Virgin Islands in St. Thomas and runs a 1-week activity camp for adults with diabetes (Camp DAVI, see RESOURCES at the end of this chapter), is the man behind some of the techniques for avoiding hypoglycemia while scuba diving.

Prosterman came up with the idea of finding the direction of the blood glucose change. "This is really more important than knowing the level of the blood glucose at the beginning of an activity," he says. "It's especially important to find out if the blood glucose is dropping."

Prosterman instructs his pupils to do a series of three blood glucose tests within 1½ h (e.g., 1 h, 30 min, and 5–10 min) before an activity. "You should be able to see if the blood glucose is stable, dropping, or rising. If it is stable, aim for a 180–190 mg/dl minimum before beginning. If it is dropping, stabilize it before beginning. You may need an extra carbohydrate snack and two more tests to ensure the blood glucose level is acceptable. If blood glucose is rising, aim for a 120–130 mg/dl minimum before beginning. But do not dive until you have stablized it." Prosterman also recommends testing after (or during, if possible) the activity.

In the unlikely event that a person experiences low blood glucose during scuba diving, Prosterman devised the "L" hand sign (using the thumb and index finger). If the sign is given, the buddy team and instructor ascend to the surface, inflate the buoyancy compensation device, and administer a fast-acting carbohydrate, such as a glucose gel. Prosterman prefers Insta-Glucose (ICN Pharmaceuticals, Costa Mesa, CA) because the packaging holds up to the effects of the sun and ocean.

"It is so important to avoid hypoglycemia while scuba diving or participating in any activity that may isolate you or that would make it difficult to treat."

fied of ensuing hypoglycemia through hand signals (such as "L" to indicate low blood glucose; see Box 33.1). When the signal is given, divers should slowly and calmly ascend. Once on the surface, the buoyancy compensation device should be inflated enough to allow the affected diver to float high in the water. Fast-acting glucose gel should be administered by either the diver himself or his buddy (Each diver should carry two tubes of glucose gel). The affected diver should leave the water.

Diabetic Complications and Diving Physiology

It is speculated that joint and capillary basement membrane thickening, increased platelet aggregation, reduced flexibility of red blood cells, and the microcirculatory changes associated with diabetes may increase the risk of DCS. But research needs to be done to confirm or refute this. DCS is generally avoidable by diving conservatively. In addition, diving may pose additional risks for people with diabetes who also have cardiovascular disease or cardiac autonomic neuropathy.

Training for Diabetes-Related Problems

All divers need certification by a reputable agency. Certification includes training in diving physiology, gas kinetics, safety, and rescue. Specifically, people with diabetes must learn how exercise affects blood glucose levels and the need for carbohydrate intake and insulin adjustments. People using insulin pumps must disconnect them when diving to depths >15 feet. Divers obviously need to be physically fit.

PRELIMINARY RECOMMENDATIONS

More research and guidelines need to be established for safety and medical screening of recreational scuba divers with diabetes. The scuba diving committee of the American Diabetes Association Council on Exercise and representatives of the Undersea Hyperbaric Medical Society have come to the following initial conclusions:

- A significant number of diabetic individuals treated with insulin or oral hypoglycemic agents are scuba diving.
- There is evidence that individuals treated with insulin or oral hypoglycemic agents are at increased risk while scuba diving, principally from hypoglycemia.
- Individuals with diabetes treated with insulin or oral hypoglycemic agents should consider that others, including companions, instructors, and families, share this risk.
- There are insufficient data to justify a blanket proscription against scuba diving for individuals with diabetes.
- Until further data become available, it seems prudent to exclude the following individuals from diving:

  Those with a history of episodes of severe hypoglycemia (i.e., loss of consciousness, seizures, or requiring the assistance of others) within 12 months before diving.

  Those with advanced secondary complications, such as proliferative retinopathy, neuropathy, or coronary artery disease.

  Those with hypoglycemia unawareness (lacking adrenergic symptoms of mild hypoglycemia).

  Those who do not have adequately controlled diabetes (as determined by their physician) or who do not have a good understanding of the relationship between diabetes and exercise.

To be considered for recreational scuba diving, individuals must *1)* have well-controlled diabetes, *2)* have a good understanding of their disease, *3)* receive suitable training, and *4)* follow a specially designed management protocol.

SUGGESTED READINGS

1. Bove AA: Medical aspects of diving. In *Exercise in Medicine*. Bove AA, Lowenthal DT, Eds. Orlando, FL, Academic, 1983
2. Strauss RH (Ed.): *Diving Medicine*. New York, Grune & Stratton, 1976
3. Melamud Y, Shupak A, Bitterman H: Medical problems associated with underwater diving. *N Engl J Med* 326:30–35, 1992
4. Bradley ME: Fitness to dive: metabolic considerations. *Proceedings From the 34th Undersea and Hyperbaric Medical Society Workshop, Bethesda, MD*
5. Department of Commerce, National Oceanic and Atmospheric Administration: *NOAA Diving Manual*. Washington, DC, U.S. Govt. Printing Office, 1979

RESOURCES

Divers Alert Network
Box 3823
Duke University Medical Center
Durham, NC 27710

Undersea Hyperbaric Medical Society
9650 Rockville Pike
Bethesda, MD 20814

Camp DAVI
The Diabetes Association of the
Virgin Islands
P.O. Box 5511
St. Thomas, VI 00803-5511

34. Mountain Hiking

Introduction

Hazards of Mountain Hiking

    Dehydration
    Sun Radiation
    Frostbite and Hypothermia
    Avalanche
    Lightning
    Mountain Sickness Syndrome

Insulin Conservation

Self-Monitoring of Blood Glucose (SMBG) Equipment

Diabetes Complications

    Hypoglycemia
    Retinopathy
    Neuropathy

Self-Management

Mountain Hiking

JEAN-JACQUES GRIMM, MD

INTRODUCTION

Mountains, like deserts and oceans, are relatively unaltered by human civilizations. They can sometimes be hostile to people, who nevertheless enjoy a sense of self-accomplishment from climbing them. Most hikers feel that they are doing more than simply exercising at high altitudes. Mountaineering is a complex experience; climbers are both exhilarated and challenged by the hazards of surviving in a demanding environment.

There are many mountain climbers with diabetes, such as the well-known Italian Vittorio Casirahgi. Their experience shows that even in this very strenuous activity, people with diabetes can still be active. However, they must take special care to monitor and manage their diabetes. There are some inherent dangers in mountaineering.

HAZARDS OF MOUNTAIN HIKING

Dehydration

Sweating and high respiratory rates at high altitudes induce substantial fluid loss. Minimal water requirements are about 2–3 liters/day in these conditions. It is often difficult to melt snow because of wind, bad weather, and time constraints. Climbers usually find it more convenient to carry a daily quantity of water that they have prepared before starting each morning.

Sun Radiation

Ultraviolet (UV) radiation can be very strong at high altitudes and increases even more in snow-covered areas. Climbers must protect their eyes with high-quality glasses and coat exposed skin areas, such as the nose, ears, neck, and scalp, with lotions offering high degrees of UV protection.

Frostbite and Hypothermia

Even the best footwear cannot prevent some moisture in the feet after a couple of hours of walking. Moisture exposes the toes and the heels to cold injuries, even when the temperature is above freezing. The same is true for fingers in wet gloves. The nose, the ears, and other exposed parts of the face are also at risk in windy conditions. Abnormal skin sensitivity at the feet or circulatory insufficiency increases the danger of frostbite. Bivouacs are often unexpected or do not happen at the planned location. Protection from wind in a rock or ice cave is often lifesaving. Additional dry underwear and an aluminum emergency sheet should be available.

Avalanche

Drifted or recently fallen snow can be unstable on certain slopes. In some mountain ranges, good information about the risk of avalanche is available via a snow information telephone number, tourist information booths, or guide company offices. This danger should be taken into account when planning a hike during the winter or spring. Generally, starting early and returning in the early afternoon, before long sun exposure on the slopes, gives climbers some security.

Lightning

During the summer months, lightning is a common threat to climbers. Some exposed areas, such as ridges and summits, must be avoided when the risk for storms is high, usually in the late afternoon.

Mountain Sickness Syndrome

When lowlanders ascend to high altitudes (over 2,500 m/8,200 ft), they often experience headache, nausea, vomiting, insomnia, and lassitude. High-altitude pulmonary edema (HAPE) is a rare but potentially fatal complication of acute exposure to high altitudes (1). Progressive acclimatization, over weeks, decreases the risk of these illnesses. No data are available for the prophylactic use of drugs (for example, acetazolamide) in people with diabetes. Nifedipine has proven to be helpful for the treatment of HAPE.

INSULIN CONSERVATION

Insulin is altered by high temperatures, light, excess agitation, and freezing (2). At 45°C, for example, a loss of up to 15% of the biological activity can be expected after 1 month, depending on the type of insulin. Moreover, at high temperatures, degradation products with unwanted immunological effects (i.e., allergy) can appear. Excess agitation increases the risk of degradation with high temperatures.

When walking in the sun, it is advisable to store insulin in an insulated box in a nonexposed place in a backpack. With cold weather or at night, placing the insulin in a location close to the body—for example, a sleeping bag—can prevent it from freezing. If despite all care the insulin freezes, a significant decrease in potency must be expected. This is particularly true for the long-acting preparations in which large aggregates are no longer soluble. Furthermore, these aggregates can also block the needle or the pump catheter. Table 36.1 provides insulin storage temperatures.

SELF-MONITORING OF BLOOD GLUCOSE (SMBG) EQUIPMENT

All the SMBG devices and their strips deliver acceptably accurate results as long as they work and are stored in the desired temperature, moisture, and oxygen pressure ranges (3). For most of these devices, these ranges are about 1–30°C (59–86°F) for temperature and 20–80% for relative humidity. At high altitudes (4,350 m/14,272 ft), some systems underestimate the blood glucose results by as much as 45%, and others overestimate it up to 35%. It is hazardous to try to correct supposed under- or overestimated values.

DIABETES COMPLICATIONS

Hypoglycemia

Exercising at high altitudes is a potent stimulation for the sympathetic nervous system, resulting in high heart rates and sweating. The recognition of hypoglycemia can be confusing in these conditions. Poor appetite and sometimes nausea are frequent at high altitudes and can compromise proper food and fluid intake, precipitating hypoglycemic attacks. Climbers must carefully plan drinking and eating schedules before getting started and monitor their blood glucose frequently. Hiking with at least one other person is very helpful as well as safer in this regard.

Retinopathy

Retinal hemorrhages have been described in people without diabetes as

---

Table 36.1. Insulin Storage

< 2°C (36° F; risk of freezing)
- Short-acting insulin (soluble): usually no damage. Nevertheless, change to a new vial as soon as possible.

- Long or intermediate-acting insulin: probable loss of biological activity. Change to a new vial as soon as possible.

2–8°C (36–46°F)
- Ideal storage temperature.

8–30°C (46–86°F)
- No significant effect on insulin activity for 1 month.

30–45°C (86–113°F)
- Acceptable for very short periods (days); loss of biological activity possible.

Check all insulins regularly for clumping or precipitation.

part of the mountain sickness syndrome (4). It seems likely that an untreated abnormal diabetic retina could be harmed by the same exposure to high altitudes. Whether a clinically normal diabetic retina is at high risk of damage is not yet known. A thorough retinal check should absolutely be performed before climbers with diabetes participate in high-altitude activities.

Neuropathy

Hikers with altered sensitivity in the lower extremities are prone to more frequent and severe foot injuries than would normally be expected. Even common blisters will be more severe because of the lack of sensation. The difficulties in maintaining adequate hygiene and, very often, the necessity to continue to walk makes wound healing a difficult challenge. Autonomic neuropathy can alter the heart rate and blood pressure adaptation to the effort and to the altitude.

SELF-MANAGEMENT

If performed during good conditions, mountain hiking is an endurance sport. The exercise is aerobic and lasts many hours to several days. Under these circumstances, insulin needs usually decrease substantially and carbohydrate consumption increases. Therefore, climbers should regularly monitor their blood glucose levels and keep a record of the duration and quality of their exercise in relation to their body's reactions. Access to aid stations may be difficult; rescue may not be available for several days. Therefore, careful self-management is essential (5).

REFERENCES

1. Tso EL, Wagner TJ: What's up in the management of high-altitude pulmonary oedema? *MD Med J* 42: 641– 45, 1993
2. Brange J: *Galenics of Insulin.* Berlin, Springer-Verlag, 1987
3. Banion CR, Klingensmith GJ: Performance of seven blood glucose testing systems at high altitude. *Diabetes Educ* 15:444–48, 1989
4. Frayser R, Houston CS, Bryan AC, Rennie ID, Gray G: Retinal hemorrhage at high altitude. *N Engl J Med* 282:1183–84, 1970
5. Auerbach PS (Ed.): *Wilderness Medicine: Management of Wilderness and Environmental Emergencies.* 3rd ed. St. Louis, MO, Mosby, 1995

35. Ice Hockey

Ice Hockey

CARL FOSTER, PhD, AND ROBERT J. HANISCH, MA, CDE

INTRODUCTION

I ce hockey can be a safe and enjoyable winter sport for people with diabetes. Ice hockey involves many comparatively brief bursts of high-speed skating interspersed with equally brief periods of rest. Although players are nominally designated as offensive, linking, or defensive, the size of the ice surface and the necessity for coordinated team play dictate that the players move as something of a unit. The rules allow considerable contact between players, including deliberate checking (running into your opponent and/or forcefully pushing your opponent into the boards surrounding the playing surface). Because of the high-speed skating, players can become fatigued rather rapidly. In serious adult competition, players may be substituted as often as every 30-40 s to minimize the consequences of fatigue (1).

MEDICAL EVALUATION

As with any high-intensity contact sport, the physician should be aware of general constitutional factors, orthopedic limitations, and overall health when evaluating potential players.

Skin

Because of the frequency of violent contact, chafing by the large amount of padding (which is often wet and an excellent medium for bacterial growth), and abrasions from the skate boot, diabetic individuals who show evidence of slow healing of cutaneous lesions will need to be particularly careful of skin hygiene.

Heart

Given the high intensity of play and the increased risk for people with diabetes to develop precocious coronary artery disease and for myocardial ischemia to be asymptomatic in diabetic individuals with evidence of autonomic neuropathy (see Chapter 18), evaluation of the adult ice hockey player should at least consider the potential for exertional myocardial ischemia.

Knees and Back

High-speed skating places particular stress on the knee joint and lower back. Diabetic or not, these areas should be carefully evaluated in all prospective players.

Eyes

Because of the frequency of violent contact, prospective hockey players should undergo a retinal examination (see Chapter 14). Even in recreational or youth leagues, where checking is restricted, the fundamental nature of ice hockey dictates that a given player is going to collide with other players, the side boards, or the ice surface several times during each practice and competition. Accordingly, trauma to the head must be considered unavoidable. In the presence of significant retinopathy, players should be discouraged from playing.

Metabolic Effects

The intensity of play in ice hockey leads to high blood lactate concentrations during play (1,2), with predictable disturbances of pH that may be important for the person with inadequately controlled diabetes. High-speed skating also leads to fairly profound levels of muscle glycogen depletion, from both type I and II muscle fibers (3). Accordingly, glucose disappearance from the blood may occur at a very high rate for several hours following practice and/or competition. This may lead to a significant incidence of late postexercise hypoglycemia if insulin dose and carbohydrate intake are not properly adjusted. Further, the tradition of significant post-game alcohol consumption may exaggerate the tendency toward late postexercise hypoglycemia.

Because of the intrinsically competitive nature of ice hockey and the potential for violent contact between players, the effects of strong emotional arousal on glucose homeostasis must be accounted for. Insulin dosages and/or carbohydrate intakes that are appropriate for equally intense exercise without emotional arousal may be completely inadequate during competitive ice hockey play.

MEDICAL INTERVENTION

The coach and teammates of the diabetic player should be informed of his or her condition, briefed on the basic problems likely to be encountered by the diabetic player, and understand the basic strategies for acute intervention.

REFERENCES

1. Cox MH: Applied physiology of ice hockey. *Sports Med* 19:184–201, 1995
2. Jacobs I: Blood lactate: implications for training and sports performance. *Sports Med* 3:10–25, 1986
3. Green HJ: Glycogen depletion patterns during continuous and intermittent ice skating. *Med Sci Sports* 10:183–87, 1978

VI. Resources and Reimbursement

Reimbursement Issues

ERIC P. DURAK, MSc

MEDICAL BILLING

Although exercise has long been touted as part of the trilogy of treatment in diabetes, its use within the current health-care system has been minimal at best. One reason for this is the lack of third party reimbursement for health education or exercise therapy services. This chapter provides information on how exercise programs may be billed through physicians' offices, clinics, or hospitals.

Most patients think of insurance as a "shared cost" in case of an emergency. With the emergence of health-care reform, how we think about insurance is changing. Managed care may dictate that certain types of services are performed less often, and other, more cost-effective, services are performed more often. Exercise therapy is an example of this latter type of service.

Because insurance companies typically recognize the services of licensed practitioners, exercise-related services should be co-signed by the physician. This helps alert insurance companies that physicians are prescribing these types of services. It is important to use the proper billing codes for reimbursement.

INTERNATIONAL CLASSIFICATION OF DISEASES, 9TH REVISION, CLINICAL MODIFICATION (ICD-9-CM) CODING

The International Classification of Diseases manual organizes and classifies known causes of morbidity and mortality. Listed below are a few examples of diseases that are pertinent to exercise therapy. These examples are based on the 1995 update.

- 250   diabetes mellitus–general coding category
- 250.0   type II diabetes mellitus, or unspecified type, not stated as uncontrolled
- 250.01   type I diabetes mellitus, not stated as uncontrolled
- 250.03   type I diabetes mellitus, uncontrolled
- 251.2   hypoglycemia, unspecified
- 278   obesity and other hyperalimentation–general coding category
- 390–398, 402   diseases of the circulatory system
- 401   essential hypertension–general coding category
- 580–89   nephritis (kidney disease)
- 646.1   weight gain in pregnancy (excessive, without hypertension)
- 648.8   gestational diabetes mellitus
- 728.2   muscular wasting and disuse atrophy, not elsewhere classified

ICD-9 diagnostic codes are usually "rank-ordered" so insurance companies understand that a more severe disease gets reimbursed first.

CURRENT PROCEDURAL TERMINOLOGY (CPT) CODING

CPT codes are published by the American Medical Association for physician and allied health services. They are used to determine charges for office visits and follow-ups. Exercise-related services would include exercise counseling, exercise therapy sessions, and exercise evaluations. Each medical group has established its own prices for services, based on the Health Insurance Association of America's usual and customary reimbursement for a particular community.

CPT codes are five-digit numbers that equate a service with a cost. They were designed by physicians to coordinate a particular service with a pricing scheme. This charge varies by geographical location. CPT codes used by allied health professionals usually fall in the physical medicine section of the coding book.

Of interest to exercise professionals are codes that apply to exercise services and wellness counseling. Some of the most common codes and new codes are highlighted below. Note that when performing these services, the physician or therapist must be with the patient at all times.

Therapeutic Exercise Code (97110)

The therapeutic exercise code is used for limited visits, such as teaching patients how to use exercise equipment, do resistance training, or perform specific types of exercise to strengthen certain areas of the body. This type of training may take place 3-5 times over a 1- or 2-week period.

Aquatic Therapy Code (97113)

The aquatic therapy code is used for any therapeutic exercise performed in the water, including aerobic work or specific muscle strengthening.

Kinetic Activities Codes (97530, 97531)

Kinetic activities codes are used for more extended visits, during which patients are taught how to use equipment and perform various home exercises and are monitored until they reach certain end-point criteria. Therapists often use the 97530 code, because it applies to many types of exercise situations.

Activities for Daily Living (ADL) Codes (97540, 97541)

ADL codes are used for single session patient visits. They are primarily designed to teach patients an activity they may have trouble performing at home (for example, getting in and out of a chair or reaching for a household appliance) as a result of their medical condi-

tion. Attempted use of ADL coding over prolonged time periods may result in denied claims.

Work Hardening Codes (97545, 97546)

Work hardening codes refer to exercises designed to help create a more ergonomically efficient worker. They may include back therapy or corrective exercises for carpal tunnel syndrome.

Extremity Testing Codes (97720, 97721)

The extremity testing codes cover assessments of muscle strength and dexterity. They are used when testing new patients or reevaluating existing patients, and they should be used only a few times during the entire patient rehabilitation.

Performance Testing Code (97750)

The performance testing code refers to a test of the musculoskeletal and cardiovascular systems. The test runs about 15 min, and the clinician provides a written report of the results.

Some codes in the 1995 CPT coding book may pertain to the clinical exercise or health education specialist working with diabetes patients. After a medical evaluation, the physician can refer patients to a health education specialist who is familiar with lifestyle counseling (diet, exercise, stress reduction, etc.), and the following codes can be used for counseling purposes:

- 99401, 99402, 99403, and 99404: Counseling and/or risk factor reduction intervention(s) provided to healthy individuals for ~15, ~30, ~45, and ~60 min, respectively.
- 99411 and 99412: Counseling and/or risk factor reduction intervention(s) provided to healthy individuals in a group setting for ~30 and ~60 min, respectively.
- 99429: Unlisted preventive medicine service

At present, Medicare does not reimburse for "wellness services." Some HMOs do reimburse for these codes, and it is anticipated that many more will in the near future. These codes can be modified for many health education situations, such as diabetes education, dietitian counseling, stress counseling, lifestyle education, and weight management programs.

CHANGES IN HEALTH CARE

There are negative and positive aspects to health-care reform in the United States. A government-regulated system is expensive, and quality of care is difficult to guarantee. However, many insurance companies are enacting their own reforms in order to provide more services to their customers and decrease their overhead costs.

By the end of the decade, HMOs may be the primary insurance reimbursement system used in this country. This system usually pays a capitated fee to providers for services rendered. For many rehabilitation specialists, this reimbursement cap means, in some instances, less money for services. This pricing structure may work well for therapeutic exercise and wellness services, which, by their nature, are less expensive than traditional rehabilitation. If quality exercise-related services can be provided to patients at a reasonable cost, they may increasingly be reimbursed within the third party/HMO system.

CONCLUDING REMARKS

In order for exercise to be routinely prescribed as part of the overall diabetes management program, it must be as reimbursable as any other medical or health procedure. To increase the likelihood of reimbursement, health-care professionals should 1) be familiar with the current reimbursement system in terms of diagnosis, coding, price structuring, letters of prior authorization, and appealing denial letters; 2) understand current changes in the health-care system and the role exercise and health promotion play in clinical practices; 3) be able to negotiate with physicians for patient referrals; and 4) demonstrate positive health outcomes in patients.

SUGGESTED READINGS

1. Boughton B: An ounce of prevention. *Northern California Medicine.* July 1993, p. 25–27
2. Burrough DJ: Insurer and health clubs form partnership. *The Business Journal* (Phoenix). January 1995, p. 1
3. Curfman G: The health benefits of exercise. *N Engl J Med* 328: 574–76, 1993
4. Dowel JR, Boltier CP, Thomas KL, Klein DA: Psychological well-being and its relationship to fitness and activity levels. *J Hum Mov Stud* 14:39, 1988
5. Durak EP, Shapiro AA: *The Ins and Outs of Medical Insurance Billing: a Resource Guide for the Fitness and Health Professional.* Santa Barbara, CA, Medical Health and Fitness, 1994
6. Eisenberg DM, Kessler RC, Foster C, Norlock FE, Calkins DR, Delbanco TL: Unconventional medicine in the United States: prevalence, costs, and patterns of use. *N Engl J Med* 328:246–52, 1993
7. Fiatarone MA, Marks EC, Ryan ND, Evans WJ: High-intensity strength training in nonagenarians: effects on skeletal muscle. *JAMA* 263:3029–34, 1990
8. Goldstein MS: *The Health Movement: Promoting Fitness in America.* Twayne Publishers, New York, 1992
9. Herzlinger RE: The simplest, best cure for our health-care crisis. *Medical Economics.* November 1991, p. 135–47
10. Leaf A: Preventive medicine for our ailing health-care system. *JAMA* 269:616–18, 1993
11. Naisbitt J: The wellness redux: the mind-body connection. *John Naisbitt's Trend Letter.* October 1994, p. 1–4

12. Quebec Task Force Study: Low back pain: causes and treatment. *Spine* 12:S-7, 1987
13. Shephard RS, Corey P, Renzland P, Cox M: The impact of changes in fitness and lifestyle upon health-care utilization. *Can J Pub Health* 74:51–54, 1983
14. Young QD: Health-care reform: a new public health movement. *Am J Pub Health* 83:945–46, 1993

Resources

AMERICAN DIABETES ASSOCIATION COUNCIL ON EXERCISE

The Council on Exercise is one of 13 Professional Section Councils of the American Diabetes Association. ADA Professional Section Council members serve on policy-making committees and task forces, write technical reviews and position statements, and act as liaisons and representatives to other organizations. Council members may also write, review, and/or edit professional and consumer books.

Professional Section Councils meet each year at the ADA Annual Meeting and are responsible for organizing and chairing Scientific Symposia and reviewing submitted abstracts for presentation at the meeting.

ADA professional members with a clinical or research interest in exercise therapy and exercise physiology may become members of the Council on Exercise. The Council on Exercise provides a forum for professional members to

- Discuss the benefits, risks, and practical problems associated with exercise in patients with diabetes.
- Disseminate new information about the effects of exercise to both medical professionals and consumers.
- Establish standards for the development of safe and effective exercise programs.
- Foster research interest in the physiology and pathophysiology of exercise and its use in the treatment of diabetes and its complications.

AMERICAN COLLEGE OF SPORTS MEDICINE

The American College of Sports Medicine (ACSM) is the largest sports medicine and exercise science organization in the world. ACSM's mission is to promote and integrate scientific research, education, and practical applications of sports medicine and exercise science to maintain and enhance physical performance, fitness, health, and quality of life.

ACSM members, who work in diverse medical specialties, allied health professions, and scientific disciplines, are committed to the diagnosis, treatment, and prevention of sports-related injuries and the advancement of the science of exercise.

Professional Membership Benefits and Services

The three main categories of professional membership in ACSM are medicine, basic and applied science, and education and allied health. Benefits and services to professional members include subscriptions to *Medicine and Science in Sports and Exercise*, ACSM's monthly scientific journal, and *Sports Medicine Bulletin*, ACSM's quarterly newsmagazine. Each year, members also receive a membership directory and a review of current research topics in exercise science published in *Exercise and Sport Sciences Reviews*. In addition, ACSM members receive discounts on meeting registration fees, certification examinations, and other products and services.

Professional Education and Certification

ACSM offers professional education programs in sports medicine and exercise science. Nearly 5,000 people attend ACSM's Annual Meeting, where more than 1,200 research studies are presented. In addition, the ACSM Team Physician^{SM} Course enhances the medical skills of physicians working with athletic teams and individual athletes.

Seeking to increase the competency of individuals involved in health and fitness and cardiovascular rehabilitative exercise programs, ACSM offers professional certification. For certification, professionals must meet specific prerequisites and successfully pass both a written and practical exam. Under review every 4 years, certified individuals must provide proof of continuing education to remain certified by ACSM.

Physician and Patient Information

ACSM provides educational videos and brochures to physicians and patients. Summaries of official ACSM Pronouncements covering a variety of topics, including anabolic steroids, youth fitness, and weight-loss programs, are also available. A complete list of educational materials may be obtained on request.

Research Grants

Research grants are available each year through the ACSM Foundation to student and professional members. Specific areas of funding include the effects of exercise on human aging, exercise and cardiovascular disease risk factors, and exercise and nutrition.

For more information about ACSM or any of these programs contact

American College of Sports Medicine
P.O. Box 1440
Indianapolis, IN 46206-1440
Tel: 317-637-9200
Fax: 317-634-7817

INTERNATIONAL DIABETIC ATHLETES ASSOCIATION

The International Diabetic Athletes Association (IDAA) is a nonprofit service organization dedicated to encouraging an active lifestyle for people with diabetes. Members include individuals with diabetes who participate in fitness activities at all levels, health-care professionals, and everyone interested in the relationship between (or special problems of) diabetes and sports.

The IDAA's mission is to enhance the quality of life for people with diabetes through exercise. To accomplish their mission, IDAA

- Educates people of all ages with diabetes and their health-care providers about the role of exercise in enhancing health.
- Creates opportunities for those with diabetes to participate in a broad range of recreational, sport, and athletic activities.
- Enhances self-care and self-management skills among sports-minded individuals with diabetes.
- Improves clinical skills and promotes a positive attitude toward exercise among health professionals working with active individuals with diabetes.
- Promotes networking, support, and sharing of experiences among physically active people with diabetes.
- Provides a forum for exchanging information and access to resources and role models.
- Increases knowledge and promotes positive attitudes about diabetes and exercise among coaches and physical education teachers.

With chapters in a dozen U.S. cities, Canada, Australia, and eight European countries, the IDAA holds forums annually. These forums include regional, national, and international conferences that provide up-to-date information from medical professionals and an opportunity to exchange ideas with athletes with practical experience. In addition, quarterly newsletters enable networking support and further sharing of experiences. Membership costs $15.00/year in the U.S., $20.00/year outside the U.S. For more information about IDAA, contact

International Diabetic Athletes Association
1647 West Bethany Home Road #B
Phoenix, AZ 85015-2507
Tel: 602-433-2113
Fax: 602-433-9331

Index

Index

E

Eccentric contraction, 8, 228
Echocardiographic stress testing, 158
Edema, 188, 190
Education
  about exercise, 272
  levels of, 253, 254
Elderly
  deterioration, insulin
        sensitivity/glucose toler-
        ance, 24
  and exercise duration, 230
  and spontaneous activity, 228–229
Electrocardiographic (ECG) moni-
        toring, 73, 86, 157,
        246–247, 285
Electromyography, 185
Electron transport chain, 9–10
Embarrassment, 219, 221
Endurance, 91
  aerobic, 17–19
  athletes, 13, 18
  exercise programs, 239, 272
Energy
  expenditure, 74, 284
  needs, 101
  systems, 9–10
Entrapment syndromes, 184–185
Ephedrine, 188
Epigastric discomfort, 188
Epinephrine, 29–32, 235
Ergogenic aids, 280–281
Erythromycin, 238
Erythropoietin, synthetic, 177–178
Estradiol, 212
Estrogen therapy, 212–213
Euglycemic clamp, 24
Exercise
  abnormal response to, 15
  adaptations, 17
  aerobic. *See* Aerobic
        exercise
  and aging, 223–232
  and amputation, 139–140
  anaerobic, 21–22
  antidepressant effect of, 61
  anxiolytic effect of, 61
  barriers to, 113, 252–253, 254

  capacity. *See* Aerobic exercise
        capacity (VO$_{2max}$)
  chair, 139
  compliance, 43, 78, 129–130, 253
    enhancing, 80, 254
  complications with NIDDM, 147
  compulsion, 62–63
  counseling, 309
  duration, 12, 38, 42, 71, 80, 113
    with coronary disease, 159
    and the elderly, 230
  equipment, 202, 231
  and foot trauma, 77, 202
  formal sessions, 130
  frequency of, 71, 77
  friend, 228
  graded, 178
  high-impact and proliferative dia-
        betic retinopathy, 149
  high-intensity, 35, 38, 113, 157
  high-resistance, 202
  hypertensive response to, abnor-
        mal, 158
  and IDDM, 36–38
    with amenorrheic athletes, 211
  intensity, 71, 75, 78–80, 93, 159,
        192–193, 230
  isometric, 156, 157
  light-to-moderate, 73–74, 170
  log, 130
  low-intensity, 12, 113
  maintenance, 128
  mode of, 71, 74–77
  moderate, 104, 157, 226, 251
  in morning
    and hypoglycemia, 191
  negative psychological effects,
        62–63
  for older people, 226–227
  physiology, 5–26
  prescription, 3, 69–82, 86–87, 309
    with neuropathy, 190–193
  programs
    adherence to, 63, 113, 129–130,
        253–254
    for adolescents, 221–222
    community-based, 257–264
    for children, 221–222
    culturally acceptable, 260

Lovastatin, 238
Lungs, perfusion of, larger, 18

M

Macrovascular complications, 72
Macular edema, 145
Magnesium levels, 235
Magnetic resonance imaging (MRI), 244
Mahler, Halafdam, 261
Malaria, severe falciparum, 239
Malate-aspartate shuttle, 20
Marathon running, 273–277
Medical
    evaluation, 86, 202
    history, complete, 71–72
Menopause, 211
Menstrual disorders, 210–211
Metabolic
    adaptations, 21–22
    control, 191
    equivalents (METS), 284
    rate, resting (RMR), 111, 209, 229
Methylpalmoxirate, 40
Metoprolol, 235
Mexican Americans, 246–247, 253–254
Mexilitine, 191
Microalbuminuria, 167, 237
Microangiopathy, 147, 155
Microvascular
    complications, 72
    disease, 80
Minority populations
    African Americans, 238, 246–247, 251–253
    Asian Americans, 251
    exercise programs for, 249–256
    Hawaiians, native, 254
    Hispanic Americans, 251, 253
    Japanese Americans, 246–247
    Latinos, 247, 251
        Urban Caribbean, 253
    Mexican Americans, 246–247, 253–254
    Native Americans, 246–247, 251, 254
    Puerto Ricans, 251

Mitochondria, 9–10
    increase in, 20
Mortality risk, 251
Motivation, 259, 262, 276–277
Motor units, 11, 12–13, 22
Mountain hiking, 299–302
Mountain sickness syndrome, 300
Muscle, skeletal
    biopsies, 178
    capillary density, 24, 127
    cellular adaptations, 17, 19–21
    contraction, 11–12, 16, 86, 228
    degeneration, natural, 202
    fibers, 10–11
    fitness, 7
    glucose uptake, 34–35, 92
    glycogen, 21, 29, 35, 92–93
        breakdown to lactic acid, 9–10, 16, 92, 304
    glycogenolysis, 33–34
    groups, large, 75
    mass, 22, 24, 127, 225, 228
    metabolism, 35
    necrosis, 238
    sensitivity to insulin, 52
    strength and power, 225
    wasting, 179, 183
Musculoskeletal
    injuries, 71, 74–75, 76, 130, 199–204
        reduced, 226
    system testing, 310
Myocardial
    contraction
        increased strength of, 15
    enlargement, 155
    infarction, 155, 156, 158, 235
        and ACE inhibitors, 237
        silent, 185, 191–192, 304
    ischemia, 74
    oxygen demand, 52
    scintigraphy, [210]T1, 285
Myogenic adaptations, 22
Myoglobinuria, 238
Myokinase, 22
Myopathy
    steroid, 237
    uremic, 178
Myosin ATPase, 8, 16

Uremia, 178
Uric acid levels, 235
Uterine contractions, 210

V

Vaginal bleeding, 209
Valsalva
  effect, 79–80
  maneuvers, 15, 85–86, 146, 149,
    230
Vascular disease, 202–203
  peripheral, 179, 203
Vasoconstrictive stimuli, 188
Vasoconstrictor responses, impaired
    peripheral, 187
Vasodilators, 158, 188
Venous return
  during exercise, 192
  systemic, inadequate, 155
Ventilation, minute, 209
Ventricular
  arrhythmias, 190
  diastolic function, left, 186–187
  filling
    increase in, 18
    left, limitation in, 155
  systolic function, left, 157, 158
  wall thickness, 18, 21
Verapamil, 237
Very-low-calorie diets (VLCDs),
    111, 112
Virilization in women, 238
Vomiting, 188

W

Waist-to-hip ratio (WHR), 244, 251,
    253
Walking, 113, 137, 139, 149
  ability, 225
  brisk, 203
  during pregnancy, 209, 210
Warm-up, 78–79, 86, 227, 275
Waterskiing, 270
Weather conditions, 286
Weight
  -bearing exercise, 212

control, 109–114, 260
lifting, 8, 12–13, 192, 279–281
loss
  and carbohydrates, 41
  and fluid loss, 106–107
  programs, 112, 251–253
training
  and the elderly, 24, 184, 280
Well-being, sense of, 62, 71
Wellness counseling, 310–311
Western lifestyle, 243, 245, 246
Wilson, Wade, 270
Women and exercise, 130, 207–216
  reduced risk of proliferative dia-
    betic retinopathy, 147
Work capacity, functional, improve-
    ment in, 52
World Health Organization, 261

Y

Yoga, 62, 290

Z

Zuni Diabetes Project, 259–260

American Diabetes Association Professional Section Membership

Two types of memberships for all kinds of health-care professionals. Choose the one that's right for you!

Category I

Designed primarily for physicians and researchers, Category I offers you the full range of benefits, plus your **choice** of the leading monthly publications, *DIABETES* or *DIABETES CARE*.

Category II

Created expressly for nurses, dietitians, educators, behaviorists, and other health-care professionals interested in diabetes education and counseling, Category II offers the full range of benefits, plus subscriptions to *DIABETES SPECTRUM* and *DIABETES FORECAST*.

Order additional journal subscriptions at low "members only" rates.

* *DIABETES CARE* — features the latest clinical research with comment on clinical trials, behavioral medicine, nutrition, complications, patient education, epidemiology, health-care delivery, and other aspects of clinical care.

* *DIABETES* — premier journal of world-wide basic diabetes research focuses on such areas as pathogenesis of diabetes and its complications, metabolism, pharmacology, and biochemical and molecular aspects of biological processes.

* *DIABETES SPECTRUM* — quarterly journal translates research into practical real-world solutions for patient education and counseling.

* *DIABETES REVIEWS* — presents comprehensive reviews on cutting-edge research and clinical findings from leading diabetes investigators.

* *CLINICAL DIABETES* — bimonthly newsletter that presents updates on treatment strategies, reimbursement, research abstracts, and other public policy issues.

* *DIABETES FORECAST* — an upbeat monthly magazine for those who live with diabetes and for their families. Emphasizes self-management.

* *SCIENTIFIC SESSIONS ABSTRACT BOOK* — brings you abstracts of research presented at ADA's Annual Scientific Sessions.

With the American Diabetes Association, you'll have more ways to make a difference.

* **FREE COUNCIL MEMBERSHIP** — Special Interest Councils give professionals from varied specialties a chance to advance in the field, learn, and work together to set standards in diabetes treatment and patient care.

* **FREE LOCAL ADA AFFILIATE MEMBERSHIP** — As a national ADA member, enjoy automatic membership in your local Affiliate where you can vote and help shape the future of ADA. Take part in locally sponsored professional and patient education programs to enrich the lives of those with diabetes.

* **UP TO 50% OFF CONFERENCE AND EDUCATION PROGRAMS** — Save on fees to ADA's Annual Scientific Sessions, Postgraduate Courses, and Research Symposia — all approved for Continuing Education credit.

* **REFERRALS AND NETWORKING** — Gain useful professional introductions and meet your peers through your ADA membership and participation in ADA meetings.

* **RESEARCH GRANTS, ADA AWARDS** — As an ADA Professional Section Member, you'll be eligible for grants for diabetes research and for annual awards honoring outstanding achievement.

* **PROFESSIONAL MEMBERSHIP DIRECTORY** — You'll be listed in the annual ADA Directory — your link to more than 12,000 experts — a Who's Who of diabetes professionals.

* **CLINICAL PRACTICE RECOMMENDATIONS** — Keep up-to-date on ADA's current guidelines on clinical practice and apply them in your own practice setting.

Additional Resources From the American Diabetes Association

To order any of the following publications or to receive a free catalog, call **1-800-ADA-ORDER**. Or, you can mail in the order form on the following page.

NEW!

The ADA Clinical Education Series on CD-ROM

The world's most comprehensive diabetes treatment information can be at your fingertips in seconds with CD-ROM technology! Presenting the first all-in-one database of diabetes treatment information. Includes: *Medical Management of Insulin-Dependent (Type I) Diabetes, 2nd Ed.*; *Medical Management of Non-Insulin-Dependent (Type II) Diabetes 3rd Ed.*; *Therapy for Diabetes Mellitus and Related Disorders, 2nd Ed.*; *Medical Management of Pregnancy Complicated by Diabetes, 2nd Ed.*; plus ADA's *Clinical Practice Recommendations 1995*. It's all on one compact disc, allowing for quick searches of key terms or phrases across all titles in the database. It also features a "hypertext link," giving you instantaneous browsing between text, references, and illustrations. Best of all, it's easy to install and use. You need no previous familiarity with CD-ROM technology. If you do need assistance, technical experts will be available to help. System requirements: *Macintosh* — 6820 or greater processor, System 7.0 or greater, 2MB RAM (4MB recommended); *Windows* — 386 or 486 processor (486 recommended), Windows 3.1 or greater, 4MB RAM. 1995. #PCDROM1. *Nonmember*: $225.00; *Member*: $179.50

NEW!

Intensive Diabetes Management

An all-inclusive "how to" on implementing tight diabetes control in your practice. Written by a team of experts with first-hand DCCT experience, this valuable guide provides you with the practical information needed to implement intensive management. *Contents*: Rationale for and Physiological Basis of Intensive Diabetes Management, The Team Approach, Diabetes Self-Management Education, Psychosocial Issues, Patient Selection and Goals of Therapy, Multiple-Component Insulin Regimens, Insulin Infusion Pump Therapy, Monitoring, Nutrition Management, Adverse Effects, and Resources. Softcover; 116 pages. #PMIDM. *Nonmember*: $37.50; *Member*: $29.95

NEW!

Medical Management of Pregnancy Complicated by Diabetes, 2nd Ed.

Just updated with the new ADA Nutrition Recommendations! A must-read for anyone involved in treating women with type I, type II, or gestational diabetes. This concise, yet comprehensive guide takes you through every aspect of pregnancy and diabetes, from prepregnancy counseling to postpartum follow-up and everything in-between. Provides precise protocols for treatment of both preexisting and gestational diabetes. Tabbed and well-indexed for easy access to important information. 1995; Softcover; 136 pages. #PMMPCD2. *Nonmember*: $37.50; *Member*: $29.95

Medical Management of Insulin-Dependent (Type I) Diabetes, 2nd Ed.

formerly: *Physician's Guide to Insulin-Dependent (Type I) Diabetes*

The DCCT proved that complications such as neuropathy, nephropathy, and retinopathy can be halted, or even prevented, with proper diabetes management. This book gives you the tools to accomplish this goal. It shows you how to take a proactive approach to managing your patients' diabetes and provides you with state-of-the-art instruction on all issues impacting type I diabetes, including: blood glucose regulation, nutrition, exercise, blood pressure, blood lipid levels, and other key elements. This book is a must if you treat patients with type I diabetes! 1994; Softcover; 163 pages. #PMMT1. *Nonmember*: $37.50; *Member*: $29.95

Medical Management of Non-Insulin-Dependent (Type II) Diabetes, 3rd Ed.

formerly: *Physician's Guide to Non-Insulin-Dependent (Type II) Diabetes*

This new book will give you the tools you need to diagnose and treat type II diabetes and other forms of glucose intolerance. Includes: revised diagnosis and classification criteria, updated information on pathogenesis, new strategies for achieving better metabolic control, new information on preventing and treating complications, as well as ADA's new nutrition recommendations and standards of medical care. 1994; Softcover; 99 pages. #PMMT2. *Nonmember*: $37.50; *Member*: $29.95

Therapy for Diabetes Mellitus and Related Disorders, 2nd Ed.

Put the knowledge of more than 50 diabetes experts right at your fingertips! Updated to reflect DCCT findings and new treatment recommendations, each chapter focuses on a different aspect of diabetes and its complications, presenting a concise, practical approach to treatment. New and updated chapters include: DCCT: Significance & Implications; Rationale for Management of Hyperglycemia; Role of the Diabetes Educator; Nutrition Management; Metformin; Antihypertensive Therapy; Noninvasive Cardiac Testing; Chronic Renal Failure; Dyslipidemia; and much more. 1994; Softcover; 384 pages. #PMT-DRD2. *Nonmember*: $34.50; *Member*: $27.50

Maximizing the Role of Nutrition in Diabetes Management

It's from our popular Clinical Education Program, available in book form or as color slides. Covers the pivotal role of medical nutrition therapy (MNT) in diabetes management. MNT integrates medical, nutritional, and behavioral sciences, recognizing the importance of each in total diabetes care. Focuses on the DCCT and its implications for nutritional management of both type I and type II diabetes, as well as other forms of impaired glucose tolerance. Topics include: exercise, insulin regimens, oral hypoglycemic agents, blood glucose monitoring, diabetes complications, and other medical conditions. Book: 1994; Softcover; 64 pages. #PMNDMB. *Nonmember*: $21.95; *Member*: $17.50. Slides: 198 color slides with talking points and printout of each slide. #PRDCEPSS. *Nonmember*: $250.00; *Member*: $200.00

NEW!

Diabetes: 1995 Vital Statistics

Coming in October 1995

Our ever-popular book of diabetes facts and figures has been revised to include the most up-to-date information available. You'll find new and expanded information on prevalence and incidence by age and race, diabetes risk factors, diabetes in minorities, complications, mortality, use of health care, costs, treatment, and more. And throughout the book, extensive charts and graphs highlight and clarify important information. Perfect for researchers, diabetes educators, or anyone interested in the latest data on diabetes and its complications. 1995; Softcover; 72 pages. #PMDVS95. *Nonmember*: $18.50; *Member*: $14.75

The Fitness Book: For People With Diabetes

The first guide to exercise specifically for the person with diabetes. Helps patients learn to incorporate exercise into their lives and maintain motivation to keep it up. Topics include: the value of exercise, getting your mind and body ready to exercise, exercising to lose weight and increase fitness, exercising with complications, and much more. #CSMFB3. *Nonmember*: $18.95; *Member*: $14.95

NEW!

Diabetes Education Goals

Features the most up-to-date advice on how to assess, plan, and evaluate patient education and counseling programs, including the newly revised content areas recommended by the National Diabetes Advisory Board. Divided into sections on IDDM, NIDDM, and gestational diabetes, the book highlights both short-term and continuing goals. It also features sections devoted to age-sensitive considerations and approaches for educating patients with special challenges to learning. More than a series of checklists, this valuable guide focuses on the education process and emphasizes assessing the unique needs of each patient. A vital addition to your library! 1995; Softcover; 64 pages. #PEDEG. *Nonmember: $21.95; Member: $17.50*

Order These Valuable Publications Today!

Title

		Qty.	Price	Total

Clinical Education Series on CD-ROM
#PMCDROM1_____@$_____each = $_____

Intensive Diabetes Management
#PMIDM _____@$_____each = $_____

Medical Management of Pregnancy
Complicated by Diabetes, 2nd Ed.
#PMMPCD2 _____@$_____each = $_____

Medical Management of Insulin-Dependent
(Type I) Diabetes, 2nd Ed.
#PMMT1 _____@$_____each = $_____

Medical Management of Non-Insulin-
Dependent (Type II) Diabetes, 3rd Ed.
#PMMT2 _____@$_____each = $_____

Therapy for Diabetes Mellitus and
Related Disorders, 2nd Ed.
#PMTDRD2 _____@$_____each = $_____

Maximizing the Role of Nutrition in
Diabetes Management (Slide Set)
#PRDCEPSS _____@$_____each = $_____

Maximizing the Role of Nutrition in
Diabetes Management (Book)
#PMNDMB _____@$_____each = $_____

Diabetes: 1995 Vital Statistics
#PMDVS95 _____@$_____each = $_____

The Fitness Book: For People With
Diabetes
#CSMFB _____@$_____each = $_____

Diabetes Education Goals
#PEDEG _____@$_____each = $_____

The Health Professional's Guide to
Diabetes and Exercise
#PMHDE_____@$_____each = $_____

Shipping & Handling Chart
Up to $30.00 . . . . add $3.00
$30.01-$50.00 . . . . . . add $4.00
Over $50.00 . . . . add 8% of order

Publications Subtotal: $_____

VA Residents Add 4.5% Sales Tax: $_____

Shipping & Handling (based on subtotal): $_____

Grand Total: $_____

Allow 2-3 weeks for shipment. Add $3.00 to shipping & handling for each additional shipping address. Add $15 to shipping & handling for each international shipment. Foreign orders must be paid in U.S. funds, drawn on a U.S. bank. Prices subject to change without notice.

Ship to:

Name_____

Address _____

City/State/Zip _____

____Enclosed is my check or money order (payable to American Diabetes Association)

____Please charge my: ❏ VISA   ❏ MC   ❏ AMEX

Account #_____Exp. Date_____

Signature_____

Call **1-800-ADA-ORDER** or mail to:
American Diabetes Association
Order Fulfillment Department
P.O. Box 930850
Atlanta, GA 31193-0850